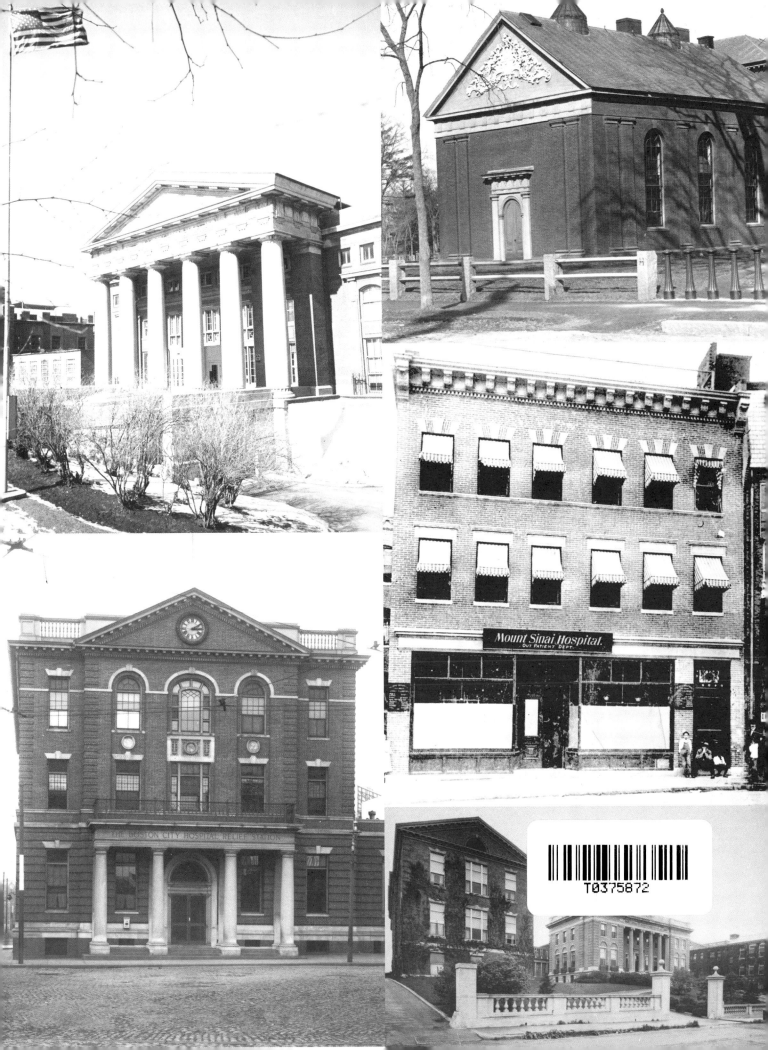

BIRTH
of a
SPECIALTY

BIRTH

of a

SPECIALTY

A History of Orthopaedics at Harvard
and Its Teaching Hospitals

VOLUME 1

by

James H. Herndon, MD, MBA

Peter E. Randall Publisher
Portsmouth, New Hampshire
2021

ISBN: 978-1-942155-36-2
Library of Congress Control Number: 2021916147

Published by
Peter E. Randall Publisher LLC
Portsmouth, NH 03801
www.perpublisher.com

Volume 1: Harvard Medical School
Volume 2: Boston Children's Hospital
Volume 3: Massachusetts General Hospital
Volume 4: Brigham and Women's Hospital, Beth Israel Deaconess Medical Center, Boston City Hospital,
   World War I, and World War II
Volume 5: Bibliography (available only in PDF form, visit www.birthofaspecialty.com)

Cover images:
Front:
   Volume 1: Boston Medical Library collection, Center for the History of Medicine in the Francis A. Countway Library.
   Volume 2: *Images of America. Children's Hospital Boston.* Charleston, SC: Arcadia Publishing, 2005. Boston Children's Hospital Archives, Boston, Massachusetts.
   Volume 3: Massachusetts General Hospital, Archives and Special Collections.
   Volume 4: Brigham and Women's Hospital Archives.

Back:
   Volumes 1–4: Warren Anatomical Museum collection, Center for the History of Medicine in the Francis A. Countway Library.

Endpaper images:
Front: **Top:** (l) Exterior view of the Old Harvard Medical School, Boston, Mass, ca. 1880. Photograph by Baldwin Coolidge. Courtesy of Historic New England; (cl) Boston Children's Hospital Archives, Boston, Massachusetts; (cr) Brigham and Women's Hospital Archives; (r) Theodore Roosevelt Collection in the Houghton Library, Harvard University.
   Center: (l) The Ruth and David Freiman Archives at Beth Israel Deaconess Medical Center; (c) Boston Children's Hospital Archives, Boston, Massachusetts; (r) The Ruth and David Freiman Archives at Beth Israel Deaconess Medical Center.
   Bottom: (l) Massachusetts General Hospital, Archives and Special Collections; (c) Boston City Archives; (r) Brigham and Women's Hospital Archives.
Back: All: Kael E. Randall/Kael Randall Images

All reasonable efforts have been made to obtain necessary copyright permissions. Grateful acknowledgment for these permissions is made at point of use (for images) and in Volume 5 (for text). Any omissions or errors are unintentional and will, if brought to the attention of the author, be resolved.

Book design by Tim Holtz

Printed in the United States of America

Contents

Volume 2 Contents

Volume 3 Contents

Volume 4 Contents

Volume 5 Contents

Volume 5 is available as an electronic version only and is included with purchase. It is available for download at www.birthofaspecialty.com.

To access link directly, go to https://pathway-book-service-cart.mypinnaclecart.com//peter-e-randall /birth-of-a-specialty-bibliography-only/

To Gerry, whose continued support has made this book possible.

Acknowledgments

No writer works alone is a commonly used statement—one that I never fully appreciated until I began the complex task of writing this book about a significant historic period in the development of orthopaedic surgery at Harvard Medical School before and following the school's conception by the Corporation of Harvard College in 1782.

Over the past 14 years, since I first conceived this book, I have had continuous assistance from others. My research began in the Center for the History of Medicine at the Countway Library of Harvard Medical School and the unique Warren Anatomical Museum. I owe special thanks to Jessica Murphy, research archivist; Jack Eckert, public service librarian; and Stephanie Krause, research archivist, for directing me to important documents and files tucked away in different areas of this large and complex center. And to Dominic Hall, curator of the Warren Anatomical Museum, for joining me as we explored various medical marvels preserved amongst its almost 10,000 artifacts.

My research travels led me to other major sources of medical history. In each, I found the staff experts and always helpful in directing me to appropriate files and primary documents. They include the Massachusetts Historical Trust, the Boston Athenaeum, Cambridge Historical Society, and Historic New England.

A special thanks to the archivists at Harvard's teaching hospitals: Lucy Ross (archivist) and Jeff Mifflin (retired archivist and curator),

Massachusetts General Hospital (MGH); Catherine Pate (archivist), Brigham and Women's Hospital (BWH); Alina Morris (archives program manager), Katie Loughrey (archivist) and James Koepfler (medical photographer), Boston Children's Hospital (BCH); and Susan Pasternack (Ruth and David Freiman Archives), Beth Israel Deaconess Medical Center (BIDMC). We worked many hours together, enabling me to sort through files, read manuscripts (letters, memoranda, minutes of numerous meetings), and select important images for the book. I need to recognize and thank Michelle Rose, medical photographer of the MGH Photography Department, for reproducing many images whose originals no longer exist. Thanks to Cheryl Miller, my administrative assistant, for the first half of this project, for typing and retyping the manuscript, and additional typing by Mulberry Studio, Yez Picardo, and Heather Saunders.

During the initial phase of research, I was able to interview many of the recently retired leaders of orthopaedics at Harvard and some current senior faculty. They include: Henry Banks (retired dean at Tufts University School of Medicine and former chief of orthopaedics at Peter Bent Brigham Hospital [PBBH]), Clement Sledge (retired chief of orthopaedics at BWH), Melvin Glimcher (retired chief at both MGH and BCH), Henry Mankin (retired chief of orthopaedics at MGH), William H. Harris (retired chief of the Harris Laboratory at MGH), James Kassar (retired chief of orthopaedics at BCH), Mike Millis (director of adolescent and young adult hip program, BCH), John Emans (chief of spine division at BCH); Lyle Micheli (director emeritus division of sports medicine at BCH), Robert Boyd (retired chief spine clinic MGH), Zeke Zimbler (retired chief pediatric orthopaedics at Tufts and retired chief of orthopaedics at Beth Israel Hospital [BIH]), and Harris Yett (retired chief of orthopaedics at BIH). Numerous other clinicians and staff, including John Burns (chief orthopaedic technician at MGH), have been generous in providing historical details to me during casual conversations in institutions' hallways or by phone.

Some individuals have provided guidance after reading parts of the book, often making significant suggestions. They include Karla Pollick (my administrative assistant in the Partners' Department of Orthopaedic Surgery), Cheryl Miller, and my wife Gerry.

During the last two years, I have had the advice and assistance of Victoria White; developmental editor, with the assistance of Andrea Klinger; and Rebekah Jordan Smith for updating and proofreading the cross-references. Victoria has been a terrific resource. I benefited from her talents to help me organize complex historical events in chronological order, allowing readers to follow numerous events in an easily understandable manner.

I am especially grateful to Deidre Randall, CEO of Peter E. Randall Publisher, who encouraged me when I first met her with my concept for this book almost 14 years ago. After returning 10 years later with a draft manuscript, she remained enthusiastic and supportive—determined to see the book published. To her staff of colleagues, I remain extremely grateful. They include Caitlin O'Brien (Rights and Permissions Specialist); Zak Johnson (Copyeditor); Tim Holtz (Book Designer); Grace Peirce (Book Designer); Melissa Hyde (Ivy Indexing); Leslie Brenner (Proofreader); and Kael Randall (Photographer and Publishing Assistant).

As we approached the completion of editing and image selection, the United States was hit by the Covid-19 pandemic. For over one year, there were forced delays in image selection, source documentation, substantiation of quotes and accuracy of events—as the Center of the History of Medicine and the hospitals' archives remained closed or provided only limited access. I owe a tremendous gratitude to everyone working together on the final phase of producing this book as we continued to push forward, despite these difficulties, to meet our publication deadline of 2021—the 100th anniversary of the Harvard Combined Orthopaedic Residency Program (HCORP).

Foreword

Birth of a Specialty is the story of orthopaedics at Harvard over the past two centuries. This is a story beautifully told in all its depth and complexity by Dr. James H. Herndon, former head of the orthopaedic departments at MGH and BWH and former director of the Harvard Combined Orthopaedic Residency Program. This four-volume history chronicles the development of the collaborative mosaic of orthopaedic departments in different hospitals—Massachusetts General Hospital (MGH), Brigham and Women's Hospital (BWH), Boston Children's Hospital (BCH), Beth Israel Deaconess Medical Center (BIDMC), and Boston City Hospital—which became the basis for the modern juggernaut of orthopaedics in Boston and played a leading role in the development and recognition of the specialty in the United States.

It has been said many times that in order to understand the future one must study the past. Dr. James Herndon has created an epic chronicle of the foundation of orthopaedics in America in its birthplace in Boston at Harvard University. These volumes are essential reading for all who seek to have perspective on the future of orthopaedics. Dr. Herndon is eminently qualified to speak with accuracy and insight about the birth of the specialty of orthopaedics, as he has painstakingly researched not only the details and history of each hospital, but of each of those individuals who contributed to this rich history of innovation and teaching. Dr. Herndon graduated from the MGH/BWH/BCH combined program at Harvard in 1970 and

went on to become the chair of three major academic orthopaedic programs during his career. The last of these was as the chairman of the Partner's Orthopaedic Department, which was the academic umbrella over all orthopaedic programs in the Harvard Hospitals.

The history at MGH began as a family affair with the Warren family and the Brown family setting the stage for the growth of this great institution. This story spans the Battle of Bunker Hill in the Revolutionary War through the development of anesthesia and many subsequent innovations in orthopaedics. Historically, at the MGH and the other major orthopaedic hospitals at Harvard, it was the general surgeons who were the innovators in musculoskeletal care. Dr. John Collins Warren at MGH, Dr. Edward H. Bradford at BCH, and many others at BWH, BIDMC, and Boston City Hospital, were general surgeons who innovated in the area of fractures and reconstruction, and who paved the way for orthopaedics to become its own specialty.

For over two centuries of musculoskeletal care at Harvard, great surgeons created innovation after innovation long before (and after) the establishment of orthopaedics as a specialty. In fact, the concept of the hospital as a place for research was a new notion even in the early part of the nineteenth century. Some notable innovations at Harvard included: the first use of ether anesthesia, the application of radiography to diagnosis and treatment of fractures and deformities, "The End-Result

Concept of Codman" (which was the progenitor of the modern concept of "Value-Based Care"), the first fracture clinic in America, new designs for total knee and hip replacement (with registries at the MGH and BWH), invention of cross-linked polyethylene; sports medicine as a specialty (first use of helmets in football, application of Bankart repair for shoulder instability, development of arthroscopy for diagnosis and treatment of knee injuries), innovations in the care of orthopaedic issues affecting children (spinal deformities, fracture care in children, management of chronic limb deformities, hip preservation in the young patient, sports medicine management of injuries in children, management of spasticity and many more), innovations and care for musculoskeletal tumors, understanding of bone metabolism and the etiology of avascular necrosis, understanding of cartilage metabolism and degeneration, development of many novel treatments of upper extremity problems including brachial plexus injuries and thoracic outlet syndrome, the first description of lumbar disc disease and its treatment, and the co-founding of the American College of Surgeons (E. A. Codman).

The evolution of all the Harvard-linked hospitals is the story of collaboration and alliances with many clinicians playing a role at more than one institution both as surgeons and as leaders. Moreover, many surgeon leaders became influential at Harvard and on the national stage including leadership roles at Harvard University and Harvard Medical School, the American Academy of Orthopaedic Surgeons, the American Board of Orthopaedic Surgery, and additional specialty societies in orthopaedics. All the Harvard hospitals contributed during the First and Second World War, and in the process, advanced orthopaedic management of musculoskeletal trauma.

Jon "JP" Warner, MD

HCORP, Class of 1987; Chief, the MGH Shoulder Service; Acting Chief, the MGH Sports Medicine Service; Chair for Quality and Safety, MGH Orthopaedic Department; Professor of Orthopaedics, Harvard Medical School; Founder, the Boston Shoulder Institute; Founder, the Codman Shoulder Society; Founder, the New England Shoulder and Elbow Society

Preface

There is a plethora of books on the history of medicine dating back to the time of Hippocrates and even before him. So why then another history book detailing events in orthopaedic surgery? I asked myself that very question many times before actually beginning the research required for a new book on orthopaedic surgery, its history and development in the United States, the birth of a specialty. Within the existing body of work, there are numerous historical contributions that detail the development of almost every specialty, including orthopaedic surgery. As I read the usual—often repetitious—historical texts about orthopaedics, I found each text had the same focus on early developments of the specialty in Europe, followed by its development in the United States. Some focused on orthopaedics as part of an individual hospital's history, with a smaller number devoted only to the history of orthopaedic surgery at a specific hospital. A few focused on the history of a particular medical school and only briefly discussed orthopaedics. Surprisingly, some traced the history of the field of surgery in general and failed to mention orthopaedic surgery at all, including many of the great contributors and leaders at their own institution. And still others focused on the contributions of specific individuals, specific cities, or regions to the broad field of orthopaedic surgery.

I have deliberately focused this book on orthopaedic surgeons at Harvard Medical School (HMS) and its major teaching hospitals because of their pivotal contributions, which began even before the recognition of orthopaedics as a surgical specialty at Harvard. Although many other great orthopaedic surgeons—at a variety of other excellent institutions in the United States—have made significant contributions to the specialty, helped shape its development, and influenced the field's history, I have not included them in this book. I do not mean to diminish their contributions or influence, but they are for others to write about in different historical contexts.

I have had the unique opportunity to access primary source documents about individual surgeons and the origins of the institutions in which they worked in the Center for the History of Medicine at the Countway Medical Library of HMS as well as in the rich archives of each hospital. After exhaustive reading of trustees' minutes, executive committee reports, personal letters, diaries, pamphlets, and publications, I synthesized over 200 years of history on orthopaedics. Each section includes unique features, such as examples of typical case reports from the surgeon; a physician snapshot of their major contribution(s) to the field; and frequent quotes to allow the reader to hear from the surgeons, their colleagues, and others through their own words. My goal is to document the significant contributions of Harvard orthopaedic surgeons and the institutions in which they worked and to provide the reader with some insights into their lives, their personalities, and their struggles as they molded a new surgical field and nurtured it to the advanced state that our specialty finds itself today. Therefore, this history begins when only general surgeons treated musculoskeletal problems, as well as other organ systems, in their practice. In the United States, these surgeons were found mainly at Harvard, in Boston, but a few were also in New York and Philadelphia at the time.

Our history begins in the late-eighteenth century, before the Revolutionary War, and before the founding of HMS. It ends at the turn of the twentieth to the twenty-first century. During this period, surgeons influenced the development and maturation of orthopaedics from a medical to a surgical specialty, led in the effort to include the treatment of fractures within orthopaedics, helped to organize orthopaedic care during the two great world wars as well as the rehabilitation of the injured soldier, and developed a modernized teaching program to include adult care and the care of children with musculoskeletal problems. They also greatly influenced the development of sports medicine as a new specialty within orthopaedics and implemented the important concepts of prevention of athletic injuries and the role of a team physician.

The first volume of this book addresses the early surgical landscape, the development of the specialization of orthopaedics, and the history of orthopaedics at HMS. The first family of surgery—the Warren family—includes a significant number of leading surgeons of their day, and many were interested in musculoskeletal problems and injuries. The Browns opened the first orthopaedic hospital in the United States, and they began

to limit their practice of surgery to orthopaedic problems. The history of HMS discusses the creation of the orthopaedic department, curriculum, residency program, the beginnings of sports medicine, as well as the infamous murder of Dr. George Parkman at the school in 1849 and contributions by surgeons to the case. The next three volumes cover the history of orthopaedics at each of Harvard's teaching hospitals. Each hospital section begins by discussing the origins of the institution; the evolution of orthopaedic department status at each hospital; the contributions of many great orthopaedic surgeons; and the transition from the twentieth to the twenty-first century, including recruitment of orthopaedic chairpersons at each of the hospitals. It ends with a discussion of the role of Harvard orthopaedic surgeons in the world wars. In volume 5, you can access the reference list, bibliography, several appendices, and a list of important publications for further reading.

Since my first days as an orthopaedic resident in Boston, I have long had an interest in the history of the specialty that I chose for my professional career. Much like my predecessors, my contemporaries, and the orthopaedic surgeons of the future, I have succeeded in and contributed to the field only because of the guidance of contemporary mentors and orthopaedic giants of history. They have provided the knowledge for new surgical advances and technology as well as a solid foundation in understanding normal and pathologic musculoskeletal conditions. I have been fortunate to study under many of these orthopaedic giants. To these individuals, I am extremely grateful.

Introduction

Before we can begin the story of orthopaedic surgery at Harvard Medical School and its teaching hospitals, some background is needed about the name of the specialty—orthopaedics—and the original contributions that established musculoskeletal deformity as an area of interest for physicians. Basic scientific research in orthopaedics and musculoskeletal tissues progressed rapidly in Europe during the eighteenth and nineteenth centuries. Many of these great advances preceded orthopaedic research in the United States.

THE EIGHTEENTH CENTURY

It is important to recognize the timeline of clinical advances and basic scientific discoveries that shaped orthopaedics in Europe. French physician Henri-Louis Duhamel (1700–1782) laid the foundation for our understanding of bone growth, discovering that the periosteum is responsible for appositional bone growth and that bone grows in length from its ends. Scottish surgeon John Hunter (1728–1793), after repeating Duhamel's experiments successfully, further discovered that bone growth results from two distinct processes—deposition and absorption—and that bone fragments could survive with a periosteal layer ("vital principle").

Recognized as the founder or grandfather of orthopaedics, French physician Nicolas Andry wrote his classic *Orthopaedia: or The Art of Correcting Deformities in Children* in 1743. In choosing the word "orthopaedics," Andry focused on the chief clinical interest of practitioners of orthopaedics at the time, which was the correction of deformities in developing children. The name orthopaedic was derived from Greek. *Orthos* means correct or straight and *paideion* means child. At the time, treatment followed a holistic approach that focused on achieving the "best function" for the individual. Andry emphasized exercise, function, and pathogenesis when he recommended specific treatments for orthopaedic conditions and even for some physical characteristics that fall to other specialties today. He did not deal at length with fractures, stating only that "their treatment is difficult, that a physician and surgeon ought [to] be consulted, but that a severe deformity is likely to result" (N. Andry 1743).

Interestingly, Andry did not write his book as a text for physicians, but rather as a guide for parents and teachers. He hoped that the contents of his book "may be put in practice by parents themselves and all such as are employed in educating children" (N. Andry 1743). He described some orthopaedic deformities in children and provided advice on correcting them. He emphasized scoliosis, stating, "When the Spine is straight, well set, and finely turned, it makes a handsome body;

and where it is crooked and ill turned, the body is Deformed" (N. Andry 1743). He instructed parents on body mechanics and how to prevent round shoulders. He advised mothers to "swaddle their Infants, so that the shoulders and chest may not be cramped or distorted" (N. Andry 1743). He recommended specific postures when sitting and the selection of special chairs as well as positions for sleeping to keep children straight while in bed. He also noted, "Shoes that are too high heeled will make the Bodies of Children crooked" (N. Andry 1743).

Medical practitioners recognized Andry's text as the encyclopedia of deformities for decades. In his American Orthopaedic Association presidential address in 1921, Robert B. Osgood stated:

> The prevention of deformity...the first clear voice which proclaims this chiefest aim is heard in France. It is that of Andry, who gave us the name "orthopaedia" in a two-volume work published in the middle of the eighteenth century [1743]...in Andry's treatment of existing deformity there is a strange mixture of tradition and commonsense...he extols exercise as the great preventer of disease and the corrector of deformity, far more important than unpleasant medicines..."Exercise is so useful and necessary that not only man, but the most inactive and indolent of the brute creation, nay even the plants themselves, cannot thrive without it"... [but] Andry was unable quite to shake off the shackles of an empirical and fanciful therapy. (R. B. Osgood 1921)

During the century following Andry's contribution, physicians and irregular practitioners (bonesetters or "rubbers") began to do more to treat some musculoskeletal deformities; clubfoot and scoliosis were the most common in children.

The first physician to treat children with abnormalities was Jean-Andrew Venel (1740–1791), who some consider the co-father of orthopaedics. In 1780, he opened the first orthopaedic

institute in Orbe, Switzerland (a small town near Lake Geneva), which included a "hospital facility, an occupational workshop, a therapeutic bath, a classroom for the patients, and a brace shop" (L. F. Peltier 1993). Venel treated clubfeet with an "active" splint and scoliosis with traction in bed at night. For both clinical problems, he used warm baths, massage, manipulation, and stretching. Treatment lasted months and, in some cases, years. Venel's Institution "later became part of the 'Hospice orthopédique de la Suisse romande' in Lausanne and served as a model for numerous orthopedic hospitals throughout Europe, which were often referred to as 'houses of the cripples'" (L. F. Peltier 1993). In England, Robert Chessler (1750–1831), recognized as the "father of English orthopedics" used methods similar to Venel, but treated the children as outpatients.

THE NINETEENTH CENTURY

In 1803, William Hey pioneered advances in biomechanics when he coined the phrase "internal derangement of the knee" while reporting cases he had treated successfully by manipulation (A. Keith 1919). Scottish anatomist John Goodsir (1814–1867) described the Haversian system (the osteon) and discovered that bone cells, not the lymphatics, were responsible for bone resorption. In 1855, John Goodsir described the "screw movement" of the knee (A. Keith 1919).

Marshall Hall (1790–1857), an English physician scientist, described important capillary circulation and discovered the spinal cord had functions that included "purposeful and yet involuntary movements" (reflex action) which were independent of the brain (A. Keith 1919). Although relevant to orthopaedics, Hall is known as the father of modern neurology. Peter Redfern (1821–1912) described the microscopic structure of cartilage; further, he discovered that, if cut, the defect filled with fibroblasts and not cartilage cells. In 1857,

Louis Xavier Edouard Leopold Ollier (1830–1900) provided the necessary principles for bone surgery when he proved that periosteum produced bone and that bone length resulted from epiphyseal growth. He successfully transplanted articular cartilage in 1868. Bone grafting was born in 1880 when Sir William Macewen proved that bone could be grafted and reproduce itself; specifically, that bone "graft could produce new bone, independently of periosteum" (A. Keith 1919). Finally, German surgeon Julius Wolff (1836–1902) was the "first to recognize that the tissue of growing bone was in a state of constant flux" (A. Keith 1919). In 1885, he completed his description of Wolff's law. This "law of osteoblasts" states that "Osteoblasts at all times build and unbuild according to the stresses to which they are subjected" (A. Keith 1919).

While these scientific discoveries were underway, Jacques-Mathieu Delpech (1777–1832), became one of the first surgeons to correct abnormalities by surgical methods. His contributions provided new opportunities within orthopaedics—as well as surgical practice in general—because he established infection control guidelines for surgery. In addition, he differentiated idiopathic scoliosis from poliomyelitis and Pott's disease, and performed the first Achilles tenotomy for a recalcitrant clubfoot in 1816, followed by a corrective splint after the wound healed. Although successful, Delpech stopped operating because of strong opposition against surgery as a form of treatment by his colleagues. Despite this opposition, Delpech became known as the virtual founder of orthopaedic surgery.

William John Little (1810–1894), the British surgeon who first described spastic diplegia in children (Little's disease; later named cerebral palsy), had a left equinus deformity as a result of poliomyelitis at age four, and he wore a brace into adulthood. In 1836, at age 26, Little had a successful left Achilles tenotomy in Germany performed by Georg Friedrich Louis Stromeyer (1804–1876). After returning to England, he performed his first subcutaneous tenotomy in London in 1837. Over the next two years, his experience with tenotomy grew, allowing him to publish "A Treatise on the Nature of Club-Foot" in 1839. He founded the first hospital in Britain for the treatment of orthopaedic problems (the Infirmary for the Cure of Club Foot and other Contractions), which was the precursor of the Royal National Orthopaedic Hospital. Little is considered by some to be the founder of orthopaedic surgery in Britain.

Throughout the nineteenth century, there were two opposing schools of thought regarding treatment of musculoskeletal problems. The British, starting with Hugh Owens Thomas (who was from a long family history of bone-setters), believed in rest and in using splints and slings to support physiologic rest, which "must be enforced, uninterrupted and prolonged" (A. Keith 1919). The French school believed in action or movement beginning with the teachings of Just Lucas-Championniere (1843–1913), who was an "uncompromising advocate of movement as curative" for injuries and accidents (A. Keith 1919). Interestingly, Andry himself also believed that action was more important in treatment than rest. He taught that exercise and massage should be followed with rest. However, the introduction of tenotomy established a whole new era of surgical specialization in Europe. It expanded rapidly during the next century in Europe and the United States. In his presidential address in 1921, Osgood also commented:

> Rest as a curative agent in disease and injuries of the bones and joints…England speaks in the person of John Hilton in the nineteenth century. "By regarding this subject of physiology and mechanical rest…the surgeon will be compelled to admit that he has no power to repair directly any injury"…it is the prerogative of nature alone to repair the waste of any structure; he will then realize that his chief duty consists in ascertaining and removing the impediments which obstruct the reparative

process…and thus enable her [nature] to restore the parts to the normal condition… And if Hilton pursued the road of "rest" after it had become a byway and not the straight, short route to the full function, he just cleared a path which had become obscured, and this path has ever since remained open for us to follow in safety until we find a more sure and expeditious way to a common goal. (R. B. Osgood 1921)

BIRTH OF A NAME

In 1843, Valentine Mott (quoted in *American Orthopedic Association Transactions* 1937) proposed the term orthopaedic surgery:

to signify the combination of mechanical and operative surgery, which, he predicted "would inaugurate a New Era in the healing art." The title was adopted at the meeting [of the American Orthopaedic Association] (in 1887) but the question, then undetermined, was which of the two components was to be the dominant factor in the final amalgamation…At the tenth session at Vienna, Shaffer presented the following definition of the Scope of the New Specialty "Orthopedic Surgery is that department of Surgery which includes the prevention, the mechanical treatment and the operative treatment of chronic or progressive deformities, for the proper treatment of which special forms of apparatus or special mechanical dressings are necessary."

In the last decade of the century, surgery was making rapid progress, and within a few years the "New Era in the healing Art" predicted by Mott had been established… Many episodes, now forgotten, are of interest because the controversy helped to establish the status of the specialty until then undetermined.

But inherent in any history of orthopaedic surgery is the inevitable debate about the name's proper spelling: orthopaedics vs. orthopedics; a confusion that dates to Nicolas Andry in 1741. Andry was French and thus titled his famous book *L'Orthopédie, ou l'art de prévenir et de corriger daus les enfans, les difformités du corps* (orthopaedics with an "e"). This translates into English as *Orthopaedia: or the Art of Correcting and Preventing Deformities in Children, by Such Means as May Be Put into Practice by Parents Themselves and All Such as Are Employed in Educating Children* (orthopaedics with an "ae"). As a result of this difference in translation, the French and others preferred the spelling with an "e," and the British preferred the spelling with an "ae."

While orthopaedics developed in the United States during the nineteenth century, the common spelling was orthopedic with an "e." The first orthopaedic hospital in the United States; the Boston Orthopedic (or *Orthopedique*) Institution, founded by John B. Brown in 1838; used the "e" spelling. Likewise, other professional bodies and publications established during this time adopted the "e" spelling, including the American Orthopedic Association (established in 1887) and the first orthopaedic publication, *Transactions of the American Orthopedic Association*. When *Transactions'* name was changed to the *American Journal of Orthopedic Surgery* in 1903, the "e" continued to be used. However, in 1919, after the American Orthopedic Association offered the use of its journal to the British Orthopaedic Association as its official journal, the name was changed to *The Journal of Orthopaedic Surgery*, thereby eliminating the word American and using "ae" in the spelling of orthopaedic. In 1922, the journal's name was changed again, for the third time, to the *Journal of Bone and Joint Surgery* (JBJS), which it remains today.

This debate continued into the early twentieth century. Walter Stern (1929), in his chairman's address to the Section on Orthopedic Surgery of the American Medical Association on July 11, 1929, stated:

> Scarcely a decade ago, a large part of an executive session of one of the major orthopedic societies was taken up in the discussion of the proper spelling and the correct derivation of our title—was it from the Greek or was it a hybrid Latin? Was it spelled with an e or an ae?

The American Academy of Orthopaedic Surgeons founded in 1933 and the American Board of Orthopaedic Surgery established 1934 both spelled orthopaedics with an "ae." It was not until 1955 that the American Orthopedic Association changed the spelling of its name to the American Orthopaedic Association following a recommendation by a special committee.

Today both spellings remain correct and are used throughout the world, including the United States and Canada. Throughout these volumes, I use the more common spelling—orthopaedics—to tell the story of orthopaedic surgery at Harvard Medical School. Quotes from original writings and publications, however, reflect the preferred spelling of the original author or organization.

Let us now turn to the late-eighteenth century, before the Revolutionary War, to Boston, to Harvard and the beginnings of the new specialty of orthopaedic surgery in the United States. Driven by my interest in the pioneers and leaders that shaped orthopaedic surgery at Harvard Medical School, this story is told through their personal stories and the opportunities they seized upon to expand their scientific knowledge and clinical skills in defining and redefining the specialty of orthopaedic surgery as we know it today. Although these were unquestionably smart, ambitious leaders, their pursuits were shaped by service to their country during war time and peace time, as well as a tireless commitment to sustaining outstanding programs in education, research and clinical care, which continues today to advance the science and practice of orthopaedic surgery.

About the Author

James H. Herndon, MD, MBA, is the William H. & Johanna A. Harris Distinguished Professor of Orthopaedic Surgery at Harvard Medical School, Massachusetts General Hospital; and chairman emeritus of the Department of Orthopaedic Surgery in Partners Healthcare System (Mass General Brigham), Boston. He has long been a leader in orthopaedics, chairing departments of orthopaedic surgery at Brown University/Rhode Island Hospital and the University of Pittsburgh Medical School and Medical Center (UPMC). He also served as vice president of medical services at UPMC and as associate senior vice chancellor for the health sciences at the University of Pittsburgh.

He has influenced the direction of orthopaedics through leadership positions with national organizations such as the American Academy of Orthopaedic Surgeons (AAOS), the American Orthopaedic Association, the *Journal of Bone and Joint Surgery*, and the Academic Orthopaedic Society.

Dr. Herndon's interest in direct patient care solidified through his work with more than 1,000 amputees at Valley Forge General Hospital during the Vietnam War. Throughout his career, he has worked closely with patients, enjoying a large practice in trauma and adult reconstructive surgery. He has served as a management consultant for diverse physician groups and hospitals. During his leadership years in the AAOS, he focused his efforts on improving patient safety; his dedication to this cause is embodied in his 2003 AAOS presidential speech titled "One More Turn of the Wrench."

As residency program director of three well-respected orthopaedic residency programs, Dr. Herndon has trained hundreds of students and residents. As president of the American Board of Orthopaedic Surgery and chairman of the Orthopaedic Residency Review Committee, he has helped residency programs across the country develop effective teaching programs. He greatly values his role as an educator, and he hopes that *Birth of a Specialty* continues the legacy he has established through his years of teaching and his myriad presentations, publications, and studies.

Section 1

The First Family *of* Surgery *in the* United States

It is good for us today to realize our indebtedness to the past.
—**Leo Mayer**, *Journal of Bone and Joint Surgery*, 1955; 37:382

He who studies medicine without books
  Sails on an unchartered sea
But he who studies medicine without patients
  Does not go to sea at all
    —**Sir William Osler**, "Aequanimitas. Books and Men," 1904

CHAPTER 1

Joseph Warren

Physician Before the Revolution

Joseph Warren, the third Joseph in the Warren family, was a patriot of the Revolutionary War who died at the Battle of Bunker Hill. He and his brother John were the first physicians in a long lineage of Warren physicians and surgeons in Boston (see Box 1.1 for additional details), and they were the only physicians in that lineage who did not attend medical school.

Their father, also named Joseph Warren, was a successful and thrifty farmer who was eventually elected a selectman, which is a member of a New England town's governing board. He developed a new strain of apple—the Roxbury or Warren Russet or simply the Roz—that is still grown today. It is "believed to be the oldest variety of apple bred in the United States" (*Wikipedia*, n.d., under "Roxbury Russet"). Joseph's farm grew until it reached 90 acres or "approximately one-tenth the area of all Boston" (R. Truax 1968). He and his wife Mary had four sons, including Joseph and John.

On October 25, 1755, while picking apples on the farm, the senior Joseph fell off his ladder. He broke his neck and died in a few minutes. His obituary in the *Boston News-Letter* reads:

> On Wednesday last, a sorrowful accident happened here. As Mr. Joseph Warren, of this town, was gathering apples from a tree, standing upon a ladder at a considerable distance from the ground, he fell from thence, broke his neck, and expired in a few minutes. He was esteemed a man of good understanding;

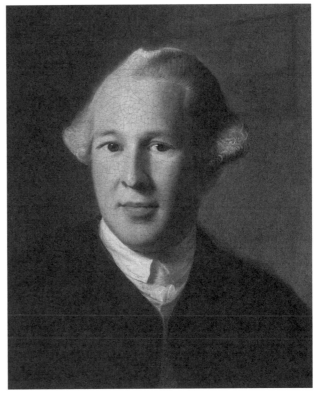

John Singleton Copley, American, 1738–1815. *Joseph Warren, about 1765*. Oil on canvas. 127 x 100.96 cm (50 x 39 ¾ in.)

Physician Snapshot

Joseph Warren

BORN: 1741

DIED: 1775

SIGNIFICANT CONTRIBUTIONS: Leader of the Revolutionary War and the first surgeon in the Warren family lineage industrious, upright, honest, and faithful; a serious, exemplary Christian; a useful member of society. He was generally respected among us, and his death is universally lamented. (quoted in R. Truax 1968)

The junior Joseph was 14 years old and his brother John ("little Jack") was two years old at the time of their father's death. Their mother, Mary, continued to run the farm and raised the four children. The youngest son became a successful farmer and another son a lawyer. Joseph

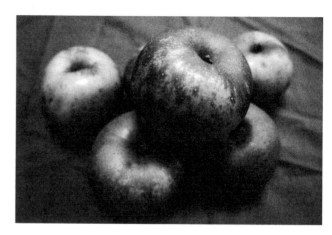

Warren or Roxbury Russet apple. Photo by author.

Box 1.1. The Early Boston Landscape and the Warren Family Tree

Boston in the early 1660s was a small island with a narrow muddy bridge of land (Shawmut Peninsula) that was barely 40 feet wide—known as the neck—and often under water, connecting the town to the mainland. Richard Warren, a merchant, was the first to arrive; he was a Pilgrim who landed in America in 1620 on the first voyage of the *Mayflower*. He was also one of the 10 members of the landing party with Myles Standish. Though nearly one-half of the 102 passengers died during a terrible winter and an influenza epidemic, Warren survived and settled with his family in Plymouth (called Plimouth). His wife, Elizabeth, and their five daughters arrived later, in 1623, aboard the ship *Anne*. They had two sons in America. Richard Warren died in 1628. Little is known about him, but it has been said that he has the most descendants (more than 14 million) of any of the other original Pilgrims. Some of his more famous descendants include Ulysses S. Grant, Franklin Delano Roosevelt, Alan Shepard, Henry Wadsworth Longfellow, the Wright Brothers, and Lavinia Warren (Mrs. Tom Thumb).

John Warren, who was possibly a brother of Richard Warren, arrived in 1630 with his wife, Margaret, and their four children aboard the ship *Arbella* (*Arabella*). The *Arabella* was one of a fleet of 11 ships organized by John Winthrop to bring 1,000 immigrants to America, who eventually founded the Massachusetts Bay Colony. The Warren family—with the entire passenger group—settled in Charlestown (then called Charlton), which, as a separate town, became the first capital of the Massachusetts Bay Colony. The entire group accepted an invitation to join others in the Shawmut Peninsula, where usable water was more abundant. Eventually the area was called Boston in homage to the city from which many of them had immigrated.

On May 18, 1631, a total of 118 people took the freeman's oath, including John Warren. John Collins Warren stated in his *Genealogy of Warren, With Some Historical Sketches* that "this John was probably the father of Peter, whose eldest son was named John, and from whom the Boston line of descent is traceable with perfect clearness and certainty" (J. C. Warren 1854). The second son of Peter Warren and Sarah Tucker (who was the first of his three wives) was Joseph Warren, a carpenter by trade. He worked in Boston until he saved enough money to purchase land outside of the cramped Boston community. He purchased six acres of land in what is now known as Roxbury, the sixth town incorporated in the colony of Massachusetts Bay. Roxbury was called Rocksbury, Rocksborough Hills, or Rocbury because of a rock outcrop in the narrow neck leading to Boston and the fields and woods of the area being generally filled with rocks. The second son of this Joseph Warren was another Joseph Warren, who was in turn the father of the first physicians in the Warren family, Joseph (the third of that name) and Jack Warren. It was common in families during the eighteenth and nineteenth centuries to reuse the same names generation after generation, and both John and Joseph were common in the Warren family. Joseph was possibly the first cousin of Colonel Gideon Warren, who fought at Ticonderoga with Ethan Allen and Benedict Arnold.

Figure 1.1 Warren Family Lineage of Physicians.*

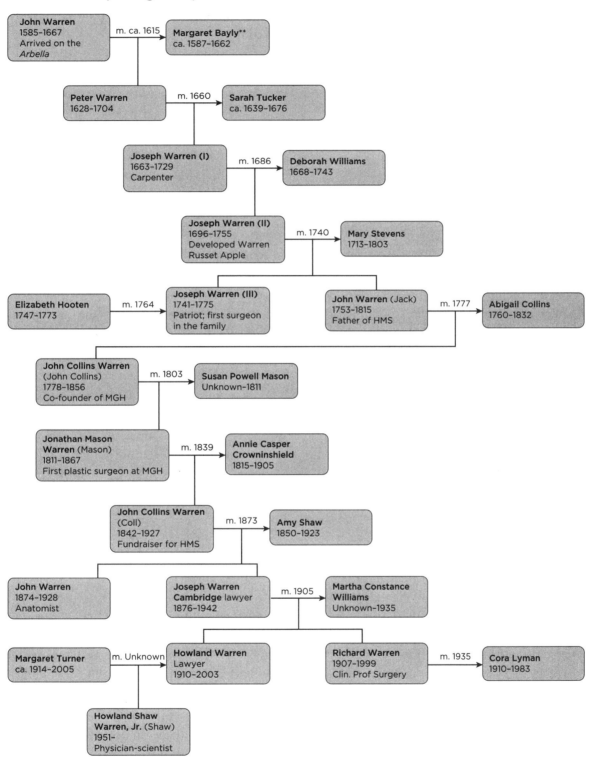

*This version of the Warren family tree is limited to the lineage of physicians in the family. Because there is large variation in the records, the total number of other children are not included. Some historians have included children who died in infancy and others have not.

**Some historian's record Margaret's surname as unknown.

Warren Family Lineage of Physicians. Compiled by the author.

and John went to Harvard and apprenticed with physicians. As a young boy, Joseph had already thought of becoming a doctor; he was probably influenced by his mother's father, Dr. Samuel Stevens of Roxbury, and later by his father's untimely death.

JOSEPH WARREN, PHYSICIAN

The year his father died, Joseph entered Harvard after graduating from the Roxbury Latin School, which is the oldest school in continuous operation in the United States today. In 1755, there were no medical classes or even premedical courses at Harvard. There were a few medical books (rare at the time) and two skeletons. There is evidence that in 1764 the leadership at Harvard began discussing the establishment of a medical school (several years after Joseph graduated), but it wasn't until 1783 that Harvard offered courses in anatomy, first held in Harvard Hall and shortly thereafter in Holden Chapel. They remained in Holden Chapel for about 33 years until Harvard moved its medical classes to Boston at the formation of the Massachusetts Medical College of Harvard University.

While at Harvard, Joseph received a partial scholarship and was granted an exception to help his mother on the farm during the busiest season. One time he stayed too long at the farm, and he was fined eight pence. A greater fine (10 shillings) was the standard custom for students who swore, cursed profanities, played cards or dice, walked or did other diversions on the Sabbath, neglected analysis of scripture or fired a gun or pistol in the Yard. Joseph, a very friendly, outgoing individual made friends easily and "managed to break a certain number of rules without being caught" (R. Truax 1968). Joseph chose a medical topic for his thesis, which was required for graduation. He took the negative position on the topic "Does all disease arise from obstruction?" He graduated in

1759 and was twenty-fifth in his class, which was determined solely on social standing. Ten boys followed him.

After graduating from Harvard, he became master of the Roxbury grammar school to make some money for his mother—34 pounds, 16 shillings—because she had to place about half of her farm as security to pay for his physician apprenticeship to Dr. James Lloyd. Joseph paid his mother back in full after practicing as a physician for one year.

Joseph left his position at Roxbury Latin to spend two years in apprenticeship to Dr. James Lloyd (1728–1810), who was a distinguished, well-respected, and popular surgeon in Boston. "In many ways [Lloyd's] course of study was typical of the pre-Revolutionary era" for physicians (H. R. Vists 1958). After early studies with an Anglican clergyman and philosopher in Stratford, Connecticut, he apprenticed in medicine in Boston. Lloyd waited several years after completing his apprenticeships to study abroad. In England, he spent a year as a dresser at Guy's Hospital and studied under the leading surgeon at the time, William Cheselden. He also studied anatomy and surgery under William Hunter. It has been assumed that while there Lloyd learned the perineal techniques for removing bladder stones as well as a "sound knowledge of anatomy, upon which all Cheselden's operations were based" (H. R. Vists 1958). Lloyd also learned the essential speed required of a surgeon before the days of anesthesia. He learned the latest techniques in managing labor and delivery and the use of forceps under William Smellie, who was famous for his courses.

After two years in England, Lloyd returned to Boston in 1752 to begin his practice of medicine. Lloyd never received a medical degree. Instead, he received certificates of attendance for each of his classes, apprenticeships, and time as a dresser. In the eighteenth century, certificates of attendance were comparable to a diploma from a university. Medical degrees were given in England and

Europe, but they were not awarded in the United States until 1768, by what is now the University of Pennsylvania Medical School. Few Americans in the mid-eighteenth century went abroad for a medical degree, and only one received a medical degree before 1750, from the University of Edinburgh in 1749.

It was during this period in the eighteenth century that the demand for physicians was increasing. Many physicians who sailed to New England from England were asked to stay. As towns became more populated, infectious diseases increased. Boston, because it was a busy port, suffered frequently from epidemics such as typhoid, yellow fever, cholera, influenza, measles, scarlet fever, diphtheria, and smallpox. At the time,

towns were overcrowded and there were serious hygiene issues. A lack of sewage systems led to pools of stagnant water and rotten vegetables and fruit in the street, where people often threw trash and sewage. Reasonable water and sewage systems were not available until the middle of the century. The first hotel in the United States to have indoor plumbing was the Tremont Hotel in Boston in 1839. The first patent for a flushing toilet was in 1775. People bathed infrequently, wore the same clothes day and night, and rarely wore underwear. People ate spoiled food and often suffered from malnutrition. There were few windows in houses, resulting in poor ventilation. Sometimes entire families slept in one room. People worked long hours and many drank heavily.

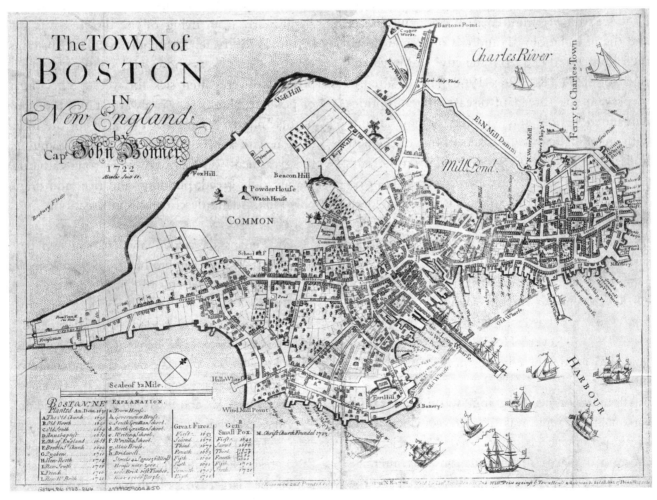

Map of Boston in 1722, *The town of Boston in New England,* by John Bonner, William Price, and Francis Dewing. Note Roxbury Flats, upper left on map. Norman B. Leventhal Map & Education Center/Boston Public Library

In the context of these times, Joseph Warren completed his apprenticeship with Lloyd in about 1761. "Without any formality, [he had become] Dr. Joseph Warren" (R. Truax 1968). He had many patients in his private practice.

A noticeable lack of physicians was obvious in the smallpox epidemic in 1764. It was devastating to the citizens of Boston; many died. Two-thirds of the blind in the Almshouse had lost their sight from smallpox. Joseph was very enthusiastic about vaccination. Death rates from smallpox were about 18%; after inoculation, the death rate was reduced to 1%–2%. Inoculations had stemmed an earlier epidemic in 1721. He had learned the inoculation method: transplanting a small portion of a smallpox pustule to the arm of a healthy person. With dry and aged material, the person would get only a mild case. But the public was extremely frightened of both the disease and the inoculation. "Hundreds of people closed their houses and fled from the city" in March and April of 1764 (R. Truax 1968). In an attempt to prevent the spread of disease, the authorities demanded people stay in their homes; anyone with smallpox had to be taken to one of the pest houses, which were empty buildings on the outskirts of town where patients received little or no medical attention. One of Paul Revere's children became sick, and Revere petitioned the selectmen of Boston to keep his child at home rather than quarantined in a pest house. They agreed but posted a guard to ensure that no one entered or left Revere's house. A white flag was hung on "the house to warn passersby that a sick person was inside" (Paul Revere House, n.d.). The Reveres remained inside their home for two months; all survived.

Because of his outgoing, warm, and caring personality, Joseph was able to convince many of his patients to be inoculated. The selectmen chose two places for inoculations to minimize contact between those recently inoculated and the well. Simultaneously with Joseph's plans to open his own inoculation hospital, the governor (Sir Francis Bernard) opened two: Castle William (a fortified island) and Point Shirley (Deer Island). Physicians agreed to only give inoculations at these two places. Joseph Warren and one other physician became assistants "in residence" to Dr. James Lloyd, Joseph's former mentor and the physician in charge of Castle William. Joseph was on duty day and night with the other physician assistant. The hospital established at Castle William was a set of barracks with 48 wards; there were 10 beds in each ward. Inoculations were free, as was room and board. The wards were filled to over-capacity, and some patients had to share a bed.

It was during this epidemic of 1764 that John Adams (in addition to Paul Revere) decided to be inoculated, after being pressured by his mother. As noted, this was no small matter because the chances of dying after the inoculation—although reduced significantly from dying of the disease—was still in the 1–2% range. Although inoculated patients were not as sick as those who contracted smallpox, they were often sick for weeks. The threat of possible blindness was always at the forefront of their minds. Adams was prepared for the inoculation with a strong emetic to induce vomiting; this treatment was followed by a strong cathartic. He ate only bread, pudding, and rice, and drank only milk. Adams described his inoculation:

> Dr. Perkins demanded my left arm and Dr. Joseph Warren my brother's. They took their Launcetts and with their Points divided the skin about a Quarter of an inch and just suffering the blood to appear, buried a thread (infected) about a Quarter of an inch long in the Channell. A little lint was then laid over the scratch and a Piece of Ragg pressed on, and then a Bandage bound over all, and I was bid go where and do what I pleased.
>
> The Doctors left us Pills red and black to take Night and Morning, and ordered my Brother, larger Doses than me, on Account of the Differences in our Constitutions. (A. Blinderman 1977)

Adams' physicians confined him to the hospital for three weeks. He "suffered headaches, backaches, kneeaches [sic], gagging fever and eruptions...[of] pock marks" (A. Blinderman 1977). Adams later revealed that he was afraid of dying when the skin eruptions developed. After leaving the hospital, Adams wrote "three weeks of Close Confinement to a House, are, according to my Estimation, no small matters" (A. Blinderman 1977). Apparently, John Adams and Joseph Warren became and remained friends after this initial meeting.

Joseph worked hard and for long hours. Contemporaries and historians noted he had extraordinary vigor and stamina, and he thoroughly enjoyed working with people. Patients who were inoculated for smallpox also received large doses of antimony and mercury—antimony to decrease the cough, mucous secretions, and fever, and mercury for congestion of the liver. Patients often remained in bed and covered with blankets that were not changed, even between patients. Recovery sometimes occurred as early as one week, but it usually took two-to-three weeks. During the first five weeks of the epidemic, 3,000 people were treated at Castle William and Point Shirley without a single death. The epidemic was under control by May, and by July life returned to normal in Boston. About 1% of those who were inoculated died. We do not know whether Joseph was inoculated or contracted smallpox, but his face apparently had no noticeable scars. According to records, "he was unmarred by any of the common disfigurements—smallpox scars" (R. Truax 1968). Because he was such a strong advocate of inoculation, Joseph and his brother John were probably inoculated.

Joseph Warren returned home from Castle Island and restarted his private practice in Boston, where he had lived for two years as an apprentice and had met Miss Elizabeth Hooton. He married Hooton shortly after the smallpox epidemic, on September 6, 1764. She was described by Warren as a kind and thoughtful person. She was also wealthy, having inherited a fortune from her deceased merchant father. Her accomplishments included the ability to read and write. She had kept her father's accounts in order and was skilled in the household chores of the day: cooking, knitting, sewing, mending, embroidering, making soap and candles, cleaning, and drying herbs and flowers. She was 18; he was 23. They were married in the Congregational Church on Brattle Street in Boston and were described as a "fairy-tale couple" (R. Truax 1968).

Joseph Warren's practice continued to grow. Many of the patients whom he had inoculated earlier sought his care for other medical problems. In each year of his first three years in practice, he added 100 patients until he had the largest practice in Boston. He remained tireless and energetic with a genuine desire to help patients. His practice was quite varied—from general medicine to surgery, obstetrics, and dentistry—which was common for physicians in the eighteenth century in the United States. His most common operation was pulling teeth. He also delivered babies and was probably the first physician in Massachusetts to devote himself to obstetrics. His "skill and gentleness made mothers prefer him to the best of midwives" (R. Truax 1968). The highest fee he ever charged for a delivery was 1£ 8s. It is hard to tell what remedies he preferred because "doctors kept their remedies and their failures to themselves" (R. Truax 1968). In addition to inoculations, he performed bleeding, which was very popular. Bleeding originated in the idea of "letting out the demons causing the disease" (R. Truax 1968). Later, during his time, people believed bleeding rid the patient of impurities in the blood. He most likely also used some of the common prescriptions of the period, including "foxglove (digitalis) for heart disease, cinchona bark (quinine) for malaria, and a tincture of alcohol and iron for a rundown condition...calomel, [preparations of] snake's skin, oil of insects, unborn puppies and unicorn's horn," elixir of camphor, and *sal votilile* (ammonium carbonate or smelling salt) among others (R. Truax 1968). Like many physicians of his day, "in the main his treatments were worse than useless" (R. Truax 1968).

He also practiced orthopaedics; he was the second surgeon in America to use ligatures, a technique he learned from Dr. Lloyd, instead of scarring wounds with hot oil. He performed amputations without anesthesia (ether was not used publicly until 1846 at the Massachusetts General Hospital). The largest fee that he entered into his day book was for 4£, which he collected after "amputating the thigh of Mr. Hale's boy" (R. Truax 1968). He completed reductions of dislocations using traction from pulleys or a ladder, similar to a torture rack, to stretch the contracted muscles. If unsuccessful, he resorted to attempting to render the patient unconscious with alcohol or laudanum (tincture of opium). Laudanum was dangerous to use because overdose and death could result from a single dose. No matter how skilled or experienced physicians were in performing reductions, they dreaded treating dislocations because of the difficulty, the pain it caused, and the uncertainty of success, especially if the muscles were in spasm or contracted. Dr. Warren was the favorite physician of Boston's Whig families, including the family of John Adams. He "saved John Quincy (John Adams's son) from losing one of his fore-fingers when it was badly fractured" (J. Parton 2003).

Joseph Warren's practice took him to Cambridge (requiring him to take the Charlestown ferry), Roxbury, Dorchester, and Brookline. He rode on horseback to his patients' homes if they preferred to see him in their home rather than in his home office, and if they could pay the extra 25 to 30 percent more than he charged for office visits. He was described as always optimistic and an excellent communicator. He was always casual in dress, leaving his "vest partially unbuttoned" (R. Truax 1968); he dusted his hair with powder but never wore a wig. As much as he was energetic, he was neither thrifty nor cautious as Puritans were at the time. His family grew to four children (each two years apart), but he was careless about collecting fees. The year 1764 was a difficult

one for more reasons than the smallpox epidemic; it was also a year of tough economic times for most. Boston's economy crashed that year following the French and Indian War, which left the colonial economies in ruins. Many had lost jobs and couldn't pay their bills with money; instead they only traded with goods. His mother, Mary, relied on his help in running the family farm. She even had to take a mortgage within a year after the crash started; there were many business bankruptcies in Boston at the time. Joseph and his family lived in a small, very modest house on Hanover Street. There are records of the inclusion of an African slave with his rented home as well as his purchase of an African slave in 1770. Some historians have said he was opposed to slavery and operated his practice in a way that mirrored that opinion. He attended to both free and enslaved patients. However, his opinions at the time were not documented and little information is available.

During this difficult period in Boston's history, many turned to politics. Joseph Warren did the same. Like many, he had been a loyal subject of the English Crown, but he was now beginning to take a different path. He had joined the Masons in 1760 and became very active in the organization by 1765. He rose rapidly through various leadership positions until finally becoming grand master of Masons in New England, where he was known as the chief at the age of 28.

THE TRUE PATRIOT: A LEADER IN THE REVOLUTION

Joseph Warren, a third-generation American, a popular figure throughout Boston, was described as a true leader with "no axes of his own to grind" (R. Truax 1968). He was "intelligent, aggressive, but good-natured with radiant health and vitality, energy and enthusiasm about things and people" (R. Truax 1968). To become the grand master of the Masons in New England, he was obviously active in their members' numerous discussions at their St. Anthony's Lodge. At the time, Masons were critical of the British-appointed governor, administrators, and Parliament. Some Masons were moderate in their views, but most tended to belong to the American Whigs, who were also called Patriots, Sons of Liberty, Radicals, Revolutionaries, Congress-Men, or Rebels. The Sons of Liberty were later called the Founding Fathers of the United States. Dr. Joseph Warren was probably the most influential Whig in Massachusetts.

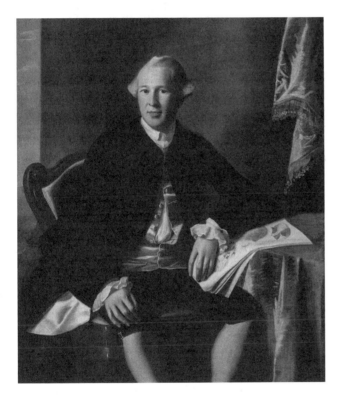

John Singleton Copley, American, 1738–1815. *Joseph Warren, about 1765*. Oil on canvas. 127 x 100.96 cm (50 x 39 ¾ in.)

On November 1, 1765—the year that Joseph was elected grand master—King George III of England and Parliament enacted the Duties in American Colonies Act, known commonly as the Stamp Act. Stamp acts had previously been very successful in raising revenue in Great Britain, and Britain's national debt had almost doubled at the end of the Seven Year's War (the French and Indian War). The British also needed to maintain individuals—especially officers—in a standing army in America. Britain's leaders argued that the costs of a military presence in America should be paid for by the colonists. The Stamp Act was a tax on stamped paper from England that the colonists were required to use for most printed materials, such as legal documents, magazines, newspapers, and other documents. It was the second tax imposed on Americans by Great Britain. The first was the Sugar Act in April 1764, which was a modification of the earlier Molasses Act of 1733. In the prior act, a tax was placed on each gallon of foreign molasses imported to Britain, effectively "giving a monopoly to molasses imported from the British West Indies" (P. D. G. Thomas 1975). Although the Stamp Act tax was small, and the colonists objected to paying it, their major concern was being taxed without their consent, which was a violation of the British Constitution. The colonists hadn't reacted to this tax by the time the stamp tax was imposed the following year.

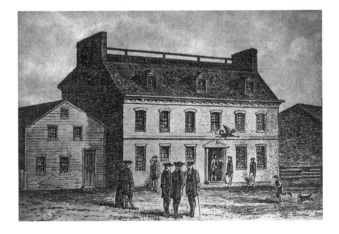

Engraving of the Green Dragon Tavern. Copy photograph from engraving by Russell, ca. 1898. Arts Department, Boston Public Library. Boston Public Library/Digital Commonwealth

The Stamp Act was expanded to include attorney licenses, court proceedings' documents, land grants, pamphlets, and even playing cards. The tax "had to be paid in valid British (sterling), not in colonial paper (currency)" (*Wikipedia*, n.d., under "Stamp Act of 1765"). The act also "allowed admiralty courts...traditionally limited to cases involved with the high seas...to have jurisdiction for trying violators" (Morgan and Morgan 1953). In addition to being taxed without representation, colonists saw this as a further attempt to replace their local courts with courts controlled by England. Ben Franklin wrote:

> That it is suppos'd an undoubted Right of Englishmen not to be taxed but by their own Consent given thro' their Representatives. That the Colonies have no representatives in Parliament. (T. Draper 1996)

Many saw the tax as a knowledge tax on the rights of the colonists to write and read freely.

Joseph Warren and others had frequent meetings in the Mason's Lodge and Boston taverns, including frequent visits to the Green Dragon Tavern (opened 1714), which remains open today. In 1766, the Green Dragon Tavern was purchased by the Freemasons. They used the first floor for meeting rooms; "the basement tavern was used by several secret groups and became known...as the Headquarters of the Revolution" (*Wikipedia*, n.d., under "Green Dragon Tavern"). As grand master, it can be assumed that Joseph Warren led many of these discussions. He wrote to a classmate friend in England:

> The strange project of levying a stamp duty, and of depriving people of the privilege of trial by jury...It is absurd to impose so cruel a yoke on a people who are so near to the state of original equality, and who look upon their liberties, not merely as arbitrary grants, but as their unalienable, eternal rights, purchased by the blood and treasure of their ancestors. (R. Truax 1968)

He also published several articles in the *Boston Gazette* under the signature "A True Patriot." Early street protests began as ordinary colonists objected to these new taxes; at the same time many different colonial legislatures were sending official protests (letters of complaints and demand) to London. In Massachusetts, a five-member committee of correspondence sent a protest to England in 1764. Joseph Warren was a member of that committee. The committee initially met at his home and then later at the Green Dragon Tavern, a few doors away from Warren's house. Nationalistic sentiments increased.

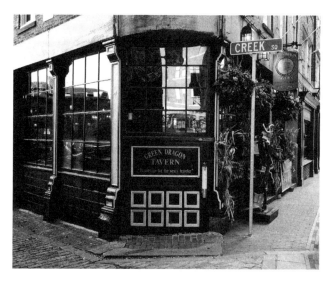

Green Dragon Tavern, 2019. Rhododendrites/Wikimedia Commons

During his short life, Dr. Joseph Warren used at least six known pseudonyms. In addition to "A True Patriot," he published articles calling for an organization of physicians in Massachusetts—similar to the Massachusetts Medical Society—to promote professionalism, ethical behavior, and clinical standards. For that he used the pseudonym of "Graph Iatroos." In a series of articles about a malpractice dispute between two colleagues, he voiced his opinion under the name of "Philo Physic." He used two other pseudonyms in various newspaper articles and letters as a staunch activist for colonial liberties, including "B. W." and "Paskalos." Editorials appearing in the *Massachusetts Spy* under the name "Mucius Scaevola" were also authored by Joseph Warren. They were pieces of fiction about a Roman patriot who attacked the king of their enemy.

On August 14, 1765, a group of militant citizens in Boston (Joseph Warren most likely included) gathered at a large elm tree near Hanover Square to protest the hated Stamp Act. They called themselves the Sons of Liberty. They hung a tax collector in effigy from the tree, which was known thereafter as the Liberty Tree. As word spread, patriots in all 13 colonies each formed a group—also called Sons of Liberty—and assembled, where possible, at a large tree in their community.

Violence and threats of violence continued in Boston. Joseph Warren became close friends with Samuel Adams, another activist and also a Son of Liberty. Membership initially included the middle and upper classes with professionals such as lawyers, doctors, traders, artists, and local politicians; however, they made appeals to lower classes in order to win local elections. Soon, the movement—often led by Samuel Adams—forced the stamp distributer in Massachusetts to resign, crowds attacked the lieutenant governor and other representatives of the crown, and others ransacked some homes and destroyed property.

In October 1765, the 27 delegates from nine colonies met in New York City at the first Stamp Act Congress. Massachusetts delegates included Samuel Adams, James Otis, Oliver Partridge, and Timothy Ruggles. They discussed three major issues: trial by jury, a right of self-taxation, and reducing admiralty courts. They adopted a Declaration of Rights and Grievances that was sent to Parliament on the same ship that had just delivered the stamps to America. Parliament rejected the colonists' petition and declared it inappropriate.

In England, citizens were beginning to feel the economic impact of the resultant diminished trade from America because many businesses were dependent on the colonial market. After many discussions and heated debate, Parliament repealed the Stamp Act, which was agreed to by the King on March 17, 1766.

The King of England and the British Parliament remained firm in their belief that they had the right to tax the colonies as they did any British citizen. Very soon after repealing the Stamp Act, Parliament began passing a series of laws including The Townshend Acts, which was a program of five laws that began in 1767 and was proposed by Chancellor of the Exchequer Charles Townshend. These acts were meant to establish the precedent that Parliament had the right to tax the colonies. They included various heavy taxes and trade regulations for the purpose of raising revenues to pay the salaries of officials such as governors and judges in the colonies and of keeping the political and judicial leadership independent of colonial rule.

It was no surprise that the colonists objected strongly to these new taxes and regulations. Francis Bernard, the royal governor of Massachusetts, requested British troops from Parliament because he feared the Sons of Liberty, who he felt were a "lawless mob" (R. J. Allison 2006). Two regiments (the 14th and 29th) arrived in Boston in October 1768 to keep the peace. But their presence only angered the colonists even more. Paul Revere, a Son of Liberty and a North-End silversmith, made an engraving of the British ship's arrival in Boston Harbor. Many church steeples were obvious in the engraving "suggesting that Bostonians were religious and orderly people who did not need troops to enforce the law" (R. J. Allison 2006). Two thousand troops arrived. Boston had 16,000 citizens at the time. Housing the troops presented a problem for Bernard. Initially he quartered them in Faneuil Hall where the colonists' leaders met. Because of the huge outcry of anger by the colonists, he soon agreed to rent several warehouses and wharves at his expense. Bernard wanted the troops in Boston to enforce the tax laws.

Samuel Adams, "a leader of Boston's town meeting and a representative to the Massachusetts Assembly, organized a boycott of the goods that Parliament had taxed: lead, paint, glass, tea, and other British manufactures" (R. J. Allison 2006). The boycott failed. Many of the merchants who remained loyal to the crown continued to supply taxed goods by setting up daily confrontations between the Sons of Liberty and these loyalist merchants. Outbreaks of violence increased daily. In one tragic incident, a loyalist's home was pelted with rocks. He responded by firing a gun into the crowd, killing an 11-year-old boy named Christopher Seider. People were outraged, and "soldiers and townspeople had begun to fight" (R. J. Allison 2006).

On the evening of March 5, 1770, a group of men and boys gathered at Dock Square in front of Faneuil Hall. They carried swords, sticks, and shovels. The crowd numbered about 300. They were angry, looking for a fight with the British troops. Rumors of isolated fights were spreading throughout the evening. The crowds grew; other smaller groups formed. One such group of about 30 men proceeded up Cornhill led by Crispus Attucks, who was a "tall, strong sailor and runaway slave" (R. J. Allison 2006). He carried "two clubs in his hand" (R. J. Allison 2006). As they reached the Custom House, the crowd had enlarged to about 60 men. They surrounded a single British sentry, threatening his life. Captain Thomas Preston formed a rescue party of seven men leaving their barracks to defend the sentry. They were pelted with "snowballs, ice and oyster shells" (R. J. Allison 2006). After reaching the Custom House, they were also surrounded by the crowd who began taunting the soldiers with insults and curses. The Riot Act allowed them to do so without fear of being shot. The punishment was a "felony for twelve rioters to continue together for an hour after the reading of a proclamation… to disperse" (R. J. Allison 2006). People yelled to the soldiers "fire, damn you, why don't you fire, you can't kill us" (R. J. Allison 2006). Someone threw a piece of wood that struck a young private in the face. As he staggered, Crispus Attucks grabbed for the private's bayonet. Raising his gun, the young private and another soldier fired simultaneously with both balls hitting Attucks in the chest. He died instantly; others were shot; several died. The Boston Massacre had occurred.

On Monday, March 12, 1770, a town meeting appointed three men, including Joseph Warren, to prepare "a particular account of the massacre in King Street so that a full and just representation could be made" (R. J. Allison 2006). The report was titled "Short Narrative of the Horrid Massacre in Boston, Perpetrated in the Evening of the Fifth Day of March 1770, By Soldiers of the 29th Regiment" (these soldiers were Redcoats, often called lobsters or bloody backs by Boston citizens). The authors of the report traced the "causes of the late horrid massacre" to the arrival of customs commissioners in November 1767 to enforce the Townshend Acts (R. J. Allison 2006). A grand jury indicted the loyalist who killed the 11-year-old boy in the earlier incident, Captain Preston and his men, and four civilians in the Custom House. The loyalist was convicted of murder but was later pardoned. All soldiers and civilians were acquitted except for the two privates who fired the first shots. They were found guilty of manslaughter. The two soldiers had been defended by John Adams and Josiah Quincy. Because they could still be hanged for manslaughter, Adams pleaded for "benefit of clergy" (R. J. Allison 2006), which was a medieval protection for priests and those who could read. He was successful. The soldiers were branded on a thumb so that they could not use this defense in future trials; they were then released afterward.

To ease tensions, the British troops were transferred to Castle Island. Joseph Warren and his committee sent their report to members of Parliament, a former governor, and Benjamin Franklin, who was in London representing three colony assemblies. Paul Revere produced another engraving (a copy of a drawing by Henry Pelham); this time the engraving represented the massacre. He named the Custom House "Butcher's Hall" in the engraving to keep the memory of the massacre alive. To continue the campaign against British rule, the colonists established a memorial lecture. The first was given on March 5, 1771. Dr. Thomas Young recalled the events of the massacre and reminded everyone that "the real treason was the threat to take away the Massachusetts provincial charter" (R. J. Allison 2006). Bells rang in Boston between 9:00 p.m. and 10:00 p.m., and Paul Revere displayed scenes of the massacre in his windows on North Square. The second annual commemorative lecture was given by Dr. Benjamin Church and the third by Dr. Joseph Warren (March 5, 1773) in the Old South Meeting Hall. Warren's speech greatly affected those attending the memorial. He said, "It had never occurred to our ancestors, that, after so many dangers in this then desolate wilderness, their hard-earned property should be at the disposal of the British Parliament, and that when Parliament realized it could not persuade them through reason and argument to forfeit their property, it seemed necessary that one act of oppression should be enforced by another, and so sent a standing army...among us in a time of peace to enforce laws that violated the Constitution" (R. J. Allison 2006). Warren gave the commemorative oration a second time on March 5, 1775; he was the only person to give two orations. They stopped after 1783 (13 years later).

As a result of the Boston Massacre, Parliament began to partially repeal some of the Townshend taxes. But the Townshend duty on tea was retained with the passage of the Tea Act in 1773; the first ships arrived with tea in Boston Harbor at the end of 1773. Warren remained active in the Sons of Liberty and—along with Samuel Adams and James Otis—became a member of the first committee of correspondence. He was also a member of the committee of safety, formed after the Boston Massacre. One of Warren's loyalist contemporaries said, "One of our most bawling demagogues and voluminous writers is a crazy doctor" (JosephWarren.com, n.d.). Warren continued to practice medicine and had been appointed physician to the Almshouse for the indigent sick and mentally ill, which was an eight-bed prototype of the modern hospital. The non-contagious sick were housed in dormitories. This appointment helped support his family. The pay was good, at £198 for his first year. The position also allowed him access to patients so that he

could teach his apprentices. As busy as he must have been during this volatile period, he is said to have treated patients 730 times in his second year at the Almshouse.

Although "radical in politics, Warren was inclined to take a moderate position in medicine" (R. Truax 1968). He was skeptical of new theories or systems of cures "and all kinds of secret nostrums" (R. Truax 1968). He organized a two-year apprenticeship and had more patients and apprentices than any other physician in Boston. His younger brother John, after graduating from Harvard, apprenticed with him for two years. According to Truax (1968), "Some historians consider Joseph Warren to have been the founder of medical education in Massachusetts." He was the first to propose that doctors have a "proper examination" before being allowed to practice physic (medicine) and surgery in order to distinguish his colleagues from quacks during this early period (R. Truax 1968). Although his proposal was known by the general public and possibly even supported by the public, his idea of an examination was unsuccessful.

The year 1773 was a difficult one for Joseph Warren. His contract with the Almshouse expired, and he was replaced by a conservative physician, Dr. Samuel Danforth. Only a few weeks after the passage of the Tea Act, his wife Elizabeth died of an unknown cause, leaving him with four children. Warren was 31. He moved to Roxbury where his mother helped him raise his children. He spent increasing time in politics with Samuel Adams, Paul Revere, and other Sons of Liberty. And finally, the shipment of tea arrived in Boston Harbor in late 1773 upon which the British imposed heavy taxes.

Tea was a popular drink in America. The colonists preferred English tea. They could not produce a local tea that was as good as the imported tea. Nevertheless, on December 16, 1773, a crowd of colonists demanded that the ship's captain return the tea to England. He refused. Other ships in New York, Philadelphia, and Charleston did return to England with the tea they had imported. There must have been many meetings at night discussing what to do in response to the tax on tea, and these meetings were probably led by Warren and Samuel Adams. The colonists not only objected to the tax but also did not believe that Parliament's authority extended to the colonies; there should be no taxation without representation. The governor of Massachusetts, however, prevented the ships in Boston from returning to England. On the night of December 16, 1773, a group of colonists (Sons of Liberty), disguised as Mohawk Indians to conceal their identity, boarded the three ships containing the tea. The group numbered from 30 to 120 men and included Joseph Warren, Paul Revere, and Samuel Adams. It took them about three hours to dump all 342 chests of tea into the water; it was a peaceful protest in contrast to the Boston Massacre three years earlier. Jubilant colonists responded with a song (R. Freedman 2012):

> Rally, Mohawks! - bring out your axes!
> And tell King George we'll pay no taxes
> On his foreign tea!
> His threats are vain-and vain to think
> To force our girls and wives to drink
> His vile Bohea!
> Then rally boys, and hasten on
> To meet our Chiefs at the Green Dragon.
> Our Warren's there, and bold Revere,
> With hands to do, and words to cheer
> For liberty and laws
> Our country's 'Braves' and firm defenders,
> Shall ne'er be left by true North-Enders,
> Fighting Freedom's cause!
> Then rally, boys and hasten on
> To meet our Chiefs at the Green Dragon

The response in England was one of shock. Even friends of the colonies were appalled by this act. The prime minister stated, "Whatever may be the consequence, we must risk something; if

we do not, all is over" (W. Cobbett 1812). The British Parliament was fed up. Early in 1774, Britain closed the port of Boston and suspended the government in Massachusetts; eventually they replaced Hutchinson with General Thomas Gage, the commander of British forces in America. Although town meetings in Massachusetts were now prohibited, colonists met in county meetings. Warren presented a series of resolutions that he wrote—the Suffolk Resolves—that stated the king had forfeited the colonists' allegiance, that any taxes collected would not be turned over to the treasurer, that towns should begin to choose their militia officers, and that if any citizens were arrested for political reasons, the colonists would hold crown officers as hostages. Paul Revere carried these resolutions from Massachusetts to the Continental Congress in 1774. All other colonies pledged support for Massachusetts if armed resistance became necessary. Warren chaired the Committee of Safety for the Provincial Congress meeting in October 1774. This committee (comprised of 12 men, including two doctors) was charged with the duty of organizing the militia and collecting weapons. The committee met frequently at Hastings House in Cambridge. Thereafter, Warren was appointed president of the Massachusetts Provincial Congress.

In 1775, Dr. Joseph Warren and Dr. Benjamin Church were the top two members of the Committee of Correspondence in Boston. Church had given the Boston Massacre memorial oration in 1772 and Warren in 1773. Now in March of 1775, Warren was asked to give it again, for the second time. As the anniversary date of March 5 approached, many of the British troops were overheard making death threats against anyone who attempted to give the oration. The evening of the oration arrived. Troops blocked every approach to the pulpit. Warren climbed a ladder and entered a window in the back of the Old South Church to give his speech. He said, "Our streets are again filled with armed men; our harbor crowded with ships of war. But these cannot intimidate us; our liberty must be preserved; it is far dearer than life" (R. J. Allison 2006). Except for the soldiers who groaned and hissed and "[held] up a handful of bullets" while holding their guns, no hostile act occurred (R. J. Allison 2006). A few weeks later on April 8, Warren was notified by his watchers that British troops were moving toward Concord to capture the colonists' arms depot. Warren planned Paul Revere's ride to warn the countryside and notify Samuel Adams and John Hancock, who were in Lexington, that British troops were coming to arrest them. Many of these planning meetings took place at the Green Dragon Tavern. Revere was sent through Charlestown; Warren asked William Dawes to also alert the people from Boston to Concord by way of Roxbury. Dawes

left Boston about 9:30 p.m.; Revere left Boston about 10:00 p.m. and was rowed across the Charles River by two friends to Charlestown. He borrowed a horse and rode to Lexington, arriving about midnight. When he arrived in Charlestown, he noticed that two lanterns had been hung in the Christ Church bell tower. It signified the British troops would not march out from Boston Neck, but would instead row by sea across the Charles River to Cambridge. Revere, because he feared that he might be retained by the British, had asked a friend to hang the lanterns.

At dawn the next day, Warren visited a patient in labor, transferred her care to his apprentice, and—after crossing to Charlestown on the ferry— rode by horseback to Lexington. The Battle of

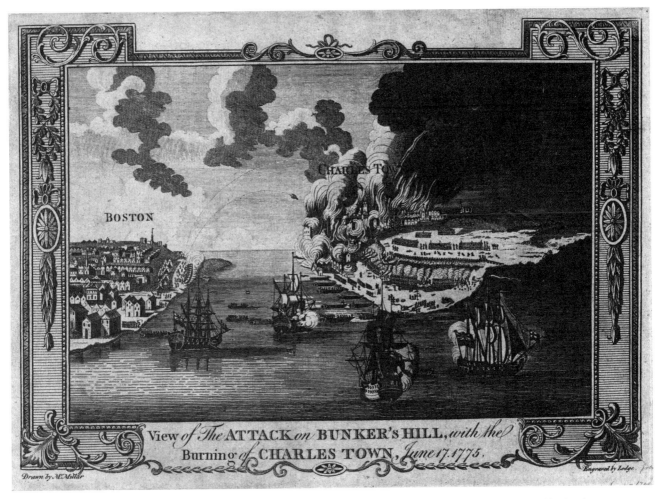

View of the attack on Bunker's Hill, with the burning of Charles Town, June 17, 1775; drawn by Millar, engraved by Lodge.
Library of Congress

Lexington and Concord occurred on April 19, 1775. British troops numbered about 1,000. They planned to confiscate and destroy the colonists' arms in Concord and arrest some of the revolutionaries in Lexington (notably John Adams and John Hancock). The militia was outnumbered as the first shots were fired at dawn in Lexington, and they withdrew to Concord. In Concord, approximately 500 militiamen inflicted heavy casualties (65 dead; 180 wounded; 27 missing) on the British, who were forced to retreat to Lexington and then back to Boston. Forty Americans died in the battle. It was during this British retreat that Joseph Warren entered the fight.

Warren joined Brigadier General William Health, who had taken command of the militia under the direction of Warren and members of the

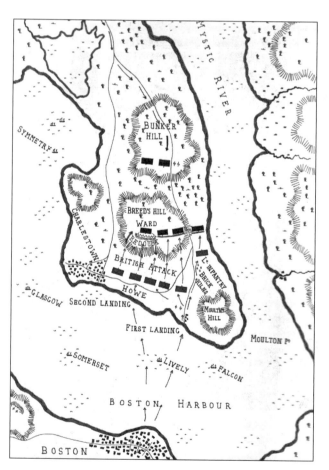

Map of the battle of Bunker Hill. Breed's Hill is where most of the fighting took place.

Massachusetts Committee of Safety. Dr. Warren cared for the injured militia, but he also fought as the British retreated. The militia continued to inflict casualties by engaging the British from their flanks throughout their march back to Boston. Warren was slightly wounded by a musket ball that grazed his ear, but he continued to fight. Battles continued in the towns of Lincoln, Menotomy (Arlington), and Cambridge. The British troops arrived and occupied the high ground of the hills of Charlestown after dark on April 19, 1775.

In recognition of Warren's leadership and numerous contributions to the freedom movement, Congress appointed him the second general (major general) in command on June 14, 1775. Two weeks prior, on May 31, 1775, he had been elected president of the Third Provincial Congress. He was "the Rebellion's executive leader of the colony" (G. C. Wildrik 2009). Only three days after his appointment, Warren volunteered to rejoin the militia at its military base on Breed's Hill (Bunker Hill), which was close to where the British had control of the high ground. Additional British troops had been assembling in Charlestown since the Battles of Lexington and Concord. The night before he joined the fighting at Bunker Hill, he was advised by a friend "not to enter the impending conflict, as, from his known ardor, he would certainly expose his life and fall a victim to his zeal" (J. C. Warren 1854). Warren replied with a quote from the Roman poet Horace: "*Dulce et decorum est pro patria mori*" or "How sweet and fitting it is to die for one's country" (Joseph Warren Monument Association 1905). Warren was asked to lead the militia, although his appointment as major general had not been finalized. Warren declined, preferring to fight as a private (without a uniform) under the direction of General Israel Putnam and Colonel William Prescott. It is said that Warren taunted the British saying, "These fellows say we won't fight! By heaven, I hope I shall die up to my knees in British blood!" (G. C. Wildrik 2009). He did; he remained in the fight until the third and final assault by the British.

He was then killed instantly by a musket ball to his head at age 34.

The British won the Battle of Bunker Hill but at great cost; there were 1,000 casualties in a garrison of about 6,000. American causalities numbered 500; "it was so costly they [British] never did what they did here again, that is, attack an entrenched position" (K. Landergan 2011). The Revolutionary War had started. The Second Continental Congress convened in 1775 and created the Continental Army. King George III issued a Proclamation of Rebellion, requiring action against the traitors. On June 19, 1775, the Continental Congress selected George Washington (1732–1799) to lead the Continental Army as commander in chief of the army of the united colonies and of all the forces who voluntarily joined the army. Some historians believe that if Joseph Warren had not been killed at Bunker Hill, he probably would have been named commander in chief of the Continental Army.

Paul Revere was a close friend of Joseph's. As a silversmith, Revere made two artificial teeth (silver bridgework) for Joseph, which was an important event that later allowed friends to identify Joseph's body after the Battle of Bunker Hill. At the time of his death, Warren was engaged to Mercy Scollay. She continued to care for his four children. Mercy and Warren's children struggled financially. Benedict Arnold gave the family $500, and through his efforts the orphans were also awarded a pension by Congress amounting to half of Joseph's army pay until they came of age. Warren's back pay at the time totaled about $7,000. Both of Warren's boys died childless in their early twenties; one daughter died without children. Only Mary, who married twice, left heirs.

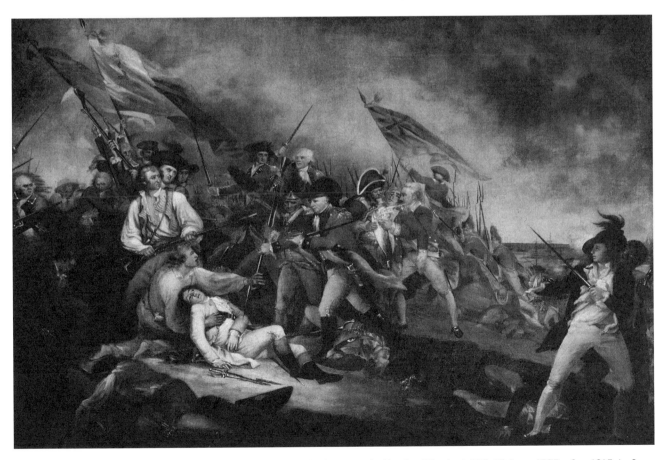

John Trumbull, American, 1756–1843. *The Death of General Warren at the Battle of Bunker's Hill, 17 June, 1775,* after 1815–before 1831. Oil on canvas. 50.16 x 75.56 cm (19 ¾ x 29 ¾ in.)

Museum of Fine Arts, Boston. Gift of Howland S. Warren, 1977.853. Photograph © 2021 Museum of Fine Arts, Boston

Dr. Joseph Warren's body was initially buried at Bunker Hill and recovered 10 months later after it was identified by his friend Paul Revere. Because Warren wore his artificial teeth on his last day, Revere was able to identify him. A statue, 35-feet high, was erected by the Masons and stood at the site where he had died. It is now located in front of the Roxbury Latin School where he had taught as a young man before becoming a physician and surgeon. He is buried in the Forest Hills Cemetery in Jamaica Plain.

Boston's Fort Warren was named in his honor in 1833. Five ships in the Continental Navy and the US Navy were named *Warren*. Fourteen states have a Warren County named in his honor, as well as 29 Warren townships. There is a Warren Street in Roxbury and a Warren Tavern, just down the hill from the Bunker Hill Monument. Dr. Warren had cared for many people as both physician and as a leader in the colonists' early fight for independence. Some historians have said he changed the direction of America.

CHAPTER 2

John Warren
Father of Harvard Medical School

John Warren, commonly called Jack, was the father of Harvard Medical School. He was 12 years younger than his brother Joseph, and he was only two when their father died. Historians described him as a "delicate child...not as emotionally or physically sturdy as Joseph" (R. Truax 1968). Somewhat slow in development, he didn't learn to read until age 10, but he then advanced rapidly, entering Harvard at age 14. He spoke Latin fluently. Although fond of people, he was "withdrawn and even depressed" (R. Truax 1968). While a student at Harvard, he joined a group called Spunkers or Spunks (formed before 1771), which was a secret anatomical society whose members studied anatomic books and a skeleton they possessed, dissected animals, and stole human bodies from graves to dissect. The society may have been founded by his brother Joseph.

Jack graduated at age 18 and then spent two years as an apprentice to his brother. He lived with Joseph, Elizabeth, and their children in their house on Hanover Street, but Elizabeth died young, at age 26 (May 3, 1773), of unknown cause during the second year of Jack's apprenticeship. Jack was 19 and his brother Joseph was 31. After completion of his apprenticeship, Jack moved to Salem to practice with the town's leading physician, Dr. Edward A. Holyoke. After Joseph unsuccessfully attempted to establish an examination for physicians and surgeons to distinguish them from what he called quacks, he asked Dr. Holyoke to examine Jack. Jack passed the examination.

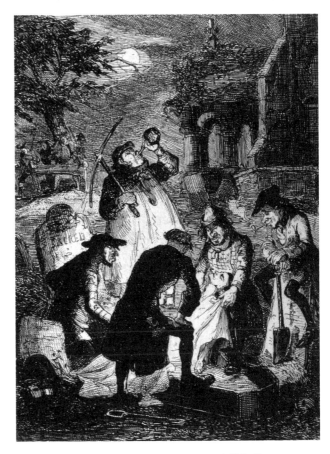

Resurrectionists by Hablot Knight Browne, 1887. Cartoon depicting grave robbers. Originally published in *The Chronicles of Crime*, Camden Pelham, 1887. Internet Archive.

Physician Snapshot

John "Jack" Warren
BORN: 1753
DEATH: 1815
SIGNIFICANT CONTRIBUTIONS: Leader in education and father of Harvard Medical School

SENIOR SURGEON OF THE REVOLUTION

Jack operated a brief—not entirely successful—general practice in Salem from 1774 to 1775. During this time, he also devoted himself to surgery. But the Revolutionary War drew him back to Boston. Some have said that Jack was also a member of the Boston Tea Party, but there is no definitive evidence to support those claims. We know that he did join a militia regiment as its surgeon, however, and volunteered in Colonel Pickering's regiment at age 22. During the Battle of Bunker Hill, Jack set out at 2:00 a.m. on Saturday (June 17, 1775) to find his brother, Joseph. Jack had heard his brother was active in the battle on Breed's Hill. We do not know whether Jack took a boat from Lechmere Point in Cambridge or approached through Charlestown Neck. Charlestown had been burned to the ground by the British. There he encountered a British sentry who refused to let him approach Breeds Hill and bayoneted him as a warning, leaving him with a permanent scar to remember the occasion.

Washington entered Cambridge on July 3, 1775. After the Battle of Bunker Hill and the Battle of Lexington and Concord, Jack's regiment marched to Cambridge; he may have served as surgeon in the temporary military hospital there. The Americans used the Ruggles-Fayerweather House, a Tory mansion. The hospital was most likely established by Congress on July 22, 1775. (The house was reclaimed by the Fayerweather family after the British evacuated Boston, and, as of 2019, it remained a private house in Cambridge.) The Americans used a total of four houses in Cambridge to care for the wounded, and Jack Warren was appointed senior surgeon for the Continental Army at age 22. His pay was approximately $1.33 per day.

It wasn't until after the British had evacuated Charlestown that Jack, Paul Revere, and some friends discovered Joseph's grave in March of

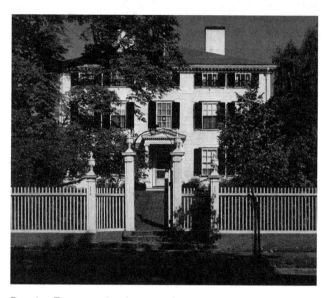

Ruggles-Fayerweather house today.
Courtesy of Cambridge Historical Society.

1776. Paul Revere identified the body (see chapter 1), and Joseph was buried in King's Chapel after a procession and funeral services led by the Masons.

After the British evacuated Boston in 1776, Jack was one of the first Americans to enter the city, where he discovered that medicine left behind in the British temporary hospital was contaminated with arsenic and was unusable by the Americans. During this same year, Jack left the Cambridge hospital to serve as surgeon of the general hospital on Long Island during General Washington's defense there. He may also have served in the Battle of Trenton and the Battle of Princeton. He returned to Boston in 1779, during which time there was a shortage of physicians and conditions were deplorable. Wound infections and illnesses were stated to have "claimed more lives than did the weapons of the enemy" (T. F. Harrington 1905a). Jack had previously declined the position of director of medical services, but upon his return to Boston—after almost two years serving as surgeon on the front lines of action—he was appointed superintendent surgeon at the Continental (military) General Established Hospital in Boston. He served there until the end of the war.

Harrington, author of *The Harvard Medical School, A History, Narrative and Documentary (1782–1905)*, explained that the surgeon's role was always subservient to physicians during the Revolution, and this resulted in delays in diagnosis or mistreatments of surgical problems. A military surgeon had a limited role, and surgical treatment was a last resort because there was no anesthesia, no aseptic techniques, no antibiotics, and no use of blood transfusions at the time. Amputations were commonly used for severe limb injuries, and limbs were often amputated in the field. Death from bleeding, or most commonly infection, resulted in most cases. Few surgeons had a university degree and very few had specific surgical skills. Chest and abdominal wounds were dressed and operations were rarely attempted. If intestines were injured and protruding, they would be sutured to the wound edges with the expectation that a colostomy or an ileostomy would form. Bloodletting always accompanied an operation, during which 16 to 24 ounces of blood was removed from an arm vein.

In addition to managing many different illnesses and infections, hospital surgeons had other major problems that Jack and some of his colleagues resolved. Prior to Jack's appointment as a hospital surgeon, discipline was lax; hospital surgeons lacked authority and were controlled by regimental surgeons, most of whom were "illiterate and untrained" and therefore inferior to hospital surgeons (T. F. Harrington 1905a); they directed hospital surgeons to admit men from the battlefield with contagious diseases, together with the wounded, as directed by regimental surgeons. George Washington called the regimental surgeons "very great rascals" (T. F. Harrington 1905a). Jack Warren and some colleagues petitioned Dr. John Morgan, who was the director of medical services as well as Jack's friend and one of the founders of the first US medical school, the College of Philadelphia. Morgan reversed the governance of military surgeons, subordinating regimental surgeons to the hospital surgeons.

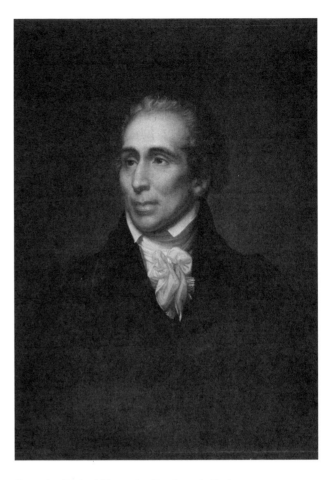

Portrait of John Warren by Rembrandt Peale.
Harvard University Portrait Collection, Gift of Dr. Richard Warren to the Harvard Medical School, 1982. Photo © President and Fellows of Harvard College.

Jack Warren was a physician who had a strong interest in anatomy that continued long after his studies at Harvard. He was intensely interested in surgery including orthopaedic surgery, although it was not named such at the time. He performed the first successful shoulder amputation in the country in 1781, which included a disarticulation for an injury of the entire arm up to the shoulder.

Anatomy is the Basis of Surgery,
It informs the Head,
Guides the hand, and
Familiarizes the heart with a kind of necessary inhumanity in
The use of cutting instruments.

—William Hunter, eighteenth century
(quoted in the *Lancet* 1829)

He also had a real fondness for teaching. He began giving lectures and human anatomy demonstrations while he was the Superintendent Surgeon at the Continental Hospital in Boston (located near what would become Massachusetts General Hospital [MGH]) at Milton and Spring Streets. At the time, it was illegal to dissect human bodies, but he felt protected because he limited himself to doing so only in the military hospital. Initially, he also only invited students and staff that he knew. He did not have to resort to robbing graves because soldiers who died without known relations were available for his dissections. J. L. Bell attributed the following statement to Jack:

> In some of the more populous towns, students were sometimes indulged with the privilege of examining the bodies of those who had died from any extraordinary disease, and in a few instances associations were formed for pursuing the business of dissection, where opportunities offered from casualties, or from public executions, for doing it in decency and safety.
> (J. L. Bell 2010)

But the Revolution was the era to which the first medical school east of Philadelphia owes its birth. The military hospitals of the United States furnished a large field for observation and experiment in the various branches of the healing art, as well as an opportunity for anatomical investigations. "Not a flashy operator" (R. Truax 1968), Warren became a very experienced surgeon during the Revolutionary War, and he remained the senior surgeon at the Military Hospital until the end of the war in 1783. He planned to remain and practice in Boston, especially after meeting Abigail Collins. Abigail, the daughter of the governor of Rhode Island, was popular among the soldiers and described as a favorite with Washington. Jack and Abigail married on November 4, 1777; she was 17 and he was 24. But 1777 in Boston, despite his happy marriage, was not a good year. Some historians have recorded it as a year with a winter as

harsh as the winter at Valley Forge. Many were without jobs. Paupers in the Almshouse often died of cold and/or starvation, and robberies became common at night. Most goods had been taken or destroyed by the British. Prices, including for food, soared. Jack and Abigail received some help from her parents, but he couldn't support both of them on his meager military salary and his limited earnings seeing private patients. That summer delivered hope when the French joined the Americans in the fight against the British, and on August 1, 1778, Jack and Abigail had their first child, whom they named John Collins Warren after her father. John Collins who was the first of an estimated 19 children; many of whom died in childhood.

When Governor Collins died, Abigail inherited two enslaved Africans, Cuff and Quaco, who were thought to be brothers. Jack had strong sentiments against slavery and the slave trade, and slavery was abolished in Massachusetts with the adoption of the state constitution in 1780; Jack's son Edward had been told that "your father was always a friend of black men" (E. Warren 1874). Cuff and Quaco remained as servants in the home of Jack and Abigail. Quaco sustained a serious head injury and died when he fell off his horse and was kicked in the head. Cuff remained an important part of Jack's home and practice until Jack's death.

Jack's practice grew steadily until he had the most popular and largest practice in Boston, but physicians continued to have business and professional difficulties. They didn't know what to charge patients. Physicians were paid little, often 50 cents for office visits or small operations, such as bleeding, tooth extraction, or opening an abscess. They were paid £1 for reducing dislocations and up to £5 for major operations. They were also concerned about malpractice and libel suits, accusations of murder and manslaughter—sometimes arising from quarrels amongst physicians, including occasional fist fights—and how to deal with what they called quacks or non-physician healers. They met frequently at the Green Dragon to establish fees and eventually to organize themselves into the Boston Medical Association on May 14, 1780 (the Massachusetts Medical Society was founded the following year). Active in organizing this group were Jack Warren, Samuel Danforth, Thomas Kast, and Isaacs Rand—all Tories except for Warren.

FATHER OF HARVARD MEDICAL SCHOOL

Soon after the Boston Medical Association formed, Warren proposed that the association start a medical institution for apprentices studying in Boston. There were about six at the time. Warren had continued his lectures and anatomic demonstrations at the Continental Hospital in Boston— his most recent ones sponsored by the Boston Medical Association, and he taught apprentices following in his brother's footsteps.

His proposal had been the first suggestion for a medical school in Boston. Warren's first anatomy course was given to army surgeons in about 1779. His third course, in 1782, was held in the Molineux House on Beacon Street. His lectures were attended by all medical students in Boston and its surrounding locale, by other literary professionals, and even by the French Fleet while in Boston harbor (Cheever 1928).

In May of 1782, Joseph Willard, the president of Harvard, met with the Fellows of the College. He—along with some members of the Harvard Corporation—had attended some of Warren's lectures and demonstrations, and he asked the Fellows to consider establishing a medical professorship. Warren was asked to write a plan for a course of medical studies to accompany the apprentice training. After consulting with Benjamin Rush and William Shippen (both had experience with the first medical school in Philadelphia), Warren presented his report to the Harvard Corporation. The corporation voted to elect three professors: Warren as professor of anatomy and surgery (November 22,

1782), a professor of theory and practice of physic and of chemistry, and a professor of materia medica (the latter two positions were selected later). Then, in 1782, the first medical school in New England was established, the Medical Institution of Harvard College (1782–1816). The Harvard Corporation voted to appoint the first dean to manage it, and on December 3, 1782, John Warren accepted the position.

The war left little money for Harvard. Dr. Ezekiel Hersey had left £1,000 in 1770 for "a professor of anatomy and physic who was to reside in Cambridge" (R. Truax 1968). Since Warren lived in Boston and, as a surgeon, was not qualified to teach physic (medicine), the Hersey family agreed with Harvard's request to split the income into two chairs. Warren received half of the income as the professor of anatomy and surgery, and Benjamin Waterhouse (who lived in Cambridge) received the other half as professor of the theory and practice of physic (December 24, 1782). Aaron Dexter was chosen to teach chemistry on May 22, 1783; the professor of materia medica was planned to be appointed later. Two issues immediately arose that could have been problematic. First, the professors were required to "declare themselves to be Protestant Christians" because of some peoples' fears that "doctors might be godless and immoral." (R. Truax 1968). The second dilemma was even greater. The newly formed Massachusetts Medical

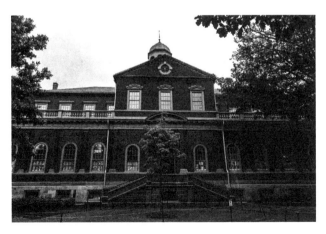

Harvard Hall, today. First home of the medical school in 1782.
Kael E. Randall/Kael Randall Images.

Society included regulation of the standards for physicians as an important part of its mission. They wanted complete control over the examination and certification process for physicians. The university, however, assumed it would have that responsibility. After many heated discussions over a lengthy period, both parties finally agreed that any physician who had a diploma from the Medical Institution of Harvard College or a certificate of approval from the Massachusetts Medical Society would be qualified to practice medicine in Massachusetts. They also required that each professor must have a BA, MA, or Doctor of Physic degree. Professors had to be qualified to see patients and were responsible for examining the students yearly in the presence of six Harvard governors and members of the Massachusetts Medical Society.

Dr. Warren's first lectures at Harvard in 1782 were in Cambridge, probably in the basement of Harvard Hall. His lectures lasted two to three hours; 20 students attended his first lecture. But in less than a year and at the end of the Revolutionary War, he moved into Holden Chapel, where all medical lectures and anatomical demonstrations were held until the Medical Institution moved

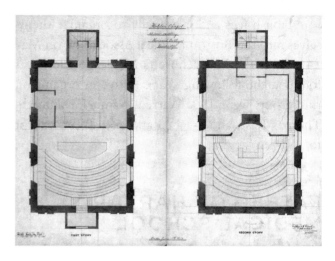

Floor plan, Holden Chapel. Anatomy lectures were on the third floor.
UAI 15.10.5 (Box 3, pages 4-5), olvwork670794. Harvard University Archives.

to Boston in 1810 (after 28 years). As of 2019, Holden Chapel remained on the Cambridge campus, used by the university's glee club. Excavations beneath the chapel have discovered bones and other artifacts from the early human dissections, which were most likely those completed by Jack Warren. Holden Chapel was built in 1744 and was the first chapel at Harvard. It was badly damaged by troops during the Revolution and functioned as Harvard's carpentry shop when Warren began his lectures there. Warren's first course included a week of lectures and demonstrations of each of the following over the course of six weeks (T. F. Harrington 1905a):

I. Osteology, or a definition of the Bones
II. Myology, of the Muscles
III. Splanchnology, of the Viscera contained in the large Cavities
IV. Angeiology, of the blood vessels and Lymphatics
V. Neurology, of the Nerves
VI. Adenology, of the Glands

By 1790, his lectures expanded to the following. His lectures began October 6 and ended November 17. Dissections began on October 15.

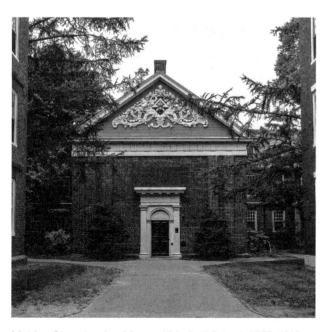

Holden Chapel today. Harvard Medical School, 1783–1810.
Kael E. Randall/Kael Randall Images.

1. Introduction: History of Anatomy.
2. General Description and Structure of Single Fibres.
3. The Five Abdominal Muscles.
4. Still on Abdominal Muscles. The Operation of Lithotomy.
5. Peritoneum and Omentum.
6. Jejunum, Ileum, Caecum, Colon, Rectum.
7. Mesentery, Stomach, Spleen, Pancreas *in situ*.
8. Abdominal Vessels, Liver, Bile and Pancreatic Ducts, with Duodenum, in situ.
9. Stomach, Duodenum and Mesentery, Liver and Spleen, removed together, to show Vessels going to each organ. Demonstrate Valoula Colica, Coats of Stomach, Structure of Spleen and Liver.
10. Brain and 10 Pairs of Nerves.
11. Rest of Abdominal Vessels, Division of Genitals, Testes, Scrotum, Tunica Vaginalis, Vas Deferens, Hernia Congenita.
12. Kidneys removed with Vessels, Ureters and Seminal Vesicles, Coats of Penis, Crura, General View of Corpus Spongiosum and Urethra.
13. Bladder removed one inch above Urethral Opening; Seminal Vesicles and Prostate exposed; open Prostatic Urethra, Caput Gallinginis; show latter in Ox also. Urethra and Cowper's glands.
14. Sphincter Ani and Levatores, structure of Urethra and Coats of Bladder dissected.
15. Female Genitals; Doctrine of Conception and Nutrition of Foetus explained.
16. Muscles of Face and Jaws. Diaphragm.
17. Muscles of Os Hyoides and of Tongue. Cartilages of Larynx demonstrated on a Preparation.
18. Lower jaw sawed in two. Pterygoid Muscles. Palate, Fauces, Eustachian Tube.
19. Five Pairs of Muscles of Head in front of Longus Colli: Muscles on Thorax, Pleura and Mediastinum, the Sternum being raised.
20. Trachea, Bronchi, Great Vessels, and General View of Circulation.

Warren was extremely popular with his students. He was an excellent teacher and apparently happiest when teaching. He never read lectures, as was common at the time, but instead spoke extemporaneously. Oliver Wendell Holmes said of Dr. Warren, "the driest bone of the human body became in his hands the subject of animated and agreeable description" (T. F. Harrington 1905a). Each of his lectures lasted two to three hours and usually included dissection. Being very knowledgeable about anatomy with years of experience in human dissection and demonstrations, as well as experienced as a surgeon, we can assume that students flocked to his lectures. Students were important to Warren, for in addition to his devotion to teaching, students had to pay a fee to attend his lectures. He made little income from the professorship, additional but variable income from his large private practice, and, therefore, needed the students' fees to help support his large family. Fees were regulated by the Corporation; £5 for BA students, 40 shillings for MA students, and £7 for all others. The first graduates from this new medical school (n=2) studied under Dr. Warren and received a bachelor of medicine degree on July 16, 1788, the only medical degree given prior to 1811. After 1811, graduates received a doctor of medicine degree.

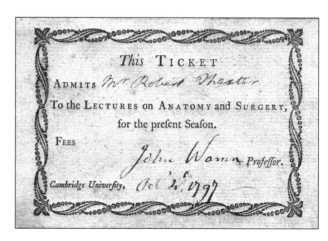

Admission ticket to John Warren's lectures on anatomy and surgery.

Boston Medical Library in the Francis A. Countway Library of Medicine.

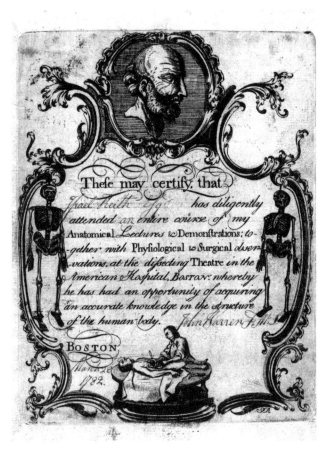

Attendance certificate: Warren's anatomy lectures. Signed by John Warren, MD, March 28, 1782. Engraver: Paul Revere. Collection of the Massachusetts Historical Society.

Lectures and demonstrations were essential to the medical students. Anatomy books were rare. Warren spoke Latin and learned French to translate the few important available books for his students. His first lecture (Osteology) was usually delivered in Latin. At his last lecture, he would give his students their certificates of completion, which were engraved by Paul Revere. He also gave a short speech and told his students that he looked forward to:

> The happy day when the Profession which has for its object the most valuable of all human blessings, will cease to be treated with neglect and indifference. (R. Truax 1968)

Warren remained very busy with a large private practice in Boston and his teaching responsibilities at Harvard. Even so, he had difficulty supporting his large family of nine children, including the four children of his brother, Joseph. It was a constant concern of his; he drove himself continuously. A typical day for Dr. Warren consisted of riding by horse early in the morning to the Charlestown ferry, which he took to Cambridge. During the winter, when the ferry wasn't operating, he rode by horseback nine miles west to Cambridge through Roxbury and Brookline. After teaching all morning, he visited soldiers in the Military Hospital in West Boston. After making house calls, he returned home where he saw private patients in a room next to his "medicine room" (R. Truax 1968). In reality his "medicine room" was a small apothecary shop where his students and apprentices studied and prepared medicines for his patients. Jack and Abigail had moved from a small house on Avon Place and Central Court to a larger house on School Street. He had a few servants including a cook, a chambermaid and two former enslaved Africans, Cuff and Quaco. According to his youngest son, Edward, who wrote Jack Warren's biography, "the back windows of the house were occupied with drying preparations of legs and arms, and other anatomical and morbid specimens prepared by Dr. Warren and forming the basis of the Warren Museum, afterwards in the Medical College" (E. Warren 1874).

But no matter how hard he worked, the decks were stacked against physicians earning a decent wage at that time. Historians muse that Charles Bulfinch—the famous architect of Boston who designed many of its major buildings, including the Bulfinch Building of the Massachusetts General Hospital—was advised by his father not to follow in his footsteps because medicine was a laborious profession and his father "had not found …[it] a profitable business" (R. Truax 1968). Eventually the Military Hospital in Boston, where Warren had also taught medical students, was closed after the war. The only other clinical facility in Boston was the Almshouse. Harvard requested

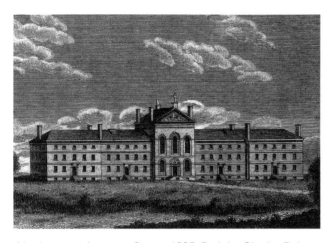

Almshouse on Leverett Street, 1825. Built by Charles Bulfinch in 1799. Engraver: Abel Bowen. Originally published in *A History of Boston* by Caleb Snow, 2nd edition, 1828.
Print Department, Boston Public Library.

that their professors be permitted to teach there, but the Massachusetts Medical Society opposed the request, believing that Warren as professor of anatomy and surgery would use his privileges for his financial advantage. But Warren "never allowed opposition to retard his efforts for what he was convinced was for the good of his patients and the profession" (E. Warren 1874). The Massachusetts Medical Society also opposed a second request of Harvard to have the state build a public infirmary for the poor in Cambridge. As a result, teaching in the Almshouse in Boston was delayed for years.

A LIFETIME OF ACCOMPLISHMENTS

John Warren had many successes and recognitions during his career. In addition to the successful shoulder dislocation he performed in 1781, he pioneered shoulder surgery. He also followed his brother in the fight against smallpox. In 1784, he and several colleagues opened a smallpox hospital at Point Shirley. In 1792, they "inoculated more than 1500 persons" (H. Stalker 1940). He successfully performed an abdominal resection in 1785 and removed the parotid gland of a patient

in 1804. In 1786, he received an honorary medical degree from Harvard while still teaching in Holden Chapel. Despite these numerous accomplishments, he published very few papers. One described the case of the abdominal desmoid tumor that he removed surgically and another most notable paper, "A View of the Mercurial Practice in Febrile Diseases," covered many of the common infectious diseases. He also published the first article in the newly founded *New England Journal of Medicine* (NEJM) in 1812.

He remained as the first Hersey Professor of Anatomy and Surgery until 1815 (32 years). Warren had established a medical board to examine competent surgeons, an idea he probably learned from his brother. The exam, a first in unofficial medical certification, consisted of anatomy, physiology, surgery and *materia medica*. Six of the 16 surgeons who took the exam failed and were rejected as military surgeons.

He followed his brother in community affairs and became the grand master of the Massachusetts Lodge of Free and Accepted Masons. At the end of the Revolutionary War in 1783, he was honored by the people of Boston when he was selected to give the first oration on July 4 to commemorate America's independence. He delivered his oration from the balcony of the State House. He also helped found the Anthology Club, was founder and president of the Massachusetts Humane Society, a fellow of the American Academy of Arts and Sciences, and a trustee of the Massachusetts Agricultural Society and the Massachusetts Charitable Society. As a trustee of the Massachusetts Humane Society, he hosted their first meeting in his home and helped raise money to eventually establish a hospital for the mentally ill (MGH). As a founder of the Massachusetts Medical Society, he became its seventh president (1804–1815).

In 1811, Warren had a slight stroke, which left him weak on his right side. For many years, he also suffered from angina pectoris. He died at age 62, on April 4, 1815, most likely of congestive heart failure. His son, John Collins Warren,

believed that his early death was a result of deliv-
ering babies late at night in the North End; Jack
had developed pleurisy at the time. John Collins
believed his father continued to work so hard in
order to increase the inheritance for his children.
It has been said that John Warren was the single
most important person in the early institutional-
ization of Boston medicine.

CHAPTER 3

John Collins Warren

Co-Founder of the Massachusetts General Hospital

John Collins Warren was born on August 1, 1778, the first son of John and Abigail Warren. He followed in his father's footsteps by co-founding Massachusetts General Hospital (MGH) with James Jackson. Collins, his middle name, was in honor of Abigail's father John Collins, a governor of Rhode Island. He was born at home, the site of the future Jordan Marsh Company in the Downtown Crossing area of Boston. At age eight, after completing his initial education at Master Vinal's Reading and Writing School on West Street, he entered the Public Latin School. Obviously a bright and competitive student, he was head of his class for seven years, sometimes alternating with one other boy. He delivered the valedictory address and received the first Franklin Medal for scholarship. The medal—named after Benjamin Franklin—was designed to honor graduates who demonstrated excellence in academics and character. Later, John Collins helped to organize the Association of Franklin Medal Scholars. His brother Edward described him as neat and reserved, probably shy. He said, "Though always delicate, he had no severe illness" (E. Warren 1860).

In 1793, at age 15, John Collins Warren entered Harvard College. He had no interest in a career in medicine while he was in college. His father wanted him to become a businessman in order not to have to deal with the complexities and stress of his own field. He enjoyed college life and

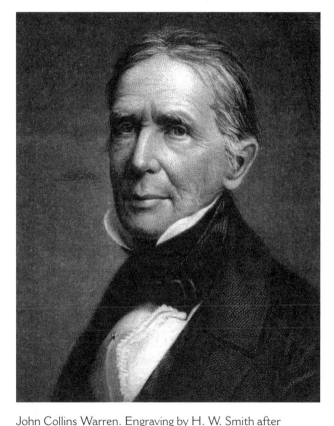

John Collins Warren. Engraving by H. W. Smith after daguerreotype by John Adams Whipple. ca. 1856.
Boston Medical Library in the Francis A. Countway Library of Medicine.

Physician snapshot

John Collins Warren

BORN: 1778

DIED: 1856

SIGNIFICANT CONTRIBUTIONS: Co-founder of the Massachusetts General Hospital; first dean of HMS; president of AMA; risk-taker was apparently "a scholar and gentleman" (E. Warren 1860). He helped found and also served as president of the Hasty Pudding Club. He did well academically and received the prize in Latin. The year prior to his graduation, he began to show some interest in medicine, and he followed in the footsteps of his father and his uncle by joining other students (Spunkers) in digging up dead bodies for dissection and study. "He began the business of getting subjects for anatomical study... At the (next) day's first class, he faced his teacher, John Warren [former Spunker and his father]...he seemed to be as much pleased as I ever saw him" after Dr. John Warren saw the excellent body that his son had helped retrieve (A. M. Menting 2009).

John Collins (circa 1796) described the incident in full (quoted in *Strangeremains* 2015):

> Having understood that a man without relations was to be buried in the North Burying-Ground, I formed a party, of which Dr. William Ingalls was one. He was a physician of Boston at that time. We reached the spot at ten o'clock at night. The night was rather light. We soon found the grave; but, after proceeding a while, were led to suspect a mistake, and went to another place. Here we found ourselves wrong, and returned to the first; and, having set watches, we proceeded rapidly, uncovering the coffin by breaking it open. We took out the body of a stout young man, put it in a bag, and carried it to the burying-ground wall. As we were going to lift it over and put it in the chaise, we saw a man walking along the edge of the wall outside, smoking. A part of us disappeared. One of the company met him, stopped him from coming on, and entered into conversation with him. This individual of our party affected to be intoxicated, while he contrived to get into a quarrel with the stranger. After he had succeeded in doing this, another of the party, approaching, pretended to side with the stranger, and ordered the other to go about his business. Taking the stranger by the

arm, he led him off in a different direction to some distance; then left him, and returned to the burying-ground. The body was then quickly taken up, and packed in the chaise between two of the parties, who drove off to Cambridge with their booty. Two of us staid to fill the grave; but my companion, being alarmed, soon left the burying-ground; and I, knowing the importance of covering up the grave and effacing the vestiges of our labor, remained, with no very agreeable sensations, to finish the work. However, I got off without further interruption; drove, with the tools to Cambridge; and arrived there just before daylight.

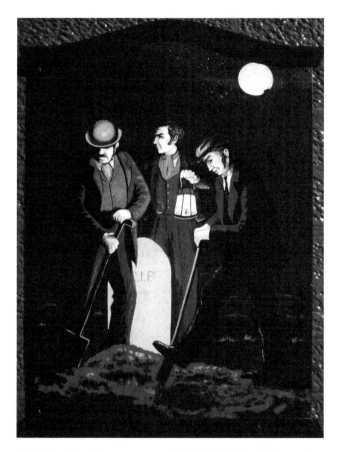

Body Snatchers. Painting on wall of the Old Crown Inn in the High Street of Penicuik in Midlothian, Scotland.
Kim Traynor/Wikimedia Commons.

> When my father [Dr. John Warren, founder of Harvard Medical School] came up in the morning to lecture, and found that I had been

engaged in this scrape, he was very much alarmed; but when the body was uncovered, and he saw what a fine, healthy subject it was, he seemed to be as much pleased as I ever saw him. The body lasted the [entire anatomy] course through.

He graduated in 1797. After graduating, he was unsuccessful in finding a job in business. He studied French for a year and then began to apprentice in medicine with his father, "who was at that period the most eminent practitioner in New England, a man of iron will, a born autocrat, who ruled the whole professional fraternity with a superb and absolute sway" (H. P. Arnold 1886). Even though his father had a busy practice and gave frequent lectures, John Collins soon became interested enough in medicine that he wanted to attend medical school. He eventually persuaded his father to allow him to travel to England to seek a more formal medical education. Despite his father's efforts to found Harvard Medical School, John Collins went to London because of its excellent reputation in medicine and medical education.

Just before turning 21, John Collins Warren arrived in England. The voyage took 24 days. It was somewhat risky to travel abroad by ship because the United States was at war with France. The crew taught all passengers to use the cannons (26 pounders) while on board the ship. They most likely did not see any hostile action, however. The ship landed in Dover; and he continued his trip to London. Before arriving in London, he had two interesting meetings that probably caused him some apprehension. He met a British captain who claimed to have fought in the Battle of Bunker Hill, where he knew his uncle had died, and on another occasion, he met Benedict Arnold and his family.

John Collins was surprised at how little the British knew about the United States. A famous surgeon asked him, "Do you have schools in America, Mr. Warren?" (quoted in R. Truax 1968). Arriving in London in mid-July, he learned that there were two types of students in hospitals:

dressers and walkers. Walkers were mere observers; they only looked at the medical/surgical care being given but did not actually care for patients. Dressers, on the other hand, took care of patients; they dressed all wounds and cared for simple cases. The tuition for walkers was £25; for dressers, it was £50. He chose to be a dresser because he knew from the beginning, "I intend to become a surgeon" and he needed the practical experience (E. Warren 1860). The medical profession in England in the eighteenth century was divided into three classes: at the top were physicians who charged high fees and carried gold-topped canes, surgeons who could bleed patients, and apothecaries at the bottom who could not bleed patients.

SURGICAL APPRENTICESHIPS

Upon his arrival in London, John Collins Warren selected Mr. William Cooper—the senior surgeon at Guy's Hospital, probably the first modern teaching and research hospital in London—as his mentor. Cooper, who was in his senior year as a surgeon and was the first surgeon to lecture in a hospital in England, placed John Collins in charge of his 40 patients. He instructed John Collins about the treatment of his patients twice weekly. John Collins also worked with one of Cooper's colleagues, a Mr. Henry Cline who had studied under John Hunter and was an excellent technical surgeon. John Collins wrote that "Mr. Cline's operations for aneurysm or hernia are grand. It is a pleasure to see him take or turn his knife" (H. P. Arnold 1886). He had never seen a hernia operation; it had not been done yet in the United States.

Cooper was in the latter years of his career and happily turned over all his patients to John Collins. He was immediately very busy because many of the patients required daily dressing changes. It must have been challenging for him, having only spent one year as an apprentice to his father. He lived in the hospital, and Cooper saw John Collins twice a week to give him instructions while making walk rounds.

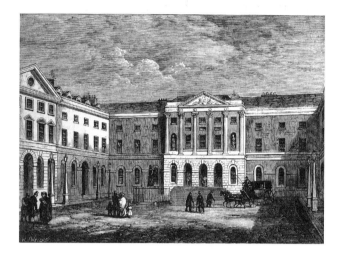

Guy's and Old St. Thomas, 1840. From *Old and New London: Vol. 6*, by Edward Walford, 1878.
University of California Libraries/Internet Archive.

Warren's experience with Mr. William Cooper was short lived. Cooper soon retired and was replaced by his nephew; Sir Astley Cooper. This change was a great opportunity for John Collins because Astley Cooper preferred surgery over some of the conservative approaches that his uncle had preferred. Warren described his mentor as "a young man of the greatest natural abilities and almost adored at the hospitals" (H. P. Arnold 1886). John Collins obviously appreciated working with a younger and more energetic surgeon.

Sir Astley Cooper had studied under Mr. William Cooper and Mr. Cline years before John Collins arrived at Guy's Hospital. Astley became fascinated—almost obsessed—with anatomy. He couldn't do enough human dissections, which he did daily. It was dangerous work because dissection of human corpses was illegal in England. If caught, grave robbing by the so-called resurrectionists was a hanging offense. Astley spent two years as a demonstrator and then became a lecturer, both while an apprentice. Initially, his only payment was student fees, but as a lecturer he received additional money (£120 per year)

from Cline. His early lectures were boring, but he enjoyed teaching and worked hard to improve them. In his lectures, he separated surgery from anatomy for the first time, which allowed him to include pathology, physiology, and other disciplines in the surgery lectures.

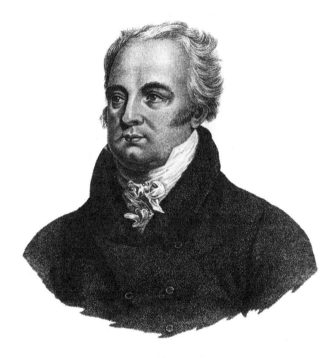

Sir Astley Cooper, Baronet. Engraver: J. Alais, 1824, after J.W. Rubidge. U.S. National Library of Medicine.

To further his education, Astley Cooper had observed Chopart operate in Paris. He learned from Chopart how to preserve anatomical dissections; a skill he later passed on to John Collins. Cooper's time in Paris was shortened because of the beginning of the French Revolution. After returning home, he continued to work on improving his lectures, developed a very large practice and continued his active daily dissections to include a variety of animals as well as humans. A typical day for Cooper began with private dissections in his house, followed by dressing, a visit from the hair dresser—his hair was powdered and included a queue—then breakfast, followed by seeing poor patients without charge for a couple of hours. The rest of the day was spent in the hospital teaching, seeing patients in his private practice, and research. Cooper's research centered on his animal dissections, and he "grew better at setting bones from having deliberately broken so many of them" (D. Burch 2007).

In 1800, Astley Cooper was elected surgeon at Guy's Hospital, a post he had strongly desired. He succeeded his uncle. At this time, he was a very popular lecturer; greatly improved from his early years as an apprentice. His income doubled immediately with his new position. Teaching rounds occurred twice weekly, lasting 30 to 45 minutes and included about 100 students. Students liked him and filled his operating room. His operations were described as elegant and rapid, but not hurried. He demonstrated compassion with his patients.

Sir Astley Cooper made many significant contributions in addition to his teaching of future surgeons. They included: successful hernia repair, rupture of the tympanic membrane for infections, successful ligation of the carotid and the femoral arteries. He developed a curved aneurysm needle that became part of a surgeon's operating kit, described the supporting (Cooper's) ligaments of the breast and the lymphatic drainage of the breast. In 1822, after dissecting two hands with Dupuytren's disease, he published the first report with his recommendation for palmar fasciotomy, 10 years before Dupuytren. Cooper's other orthopaedic contributions included teaching the "heel in axilla" method for reducing dislocated shoulders. He performed the first successful hip disarticulation, and he recognized the importance of

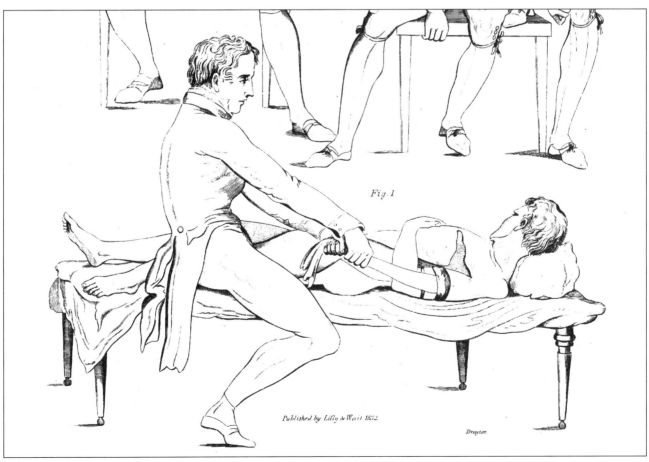

Heel in axilla method of reducing a dislocated shoulder. From *A Treatise on Dislocations and Fractures of Joints* by Sir Astley Cooper, 1832. U.S. National Library of Medicine.

the blood supply to the femoral head and bone fragility in the elderly. He published two classic books—*Dislocations and Fractures* and *Anatomical and Surgical Treatment of Hernia*—as well as four others, including *Anatomy of the Thymus Gland* and *Anatomy of the Breast*. Interestingly, John Keats, the famous English romantic poet, was his apprentice for one year before leaving medicine to write poetry. Cooper also had many honors. To name only a few, he was elected president of the Royal College of Surgeons twice and as a Fellow of the Royal Society; he also received a baronetcy by King George IV and became the official court surgeon to George IV, William IV, and Queen Victoria. His colleagues referred to him as "the Napoleon of surgery" (H. P. Arnold 1886).

Sir Astley Cooper probably exerted great influence on John Collins' devotion to surgery and orthopaedics. In a letter to his parents, John Collins enthused:

> I am the luckiest dog in life! I was called away… to a dislocated shoulder, which I have reduced in very handsome style. Within the first three days of my work, I have had one fracture and one injury of the cranium; one fractured leg, and another that we thought was fractured at first; one fracture of the ribs and this dislocation; besides two or three trifling accidents. I have been extremely fortunate in every way, and I verily begin to think I shall be famous.
> (quoted in R. Truax 1968)

John Collins recognized that surgery was becoming a respected scientific field in medicine, and he observed many of the great surgeons of the day including William Cheselden. He considered Cheselden the most skilled; Cheselden could perform an amputation or remove bladder stones in less than one minute. The surgeon had to be fast because there was no anesthesia.

John Collins learned valuable approaches to a patient about to undergo surgery from his English mentors. Many were profoundly affected by the

pain they inflicted. Cheselden became "gray and drawn" at the end of an operation (R. Truax 1968). John Hunter "went white and shook with terror when an operation approached" (D. Burch 2007). Astley Cooper "ignored the protests of his patients once an operation had begun" when they "instructed him to stop, he carried on regardless" (D. Burch 2007). It is said he became immune to the daily pain. In his biography of Astley Cooper, Burch describes his feelings about this issue. Cooper would recall a case of his uncle's (William) to his students. He felt that his uncle had too much sensitivity to be a surgeon. When about to start an amputation, the patient jumped off the table and left the operating room. William didn't catch the patient and stated he was happy the patient had left. Astley Cooper did not respect his uncle's approach, because he felt the surgeon had a responsibility to the patient. He believed that enduring the pain was necessary when ensuring the best outcome for the patient; he thought his uncle's response was cowardly, not compassionate. John Collins continued this practice after returning to Boston and never forgot Cooper's wisdom. He remembered what Astley Cooper had taught him: "tolerating pain was essential if men and women were to be helped" and a surgeon requires "an eagle's eye, a lady's hand and a lion's heart" (quoted in D. Burch 2007). As a patient was brought into the operating room (before the use of ether), John Collins would ask the patient if they wanted to proceed with the operation. If they declined, he asked them to leave. If they agreed, they were immediately held by multiple attendants and totally immobilized for the procedure. He then carried out the operation as quickly as possible, not stopping even if the patient requested.

EXPERIENCE AS A DRESSER

As a dresser, John Collins worked and slept at the hospital for a seven-day period every three months.

The on-call dresser saw all surgical emergencies presenting to the hospital during this seven-day period. He would clean and dress wounds, sometimes using plasters or poultices, bleed patients, pull teeth, reduce dislocations, immobilize fractures, perform minor operations, and use leeches or cupping on some patients. He attended lectures and made rounds with Astley Cooper, who was also accompanied by other students.

When not on call for emergencies (11 of the 12 weeks), Warren wrote: "In the morning, I went through my dressings; at noon attended Cooper's lectures; dissected in the afternoon; and wrote off my notes at night" (E. Warren 1860). James Jackson, a former Harvard student, one year ahead of Warren, was also studying in London. Their close friendship increased while in England and lasted the rest of their lives. Warren studied from copies of John Hunter's lectures, and both Astley Cooper and Cline were disciples of Hunter. It was apparent that John Hunter's scientific legacy and his approach to surgery greatly influenced John Collins Warren during his career as a surgeon in Boston.

After spending about one-and-a-half years at Guy's and St. Thomas's Hospitals, John Collins went to Edinburgh where he spent another year in training. Sir Charles Bell also heavily influenced him. Bell taught John Collins a new method of teaching by explaining what he was doing while operating while simultaneously questioning students, and he also kept them on their toes by including them as assistants. It was during his time with John Bell and Charles Bell that he considered following his father's footsteps in academia. A typical day consisted of lectures until noon (including those from John and Charles Bell), infirmary at noon, anatomy and surgery at 1:00 p.m., and returning home at 3:00 p.m. He spent his evenings writing notes from his lectures that day.

In the summer of 1801, Warren left Edinburgh for Paris. He wanted to further his studies in anatomy and to study chemistry. He stayed for one year and studied chemistry with Vanqualin and anatomy with Chavasier, Dupuytren, and Sabbatier, "whose anatomy was the favorite work of my father" (E. Warren 1860). He studied osteology with Gavard and midwifery with Dubois. In addition to lectures he worked in two hospitals, La Charité and Hôtel-Dieu. The French surgeons taught the new and popular discovery of percussion—called thumping—to feel and determine the presence of fluid or a mass. Records indicate Warren became very skilled at thumping.

LEADER IN SURGERY AND EDUCATION

During his time in Paris, the war between France and England continued. One historian wrote that John Collins was offered a position as a surgeon in Napoleon's army. He refused, returning briefly to London. After six weeks in London, leaving on October 17, 1802, he returned to Boston. The trip across the Atlantic took 50 days. He had been away from home, studying medicine and surgery for almost three-and-a-half years. He had received certificates of completion of his courses of study and as a dresser—equivalent to a medical degree from a university—and an honorary medical degree from St. Andrews University in Scotland.

By the time John Collins returned to Boston, his father was approaching 50. His father had a large practice, including midwifery, but he was having difficulty caring for all his patients, probably as a result of a recent stroke. John Collins immediately helped his father and assumed the care of many of his father's patients, beginning his practice within a couple of days of arriving in Boston. John Collins took over the large midwifery practice which included many poor patients, making up to 50 patient visits each day. He wrote, "In the course of that summer, I was left with the whole practice—medical, surgical and obstetrical" (E. Warren 1860). This allowed his father to spend more time at his farm.

Warren also met Susan Powell Mason, the daughter of a wealthy businessman, who owned a large part of Beacon Hill. They became engaged a few months after his return and were married on November 17, 1803. Susan, at 21 years old, was witty and direct but also kind and creative. After living on Tremont Street for a year, they moved into a large and grand house designed by Bulfinch, Number 2 Park Street. It was a gift from

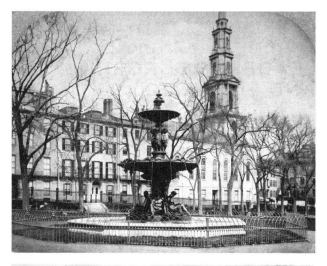

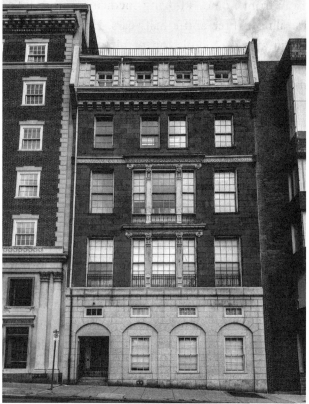

No. 2 Park Street, home of John Collins Warren (top, ca. 1860s; bottom, 2020).

Boston Athenæum (t); Kael E. Randall/Kael Randall Images (b)

his father-in-law, Jonathan Mason. They had six children, including Jonathan Mason Warren, who would follow in his father's, grandfather's, and granduncle's profession of medicine and surgery.

The fall of 1803 was a busy time for John Collins. In addition to caring for his father's patients and getting married, he started to assist his father at Harvard. He began to do the human dissections for the lectures in Holden Chapel. Originally built in 1774, John Warren convinced Harvard to use the site of the chapel for medical instruction. Both he and his son, John Collins, taught anatomy there with lectures and cadaver dissections. These instructions continued until at least 1862. During the remodeling of the chapel for choral students in 1999, excavations in the basement revealed many artifacts, including bones (femur, hips, clavicles, tibias, humeri, radii, and ulnas) from 784 adults and 34 children. Arsenic had been used as a preservative. The collection is housed in the Peabody Museum at Harvard.

At the time, the dissections took a long time, as did John Collins' travel to and from Cambridge. He was also admitted to the Massachusetts Medical Society in 1803. Warren coauthored with James Jackson a pharmacopeia for the Massachusetts Medical Society, and they formed the Boston Medical Association, "an institution invaluable for the harmony and union it has promoted for fifty years among the medical men of Boston" (E. Warren 1860). The Association had a "code of medical policy for the regulation of its members…encouraged consultations in different and protracted cases…recommended measures for avoiding the slightest attempts to deprecate the character of any other physician…use of quack medicines is forbidden…a fee-table is established" (E. Warren 1860).

In 1806, John Collins was given the title of adjunct professor of surgery, as an assistant to his father. John Collins began a common trend in his career: joining or founding educational organizations. Such organizations included a private society for the study of natural philosophy, to which Warren gave 10 lectures a year on anatomy and physiology; the Monthly Anthology Club, which published a monthly magazine of short stories (Warren was coeditor) that would eventually become the Boston Athenaeum; the Improvement Society (later called the Warren Club or the Thursday Evening Club), a private medical society that met Thursday evenings in the homes of its members to discuss medical papers and that would eventually become the Boston Medical Library; a Friday evening society in which each member read a scientific article after supper; the Society of Natural History, the Temperance Society (he was known as "an inveterate crusader against alcoholic beverages" [quoted in *Journal of the American Medical Association* 1970]); and the Humane Society for aiding sailors lost at sea. He played a leading role in the formation of the *New England Journal of Medicine and Surgery* and the *Collateral Branches of Science*, where papers were read and criticized. The initiating committee included Jackson, Gorham, Bigelow, and Channing. The *Journal* began publishing papers quarterly in 1812. It received the last paper of Warren's in 1823. It was succeeded by the *New-England Medical Review and Journal* in 1827. After one year it merged with the *Boston Medical Intelligence* (founded in 1823) to become the *Boston Medical and Surgical*

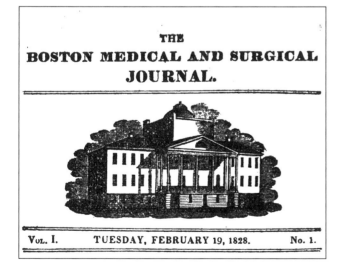

Cover of the first volume of the *Boston Medical and Surgical Journal*, February 19, 1828. The Bulfinch building is prominently displayed. Google Books.

Journal, which published papers for 100 years. In 1928, it became the current popular and prestigious *New England Journal of Medicine*.

Dr. John Collins Warren had become "very respectable" in 1806 with a large medical and surgical clinical practice (E. Warren 1860). He remained busy in multiple organizations, giving numerous lectures and demonstrations to the Harvard students in Cambridge with his father, while contributing papers to the medical society, publishing papers, co-authoring writings with Jackson, remaining active in political affairs, and beginning to give private anatomy demonstrations and lectures in Boston above White's Apothecary Shop at 49 Marlborough Street. He worked very hard, never wasting any time. Others described him as having "unwearied energy" (E. Warren 1860). He was a thrifty man who held high standards for himself and others, but compromise was not of his liking. He prepared for each operation meticulously. By age 40, he was the leading surgeon in Massachusetts and had turned down an offer to become the Professor of Anatomy at the University of Pennsylvania following the death of Casper Wistar. He also later turned down an offer of a professorship at King's College (which later became Columbia University) in New York.

Warren's day began at dawn. He ate breakfast by candlelight. He worked steadily: visiting patients until dinner at 1:00 p.m. and eating quickly in about 10 to 20 minutes. He saw patients in his house between 1:00 and 2:00 p.m., and then rested one hour. Resuming work, he continued to see patients who required continued care until 7:00 p.m., when he ate a light supper and drank tea. The evening was spent reading, writing, and preparing lectures for hours, commonly until about two in the morning. Warren was a very thin man with strong dietary beliefs—especially around anything that might affect constipation, which he believed was connected to other illnesses. He scrupulously followed a diet avoiding both alcohol and rich foods. Active as an Episcopalian, he was warden of St. Paul's Church for almost two decades. He had a real fondness for Latin, reading prayers daily in Latin. He strongly supported exercise, including a public gymnasium in Boston. He believed that "the habitual use of wine is neither necessary or salutary" (E. Warren 1860); he eventually assumed the presidency of the Temperance Society in Boston.

THE MEDICAL PROGRAM IN CAMBRIDGE MOVES TO BOSTON

By 1806, the medical faculty at Harvard had increased to six. Harvard College had only 11 faculty at the time. Anatomy and surgery were taught by John Warren, assisted by his son John Collins Warren. The teaching program in medicine was obviously growing. During this first decade of the nineteenth century, plans were developing for private medical schools throughout the United States. Boston was no different. Dr. Samuel Danforth, with the support of Professor Benjamin Waterhouse, petitioned for a private medical school in Boston, not affiliated with a university. The proposal was rejected by the legislature. Dr. John Collins Warren had begun demonstrations and lectures in Boston above White's Apothecary Shop. Although a bridge across the Charles River to Cambridge had been completed in 1786, the trip to Cambridge was time consuming and inconvenient to John Collins Warren, as well as to other teachers and students who lived in Boston. Some also objected to the attendance of undergraduate students to lectures in Cambridge specifically prepared for medical students. A final problem with the Cambridge location was recognized by both Warrens: the lack of a clinical facility for teaching. Boston had two, including the Almshouse for the poor and the Boston Dispensary for sick prison inmates. John Collins Warren had obtained approval for professors and students to use the patients in the Almshouse for teaching purposes while managing their medical care.

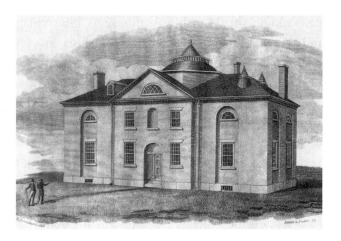

Massachusetts Medical College of Harvard University, 1816–1846. No photographs remain.
Harvard Medical Library in the Francis A. Countway Library of Medicine.

The medical professors at Harvard petitioned the Harvard Corporation for permission to move the school to Boston. Approval was given in 1810. Other professors began to give lectures at 49 Marlborough Street; John Collins Warren continued his dissections there. Because some students still preferred Cambridge over Boston for their courses, Harvard continued medical classes in both Cambridge and Boston; 70 students remained in Cambridge and 50 students attended classes in Boston. The new location in Boston, however, delayed the early threat of a competing medical school in Boston in the early nineteenth century.

Lectures at the new medical school site in Boston continued for several years until there were far too many students for the small available space. John Collins Warren and James Jackson, his friend and colleague and Hersey Professor of the Theory and Practice of Physic, led an effort to build a new medical school building in Boston. They raised money by appealing to the Harvard University Corporation and applied to the state for additional money. They were not immediately successful because the War of 1812 had caused financial hardships in New England. But in 1814, after the state approved limited funding, a new building was erected on Mason Street. It was named the Massachusetts Medical College because it had received state support. John Warren, a strong supporter of the new building, died in 1815 before the building was completed in 1816.

NEW HOSPITAL IN BOSTON

The Almshouse—located on Leverett Street and near the future site of the Massachusetts General Hospital (MGH)—was small, with only eight beds. It was neither large enough to care for the sick and poor of Boston nor large enough for John Collins' growing surgical practice. It probably was inadequate as a teaching facility because of the increasing number of students at Harvard interested in medicine. And, without a hospital in Boston, the medical school surely couldn't compete with the Pennsylvania Hospital, affiliated with the University of Pennsylvania, or New York Hospital, affiliated with King's College, later to become Columbia University.

At the time, hospitals were unpopular. People feared them and were prejudiced against them. Those with physical illnesses often shared space with those with mental health disorders or dementia in addition to criminals. Nurses were often untrained poor women or recovering patients themselves. Those in the Almshouse sometimes died not from their illness or injury but because their basic needs—food and proper heat—were unmet. Those with the means had their medical and surgical care in their own homes. A citizen, William Phillips, saw a need for a modern hospital in Boston for the care of patients in an improved environment. In 1801, he donated $5,000, a large sum at the time, for a new kind of hospital. Before John Warren's death, he and John Collins had been discussing the need for a hospital in Boston patterned after the hospitals John Collins had worked in while training in England and Europe. After John Warren's death, John Collins continued those discussions with his friend and colleague, James Jackson. Jackson agreed with the need and the British and European models. They envisioned not another almshouse, but a hospital for patients of "good" social standing where medical students could train and where patients could find both the comforts of home (such as baths) and trained medical staff. Both John Collins and James Jackson had learned firsthand from their experiences in England and France that a hospital is essential to a properly run medical school. Educating future doctors was a main concern of theirs.

Fundraising for the new hospital was renewed in 1810. Reverend John Bartlett (the chaplain of the Almshouse), John Collins Warren, and James Jackson solicited donations with a letter they sent to the wealthiest citizens of Boston (see chapter 29). They were clear in their request arguing that such a hospital was needed for the poor as well as the wealthy because "the poor patient was sure of receiving all the care and attention…equally with the rich" (E. Warren 1860). Both doctors argued that a hospital would improve medical education. A charter and funding for the new hospital was granted by the state within a single year in 1811. But the War of 1812 stalled further plans. After the war, land on the Charles River was chosen as the site for the new hospital. It was near the bridge—giving easy access to Cambridge—and the river location would allow easy delivery of needed supplies.

The famous architect Charles Bulfinch was chosen to design and build the hospital. Convicts,

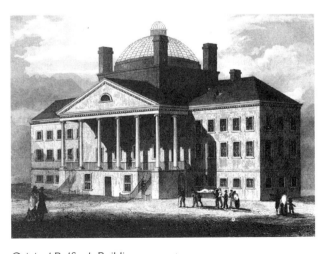

Original Bulfinch Building.
Massachusetts General Hospital, Archives and Special Collections.

in order to save money, were used to install the stones. The cornerstone was laid on July 14, 1818. Jackson admitted the first patient with syphilis on September 1, 1821. Warren admitted the next patient on September 12, 1821. During the first year, the hospital admitted five cases for surgery to treat hemorrhoids, a bladder stone, fistula-in-ano, popliteal aneurysm, and a dislocation, the latter of which was treated unsuccessfully. The hospital had 60 beds.

FIRST ORTHOPAEDIC CASE AT MASSACHUSETTS GENERAL HOSPITAL

Charles Lowell, a day laborer who owned a country store, traveled 250 miles from Lubec, Maine, in December of 1821 for a consultation with

A

TREATISE

ON

DISLOCATIONS

AND

FRACTURES

OF THE

JOINTS

BY SIR ASTLEY COOPER, BART F.R.S

SERGEANT-SURGEON TO THE KING, &c. &c. &c.

SIXTH EDITION.

LONDON:

SOLD BY MESSRS. LONGMAN, REES, ORME, BROWN, AND GREEN, PATERNOSTER ROW;
S. HIGHLEY, 174, FLEET STREET; T. AND G. UNDERWOOD, 32, FLEET STREET;
AND THE MEDICAL BOOKSELLERS IN LONDON, DUBLIN & EDINBURGH.

MDCCCXXIX.

Title page of *A Treatise on Dislocations and Fractures of the Joints*, Sixth Edition, by Sir Astley Cooper, 1829.
Open Library/Internet Archive.

John Collins in Boston. It had been a long trip, and Lowell arrived using crutches. John Collins met Lowell in a local tavern and learned that Lowell had fallen off a horse, the animal "falling back upon him and between his legs," on September 7, 1821 (J. A. Spalding 1910). Initially, in Maine, Dr. John Faxon, a physician, was called to see Lowell who, unable to walk, had been carried to a nearby house. Faxon diagnosed a dislocated left hip but was unable to reduce it. He called Dr. Micajah Hawkes, a surgeon, in consultation. Together both doctors believed that they successfully reduced the hip because "the rotation and motion of the left leg seemed as perfect as that of the right" (J. A. Spalding 1910). They wrapped Lowell's legs together and asked him to remain in bed for four weeks. Faxon then bled Lowell and gave him a sedative; afterwards, the doctors left. Lowell apparently walked home one or two weeks later. Approximately four to six weeks later, Hawkes re-visited Lowell. He found that Lowell's leg remained deformed and told Lowell that nothing more could be done for his hip. In response, "Mr. Lowell burst out in anger, swore vengeance on the men who ruined him, and started for Eastport to catch a vessel for Boston" (J. A. Spalding 1910).

Three months after his injury, Charles Lowell was thoroughly examined by Dr. John Collins Warren. After spending considerable time with Lowell, John Collins was apparently unsure of the diagnosis. He needed time to think and research his findings. He went home while considering the findings from Lowell's physical examination, and he stated in his pamphlet that he studied previous cases and Sir Astley Cooper's book on surgery most of the night. Returning to the tavern the next day, he told Lowell that his diagnosis was a "dislocation of the femur downward and backward into the ischiatic notch" (J. C. Warren 1826). John Collins couldn't "find head... in front" of the acetabulum (J. C. Warren 1826). He told Lowell to return home; he couldn't help him. Lowell pleaded for John Collins to treat him.

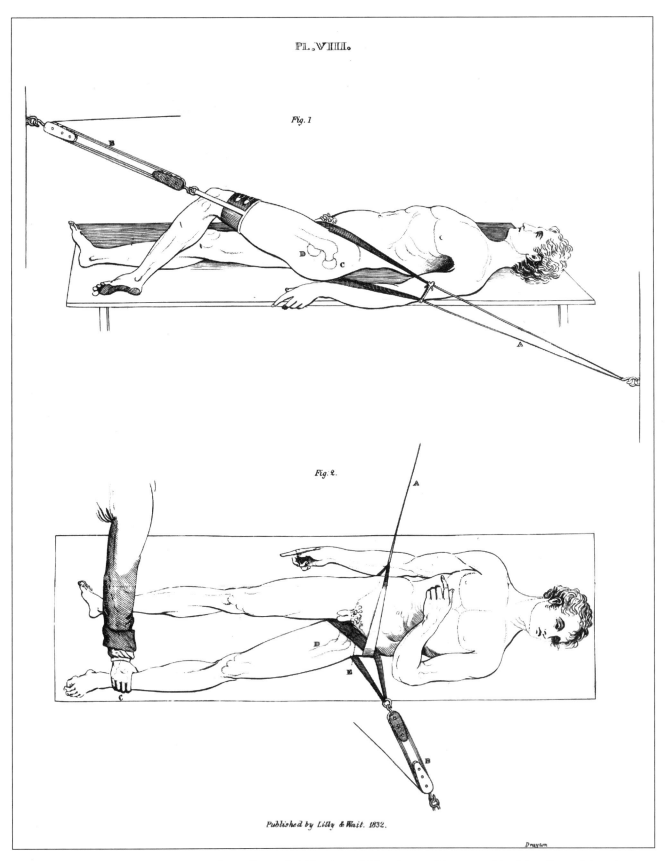

Use of traction to reduce a dislocated hip. From Cooper's *A Treatise on Dislocations and Fractures of the Joints*, Second American Edition, 1832. U.S. National Library of Medicine.

John Collins arranged for consultations with four other well-known physicians—Manor, Spooner, Townsend and Welsh—and all agreed that treatment was impossible.

After continued pleadings for help, John Collins agreed to admit Lowell to the Massachusetts General Hospital on December 7, 1821, for an attempt at reduction of his hip with the use of traction and pulleys. Lowell, with his chronic dislocated left hip, was the sixth admission of John Collins to MGH since its opening on September 1, 1821, and it was the first orthopaedic case in the new hospital. According to the MGH records, before 125 physicians and students, Lowell was bled 16 ounces, given a hot bath to relax his muscles, given magnesium sulfate to induce vomiting, and a sedative. The operation—an attempt at closed reduction with the use of traction and pulleys—was tried for approximately two hours but without success. Lowell was discharged from the hospital with his hip still dislocated.

Over the next several days, Lowell consulted with other doctors and even a bone-setter. One additional attempt at reduction also failed. He ran into John Collins while on his rounds, and told him that he was returning home to sue his doctors in Maine who had "ruined him" (J. A. Spalding 1910). John Collins, who hated malpractice suits, tried to change Lowell's opinion arguing "the rarity of such cases, the extreme difficulty of their diagnosis, the obstacles to reduction, and the impossibility of country doctors ever seeing enough injuries of this sort to be able to diagnosticate or to treat them at all" (J. A. Spalding 1910). He was also concerned that he would be forced to testify against another physician.

Lowell sued Faxon and Hawkes for $10,000. He sued Faxon "for trying to do anything with a dislocation of which he knew nothing" and Hawkes "for not reducing the dislocation originally, and for neglecting it afterward" (J. A. Spalding 1910). The verdict for Lowell was for $1,962. Both defendants appealed. The second trial was dismissed after a hung jury. Lowell sued again.

During the third trial, John Collins and other Boston physicians had to testify. During cross-examination John Collins stated he had only seen nine cases of hip dislocations; other consultants had seen far fewer cases or no cases at all of hip dislocation. The Boston physicians, including John Collins, believed that pulleys were indispensable. None of them wanted to testify against other physicians. Also, they were reluctant to testify specifically against a Maine physician because the citizens of the Commonwealth of Massachusetts had opposed the proposal that Maine be recognized as its own independent state.

At the end of the trial, Lowell was asked to strip down to his underwear and show his deformity to the jury. They were able to see that "his left leg being longer than the right, turned out a little from the body, and the foot turned outward also" (J. A. Spalding 1910). Lowell and his attorneys argued that John Collins' diagnosis was correct; it was a posterior dislocation into the sciatic notch and treatment with pulleys and traction was indispensable, neither of which Faxon nor Hawkes had or used. The diagnosis remained a major concern. Experts differed on both sides with disagreements about the position of the foot with different dislocations. Sir Astley Cooper's textbook on surgery at the time did not mention a dislocation of this type, and the plaintiff's attorneys referred to this book and the fact that John Collins, as editor, had accepted its review in the *New England Medical and Surgical Journal*.

Near the end of the trial, Chief Justice Nathan Weston stated, "personally I believe that the head of the bone is in the foramen ovale. I do not believe it is in the Ischiatic notch" (J. A. Spalding 1910). The jury promptly acquitted Faxon and, after one juror became ill, and, not wanting a fourth trial, the suit ended with the court recommending the "plaintiff to accept a non-suit and the defendant to take no costs" (J. A. Spalding 1910).

Lowell remained angered. He began bitter attacks on Judge Weston, demanding his impeachment. Throughout the long period of trials, he also repeatedly attacked his physicians and consultants in the press. Anonymous slanderous letters were sent to John Collins; many were also published in newspapers. Pamphlets, common at that time, were written by Lowell and his attorneys accusing John Collins of "ignorance of anatomy and surgery" (J. A. Spalding 1910). Friends of Judge Weston wrote their own public pamphlet defending his actions and judgment, but also included negative comments about Boston physicians. The next year, in 1826, John Collins published his own pamphlet for Isaac Parker, the chief justice of the Supreme Court of Massachusetts and defended his diagnosis and management of Charles Lowell.

John Collins' pamphlet was very long and detailed, 142 pages. He included a description of the case, depositions, court testimony, interrogatories, publications of personal letters and different newspaper articles, results of all three trials, attorneys' letters and public reports, a defense of his diagnosis, the use of pulleys, Sir Astley Cooper's experience with dislocations, a detailed discussion of the appearance of a leg with different types of hip dislocations, detailed ink drawings of the different types of hip dislocations, his personal rebuttals against the testimony of the plaintiff's experts, references to anatomical texts of the day, and finally he concluded with a case report of a man who died after severe injuries after Lowell's suits were finished in which John Collins found at autopsy a "dislocation into the ischiatic notch" (J. C. Warren 1826).

"A Letter to the Honorable Isaac Parker." Pamphlet by John Collins Warren, 1826.

Harvard Medical Library in the Francis A. Countway Library of Medicine.

Letter of support for Charles Lowell, handwritten by John Collins Warren.

Harvard Medical Library in the Francis A. Countway Library of Medicine.

Warren stated in his pamphlet that the report of the defendant's attorney contained "statements and representations calculated to produce unfavorable and erroneous impressions in regard to the professional conduct of my colleagues and myself, and to bring ridicule on the institutions, with which we are connected...the medical school and University of this vicinity" (J. C. Warren 1826). He went on to complain that these reports were "widely circulated...and most eagerly read" and that Lowell printed a pamphlet "in the form of an appeal to the public, in order to convince them of his true condition" (J. C. Warren 1826). It is easy to understand John Collins' frustration and anger and why he felt obliged to defend himself, his colleagues, the hospital, and the medical school publicly with a letter to the chief justice in Massachusetts.

Pl. I.

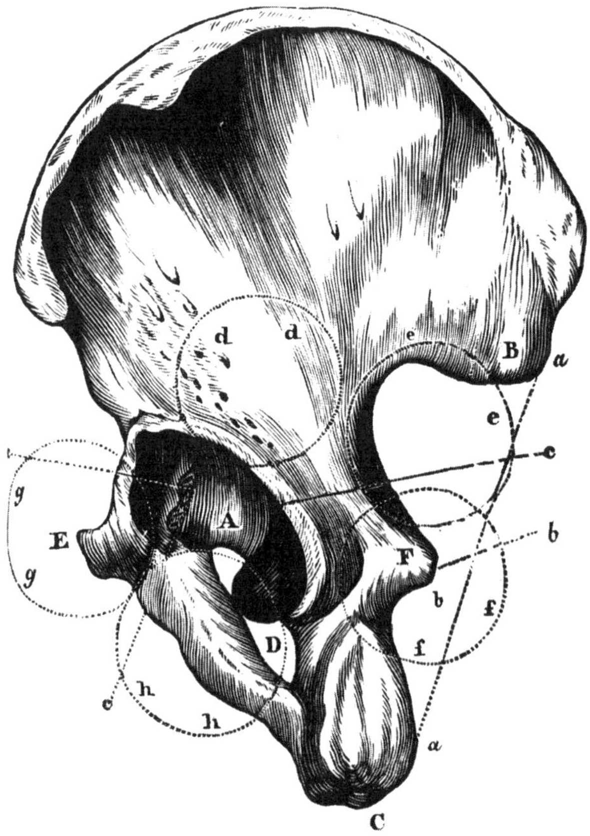

Ink drawing of the known types of dislocated hips, by John Collins Warren. Printed in his 1826 pamphlet, "A Letter to the Honorable Isaac Parker."
Harvard Medical Library in the Francis A. Countway Library of Medicine.

I do not see any reference to this case (other than his pamphlet) in any other of John Collins' writings, including his journal publications, books, lectures, and his autobiography. Nor is there mention of this case and its impact on Warren in Truax's book, *The Doctors Warren of Boston*, or in Churchill's book, *To Work in the Vineyard of Surgery: The Reminiscences of J. Collins Warren*. The medical record of Lowell remains in the archives of the MGH.

Edward Warren (not a relative), in his biography, *The Life of John Collins Warren*, refers to the "remarkable publication," the lengthy pamphlet that Dr. Warren wrote to Judge Parker (E. Warren 1860). He briefly mentions that the pamphlet contains detailed descriptions of hip dislocations "which are often the most complicated and difficult to recognize of any that occur in the human body." Warren further supports the diagnosis stating:

> He proves the possibility of a species of dislocation whose existence had been denied by Sir Astley Cooper, though recognized by some of the most distinguished Continental Surgeons. The occasional occurrence of this form of dislocation has since been proved by a specimen in St. Bartholomew's Hospital, and by cases published in the American edition of Sir Astley Cooper's work on dislocations. (E. Warren 1860)

Edward Warren's book was published in 1860, two years after Lowell's death and autopsy.

Oliver Wendell Holmes in his introductory lecture to the entering first-year class at Harvard Medical School on September 26, 1879, refers to the Lowell case without mentioning names. He states:

> Here is a dislocation of the femur, — do you remember what happened in that famous case in Maine, the legal consequences of which filled a volume? Can you afford — not merely for your patient's sake, but for your own — to take any chance of consequences which may be utter ruin? (quoted in Podolsky and Bryan 2009)

Dr. James Alfred Spalding also researched the Lowell case, including the findings at his autopsy and presented details at the annual meeting of the American Academy of Medicine in Atlantic City on June 7, 1909. He published the next year in the academy's journal. Detailed descriptions of the three trials were published by Kenneth Allen De Ville in his book *Medical Malpractice in Nineteenth-Century America*. But it was John Collins Warren's son, J. Mason Warren, who first published the findings of Lowell's autopsy in his book *Surgical Observation with Cases and Operations*, which was published in 1867, nine years after Charles Lowell died.

According to Mason, Lowell endured the painful treatment with pulleys without complaint. But in the closing speech of the plaintiff's attorney, Lowell's treatment in Boston was called "barbarous" (J. A. Spalding 1910). Most likely, Lowell was depressed and extremely angry when he returned home, and he strongly believed his continued disability was from his physicians' obtuseness and neglect. During and after the trials, Lowell continued to publicly complain about his treatment and continued his *ad hominem* attacks on his physicians, including John Collins. There was more literature produced for this case than any other prior case that century; it captured the public interest and affected the interested parties for years to come. Lowell often demanded publicly that an autopsy be done at his death to prove that his doctors were wrong and therefore negligent in his care.

Lowell eventually moved to New York, became a lawyer, a bill collector, and even started a few newspapers. According to Dr. Greeley, his personal physician, Lowell "limped on a cane, grew stout and suffered greatly for thirty-seven years" (J. A. Spalding 1910). Lowell died on October 19, 1858, at age 65, two years after John Collins died. In September 1858, Dr. J. Mason Warren stated that he received a letter from Dr. Greeley in Ellsworth, Maine, asking that an autopsy be done on Lowell at the request of Lowell as well as some of his friends. After Mason received notice of Lowell's death, he asked a colleague, Dr. H. K. Oliver, to travel to Ellsworth and perform the autopsy. Mason Warren states:

> After taking note of the external appearances of the body, separated the pelvis and the upper third of the thighs, and, by permission of his family (it being impossible to make a satisfactory investigation on the spot), brought the portions thus removed to Boston. (J. M. Warren 1867)

After returning to Boston, Oliver dissected and then removed the soft tissues to examine the bones. His report to Mason (J. M. Warren 1867) included the following statements:

> The lower extremities were on a line with the body; the heels being together, and on the same level. The limbs were therefore, to the eye, of equal length. The right side of the pelvis appeared to be somewhat lower than the left. The right foot varied but slightly from the perpendicular; the left turned out at an angle of 25° or 30°. The left knee was raised, so that the thigh made with the plane of the bed an angle of about 15°. The right knee being raised to the level of the left, a difference of about two inches in the length of the limbs was noticeable…The movements of the left thigh were limited, and confined exclusively to flexion and extension; no motion whatever being perceived in attempts at abduction or adduction. Extension of the leg was impossible, even after division of the tendons of the flexor muscles of the thigh…On the upper and inner part of the thigh, a large, hard mass could be felt, not existing in the corresponding location on the right side. This was subsequently found to be the new bony socket…the trochanter major, was felt lying rather deep below the level of the trochanter of the right side…the left hip all, of the muscles…belonging to this region were found, but noticeably less full in substance, and of less healthy color, than those of

the right side. The change in direction taken by them…was of course apparent…the cartilaginous, and, apparently, part of the osseous, rim of the acetabulum was absorbed. Stretched over what remained of the cavity was what appeared to part of the old capsular ligament, still partially enclosing the neck of the displaced bone. Beneath this ligament, and filling up the acetabulum was a dense mass of adipose and fibrous tissue…The articular cartilage of the new socket was wanting in that smooth, shining appearance, characteristic of articular surfaces generally. That of the head of the bone was much less uneven…the thyroid foramen was found to be nearly obliterated by the rounded base of the new socket…an adventitious socket for the head of the thigh-bone is formed below, and a little in advance of the acetabulum on the left side. This socket fills up the greater portion of the thyroid foramen, and is bounded as follows: Superiorly, by the body of the pubes and the acetabulum…posteriorly, by the body of the ischium, upon which the socket rests without leaving any part of the thyroid foramen visible; inferiorly, by the rami of the ischium and pubes, leaving no part of the thyroid foramen visible there; anteriorly, by an irregular, crescent-shaped portion of the foramen, one and three-quarter inches in length, by an average breadth of one-quarter of an inch. The major part of the socket is of one piece; but there are four separate pieces of bone of different sizes…The head of the left femur is much larger than its fellow of the opposite side, and its surface quite rough. From the head of the bone, along the neck anteriorly and superiorly, is thrown a ridge of bone nearly reaching the trochanter major. The most careful scrutiny fails to detect signs of previous fracture anywhere, either in the pelvis or in the femur.

Mason then confirmed that his father, John Collins, was correct. The hip was dislocated, a fact which contrasted with other experts' testimony at

trial that there was no dislocation or that the injury was a fracture. He said, "The injury was what Dr. Warren supposed it to be, — a simple dislocation" (J. M. Warren 1867). He then defended his father's diagnosis of a posterior-inferior dislocation in the ischiatic notch and argued that in subsequent editions of Dr. Cooper's book several of these dislocations were described and that he had also seen one such case in his own practice. He discussed the difficulty in making the correct diagnosis from the patient's leg and foot position as well as the difficulty in palpating the femoral head. He concluded:

> The dislocation as it now appears is not as it was described by Dr. Warren, but the socket for the head of the bone lies almost immediately under the old acetabulum, perhaps a little forward of it. The cause of the deception… lies in the fact that the head of the bone found its resting-place almost immediately under the acetabulum…Such a position of the head would render its detection anteriorly quite difficult, even in very thin persons. (J. M. Warren 1867)

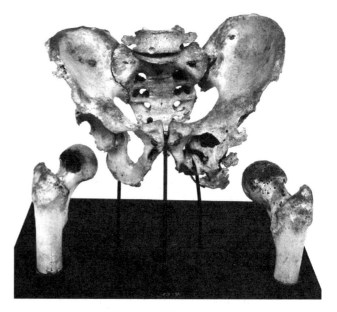

Pelvis and proximal femurs of Charles Lowell. Mounted on a wood frame and preserved in the Warren Museum.

Mason kept the pelvis and proximal femurs of Charles Lowell with John Collins' collection mounted on a wooden stand. It was eventually given to the Warren Museum by J. Collins Warren (John Collins Warren's grandson). This fact was lost for over 50 years. In about 1870, the Maine Medical Society appointed a committee to investigate the rumor that an autopsy had been performed on Lowell; they found no information.

Dr. James Alfred Spalding from Portland, Maine, became interested in this case, which had been described as a myth, about 50 years after Lowell's death while reviewing the lives of deceased physicians in Maine, including Dr. Micajah Hawkes. After reading the three major pamphlets that had been written about the Lowell case, including that of John Collins Warren, he traced Mr. Lowell's moves and discovered that he had died in Ellsworth, Maine. Continuing his research, he discovered the diary of Dr. Greely, Lowell's deceased physician. It contained notes about the autopsy of Lowell by Dr. Henry K. Oliver "at the request of Dr. John Mason Warren" (J. A. Spalding 1910). Spalding met with Dr. Oliver, who was

Box 3.1. A Modern Imaging Assessment 189 Years Later

It is remarkable that Dr. Spalding did not take any x-rays of Lowell's pelvis and proximal femurs. Roentgen had made his important discovery in 1895 and Spaulding's paper was published in 1910, 52 years after Lowell's death. While beginning research on this book, I discovered the bony specimens in the Warren Museum while reading the pamphlet of John Collins Warren. The curator of the museum brought it to my attention. With permission of the Countway Library of Harvard Medical School, we x-rayed the pelvis and proximal femurs and did a computed tomographic (CT) scan, 152 years after Lowell's death and 189 years after his injury. As stated in Dr. Oliver's report of the autopsy, Lowell had sustained an anterior obturator dislocation of his left hip without any evidence of fractures. Reviewing the skeleton today, it remains unknown—although doubtful—that the acetabular rim was fractured or that there was a depression fracture of the femoral head.

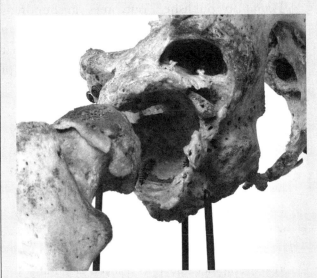

Close-up photo of Lowell's left hip. A false acetabulum, in the foramen ovale, is inferior to the empty true acetabulum.
Warren Anatomical Museum in the Francis A. Countway Library of Medicine.

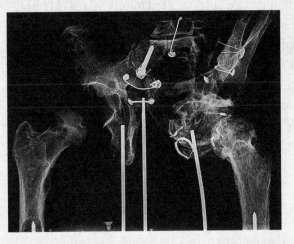

X-ray of Lowell's pelvis and hips (June 1, 2010). Specimen courtesy of the Warren Museum, x-rayed at the author's request by Brigham and Women's Hospital for publication in "An Orthopaedic Case Contributed Substantially to the First Malpractice Crisis in the United States in the Nineteenth Century," *Journal of Bone and Joint Surgery*, 2012; 94 (17): e 1291–1297.
Brigham and Women's Hospital/Warren Anatomical Museum in the Francis A. Countway Library of Medicine.

still alive. Oliver told him about the bone speci-mens in the Warren Museum and the description of his findings in J. Mason Warren's book on sur-gical cases. After reviewing and photographing the pelvis and femur of Lowell, Spalding continued his research about Lowell's life and malpractice trials. According to Spalding, "the time, correspondence and patience involved were enormous" (J. A. Spalding 1910). Pleased with himself, Spalding was "glad because the necropsy considerably vin-dicated the defendant physicians" (J. A. Spalding 1910). Ironically, a postmortem examination of Lowell's injury revealed that all of the diagnoses offered at the trial had been wrong, except that of Judge Weston. Spalding presented his findings in a paper he read before the American Acad-emy of Medicine in 1909, commenting that "it is remarkable that a suit should contain so many years, and unique that an examination should fol-low thirty years after litigation had ceased" (J. A. Spalding 1910).

This interesting case—of mythic proportions in the eighteenth century—became the tipping point for an overwhelming increase in the number of malpractice suits in the United States. Malprac-tice suits before 1830 were almost unheard of and usually brought for the following reasons: death, smallpox vaccinations, obstetrical problems, and amputations. For the next 25 to 50 years—after the enormously public display of the three Lowell malpractice trials and the awful public *ad hominem* attacks by Lowell, attorneys on both sides, and the press—malpractice suits not only increased, but the usual causes for the suits changed. Mal-practice suits during this period increased 950% and marked this period as the first malpractice cri-sis in the United States. Reasons that suits were initiated now began to focus on orthopaedics, including angular and rotation deformities after fractures, stiff joints after injury, shortened limbs after fractures (especially legs), and amputations after fractures. Up to 90% of suits involved frac-tures or dislocations. Suits were becoming public prosecutions.

By the mid-nineteenth century Dr. Frank H. Hamilton—a Buffalo, New York, surgeon and fre-quent witness—claimed that 90% of western New York physicians had to defend against charges of malpractice at some point throughout their careers. He grew concerned at the discrepancy between an increasing number of suits resulting from deformi-ties after fractures and his own contradictory obser-vations that physicians often proclaimed that their results of fracture treatment were always excellent. He collected cases of fractures and evaluated their outcomes more than 50 years before Codman did so, publishing his results in 1855:

I propose to deduce from my own experience, and from the experience of other surgeons, as recorded in this report, the true prognosis of fractures. This I shall endeavor to do with care and fidelity, avoiding, on the one hand, if pos-sible, the error of encouraging the practitioner with a prognosis too favorable, and, on the other, the equal wrong of leaving him to expect too little. (F. H. Hamilton 1855)

Hamilton published outcomes in hundreds of fracture cases in *Transactions of the American Medical Association* and his book. He noted that before his effort to determine the final results of these cases, previous publications did not

make any reference to a shortening or to any degree of deformity which may have occurred in the cases reported as cured. Dr. Pierson, in his report of the statistical tables of all the frac-tures which had occurred in the Massachu-setts General Hospital up to the year 1840... [recorded], under the head of Remarks, many interesting facts, such as delayed or nonunion, the occurrence of ulcers, gangrene, etc. etc... but there is nothing exactly pertinent to the subject of our inquiry. (F. H. Hamilton 1855)

Hamilton often appeared in court as an expert defense witness; other experts relied on his publications, and his publications were often quoted by defense attorneys. Some hoped that his work would become a standard for treatment, outcomes and legal defense, but treatment approaches for fractures continued to be unpredictable. The malpractice crisis continued until the turn of the next century. It was also in the early twentieth century that malpractice insurance carriers began to form, another consequence of the first malpractice crisis in the United States.

EXPANDING REPUTATION OF JOHN COLLINS WARREN

John Collins' surgical practice continued to grow. According to Edward Warren, "no one will ever… have so exclusively the command of all the most important surgical operations" (E. Warren 1860). He had an excellent reputation as a surgeon and was widely known because of his Harvard and

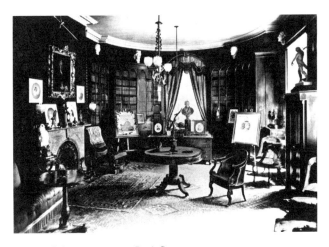

Warren's living room on Park Street.
Boston Medical Library in the Francis A. Countway Library of Medicine.

MGH positions. He remained extremely interested in dissection and skeletons of humans and other vertebrates. He even purchased an entire skeleton of an American mastodon, discovered in 1845 in a bog on the Hudson River about 100 miles from New York City. He had the mastodon skeleton assembled and exhibited in Boston; it is unclear whether he housed it for a brief period

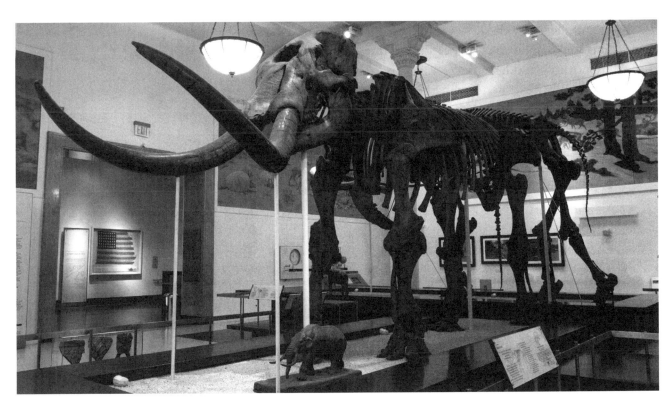

Warren Mastodon, American Museum of Natural History, New York. D. Finnin/AMNH.

in his home with other animal and human skeletons, before placing it in the Warren Museum of National History on Chestnut Street. He wrote an entire book, *Description of a Skeleton of the Mastodon Giganeus of North America*, about the skeleton. Apparently, the tusks were more than 10 feet long. Eventually, the American Museum of Natural History acquired the now-named Warren Mastodon in 1925. It remains in New York today.

The MGH had space for clinical instruction, which Warren used in addition to the space on Marlborough Street. However, it remained against the law to perform human dissections/demonstrations, and he was concerned that medical students might be hurt as a result. On one occasion he had given students refuge in his home as they were pursued by an angry mob. He feared that he might even be attacked himself. Along with the support of his colleagues, Warren lobbied for new legislation. They were successful; obtaining bodies and human dissection became legalized. The first Anatomy Act was passed in Massachusetts in 1830, followed by England in 1832.

By age 50, he was well-known for many operations, including reducing dislocations, amputations, removing bladder stones, cataracts and ligating aneurysms. He performed the first successful case of a strangulated hernia. In 1828, he published a case of

the reduction of a fracture-dislocation of the upper end of the humerus...at the MGH four weeks after injury. The patient was confined by a sheet and bands to staples in the wall of the operating room; pulleys were attached to the injured arm and as traction was made the family physician who was present was directed to bleed the patient from his sound arm until he was faint; increasing traction was made for half an hour, when the patient asked for mercy. Nevertheless, the power was increased till it regained the whole strength of one person to draw the cord of the pulleys. Then

Dr. Warren placed his knee beneath the head of the humerus in the axilla and used it as a fulcrum to raise the head of the bone. At the same time that the traction was released, adhesions were heard to crack and the bone came into its socket with an audible noise "to the great satisfaction of the patient who made a good recovery." (D. Cheever 1912)

However, he was more famous for his diagnostic and postsurgical treatment skills. Many, even in Europe, came to Boston because they had "so much more confidence in the after-treatment" because "Dr. Warren never made up his mind to perform an operation until all probable means of cure had been fully tried" (E. Warren 1860). Before surgery, "he prepared himself deliberately" and in meticulous detail by reviewing the surgical technique and the instruments needed as well as

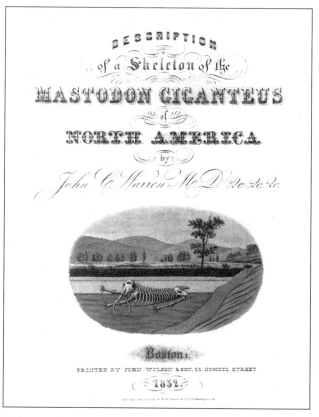

Title page, *Description of a Skeleton of the Mastodon Giganteus of North America* by John Collins Warren, 1852.
Smithsonian Libraries.

preparing a written list of contingencies or adverse events that could occur (E. Warren 1860). He frequently consulted other authorities, books, and articles, and he would often practice the operation in the dissecting room before the actual surgery. He also clearly obtained patient consent for his procedures. Years after watching Dr. Warren operate during an amputation, a surgeon told Dr. Warren's grandson that:

> Your grandfather would stand behind his back and say to the patient, "Will you have your leg off, or will you not have it off?" If the patient lost his courage and said "No," he had decided not to have the leg amputated, he was at once carried to his bed in the ward. If, however, he said "Yes," he was immediately taken firmly in hand by a number of strong assistants and the operation went on regardless of what he might say thereafter. If his courage failed him after this crucial moment, it was too late and no attention was paid to his cries of protest. (quoted in R. Truax 1968)

An excellent observer, Warren paid attention to every detail, noticing "the slightest unfavorable change, either during the operation or afterwards" (E. Warren 1860). Applying dressings "was also a science;" one of his innovations was "the use of adhesive straps" to avoid using sutures (E. Warren 1860). Warren worked continuously hard: operating, caring for patients, making hospital rounds, lecturing, performing dissecting/demonstrations, writing, and studying. Medicine, surgery and teaching were his life, and "the chair of anatomy and surgery had no soft cushion in his or his father's [John Warren's] time" (E. Warren 1860). In 1833, John Collins' published one paper in *The Journal of Medical Sciences* (13th volume), an orthopaedic case report titled "Removal of the Clavicle in a State of Osteo-sarcoma." It analyzed an orthopaedic case involving the trunk, which is riskier and an area not frequently operated upon in comparison to the extremities.

During this period, his mother was quite ill and required his daily care. She died in 1832 at age 72. By 1835, his son Mason returned from Europe, where he had studied medicine, and joined his father in practice. Two years later he was comfortable enough to leave his son in charge of his practice and returned to Europe for a second visit. In 1837 and before his vacation, he turned over a surgical case in the operating room to Mason. Dr. Henry I. Bowditch had referred the child to John Collins for surgery, but John Collins brought his son Mason with him. Although Mason did not have operating privileges nor a staff appointment at the time at MGH, John Collins gave the scalpel to him, asking him to perform the operation. The surgery went well, but Bowditch was outraged by and furious at the senior Warren. Another patient sent a letter to the *Boston Post* on April 10, 1837:

> To the Trustees of the MGH. Gentlemen—I entered your institution under the delusion that I was to receive the professional attendance of one of the surgeons of the Hospital. How is it that a very young man, who holds no appointment whatever there, has, for the last two weeks been allowed to exercise the very vitally important duties of the surgical officer much to the patients and I trust, quite unauthorized by your Board.
>
> If neither of the regular officers can attend, perhaps some practitioner in The Commonwealth can be found, who, possibly, could fill this important station and relieve the anxiety of
> One of the Patients

The trustees were upset, even though they suspected another surgeon or enemy of John Collins had written the letter. They were upset because of the adverse publicity for the MGH. They sent John Collins a censure letter.

That June, John Collins and his family left for Europe on a rare vacation. He turned his practice over to Mason and his duties as senior surgeon at

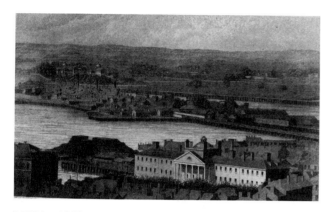

MGH in 1840. Engraving by J.W. Watts, from a daguerreotype by Southworth & Hayes, 1840. Published in *A History of Massachusetts General Hospital*, Second Edition, by Nathaniel I. Bowditch, 1872.
University of California Libraries/Internet Archive.

the MGH to Dr. Hayward. This time he took his wife and some of his six children to Europe with him. He wanted to learn new practices in medicine and surgery and obtain new information in order to modernize his teaching. On the ship, which took 30 days to reach England, he treated a patient with a fractured fibula. He spent time with Sir Astley Cooper and his eighteen-year-old daughter, Emily, who had contracted smallpox while in London. Queen Victoria's personal physician cared for her daily. She recovered fully without any scarring. The Warrens visited Scotland, Wales, Ireland, Paris, Marseilles, Italy, Munich, Frankfort, and Belgium. It was the first major vacation for them. In addition, John Collins visited many hospitals, public institutions, and doctors. He practiced operations on cadavers, studied methods to preserve bodies, obtained many anatomical preparations for his private collection (later to become the Warren Anatomical Museum), and often found himself caring for many American patients. In orthopaedics, he learned how to apply bandages after division of the Achilles tendon, studied with M. Martin—an orthopaedist and "inventor of bandages and apparatus for club-feet and distortions" (E. Warren 1860), and visited the hospital of M. Guerin who treated musculoskeletal deformities with exercises. He had been interested in exercises for years

and strongly supported exercise, along with Daniel Webster. It was Daniel Webster who in 1825 wanted a gymnasium built in Boston. John Collins returned to Boston with his family almost 14 months later, arriving on August 31, 1838.

While in charge at MGH, Hayward produced the first outcome report, of any hospital, from the MGH surgical service. According to this report, between May 12, 1837, and May 12, 1838, surgeons treated 222 patients. The report included seven categories analyzed in **Table 3.1** (L. Ottinger 2002).

Table 3.1. Treatment Categories

Discharge Status	Patients
Well	86
Much Relieved	40
Relieved	38
Not Relieved	22
Died	13
Unfit	3
Eloped	1

He listed all 53 operations (operations probably performed by Dr. Hayward, Dr. Mason Warren, and Dr. John Collins Warren) and discussed the diseases and injuries in detail. I believe this is the first public report on the outcomes of medical/surgical care in the United States.

When John Collins Warren returned from Europe, he immediately resumed practicing medicine and surgery, including his duties at MGH as chief surgeon in September 1838. He had previously appointed a person (probably a house pupil) to maintain detailed surgical records before Hayward's outcomes report. He continued with the house pupil; using these for future publications like clinical pathological conferences (CPCs) where he often commented on the cases. Many dealt with orthopaedics, including a case of a fracture dislocation of the humerus, a compound fracture requiring amputation, and a wound of the hand. He described one interesting orthopaedic operation he performed when he wrote,

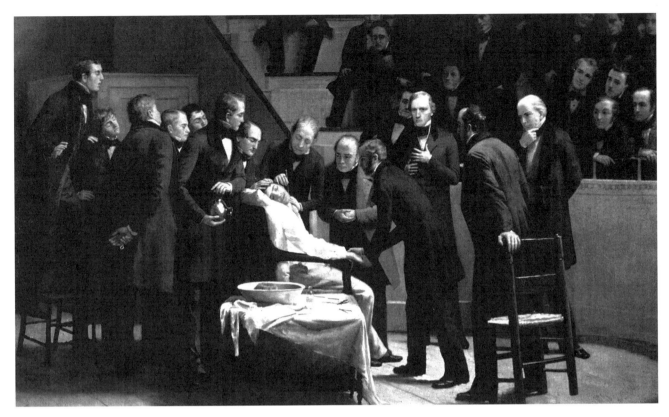

First Operation Under Ether. Painting by Robert C. Hinckley, 1882–1893. Boston Medical Library in the Francis A. Countway Library of Medicine.

"anchylosis of the right arm from fracture of the external condyle; removed under the influence of ether" (E. Warren 1860).

Following his return from Europe, he continued his busy surgical practice, but stated "as has been common to surgeons, I have been less in favor of surgical operations in the latter part of my life" (E. Warren 1860). He became so busy that it was as if he had never left his practice. In 1839, he purchased a farm and planted potatoes as well as plum and pear trees. Two years later, his wife began to have severe abdominal pains, not relieved by opiates. She died after an illness of one month on June 3, 1841, at age 59. John Collins Warren was 63. His father had died at the same age. The following year, John Collins wrote several reports, including cases of fractures of the femur, humerus and forearm. In 1843, at age 65, he got remarried to Miss Anne Winthrop, who was the daughter of the lieutenant governor and a former patient of John Collins. They never had children.

ETHER CHANGES SURGERY FOREVER

In his diary dated October 16, 1846, he wrote, "Did an interesting operation at the hospital this morning, while the patient was under the influence of Dr. Morton's preparation to prevent pain. The substance employed was sulfuric ether" (E. Warren 1860). Warren was 68 years of age and nearing retirement on October 16, 1846, what would become known as Ether Day. The successful use of ether—a pioneering step toward the new field of anesthesia and American's most important contribution to the field at the time—was the third major advance in surgery. The first was the discovery of the ligature by Ambrose Paré in the sixteenth century (first introduced in America by James Lloyd and Joseph Warren); the second was the introduction of the tourniquet by Petit in 1718. The fourth was the later discovery of antisepsis, first used by Joseph Lister in 1865.

This momentous event changed surgery forever, heralding a new specialty of medicine, later to be called anesthesia by Oliver Wendell Holmes. It surprised the medical world and yet ether as well as nitrous oxide were already known to diminish pain. Predecessors—both physicians and scientists—had studied these two anesthetics. Some had used hypnosis in the early nineteenth century, but "Warren states that mesmerism had never succeeded under his inspection" (J. C. Warren 1900).

> Wilson's recollection of his Syme's amputation by James Syme in 1843.
>
> The horror of great darkness, and the sense of desertion by God and man, bordering close on despair, which swept through my mind and overwhelmed my heart, I can never forget, however gladly I would do so. During the operation, in spite of the pain it occasioned, my senses were preternaturally acute, as I have been told they generally are in patients in such circumstances. I still recall with unwelcome vividness the spreading out of the instruments, the twisting of the tourniquet; the first incision: the fingering of the sawed bone: the sponge pressed on the flap: the tying of the blood vessels; the stitching of the skin; the bloody dismembered limb lying on the floor.
> —Professor George Wilson
> (quoted in H. R. Robertson 1989)

Sir Humphrey Davy studied nitrous oxide in the laboratory, and after two years, he published an article in 1800 describing its effects. It was originally discovered by Joseph Priestley, who called it "laughing gas" because of the behavior of individuals inhaling small amounts. Davy wrote, "as nitrous oxide in its extensive operation appears capable of destroying physical pain, it may probably be used with advantage during surgical operations in which no great effusion of blood takes place" (J. C. Warren 1900). Surgeons didn't recognize the importance of the discovery, however. Chemistry teachers (including Davy) used it in small amounts for their students at the end of classes to maintain their popularity. Laughing

gas exhibitions eventually spread to America. Henry Jacob Bigelow, a teenager at Harvard, was an active member of the Rumsford Chemical Society. He helped prepare nitrous oxide for the society's annual party. Gardner Quincy Colton began giving public demonstrations of laughing gas; in December 1844 Horace Wells, a Hartford dentist, attended one of Colton's lectures. He believed the gas could be used for painless tooth extraction because he had witnessed an individual—after inhaling nitrous oxide—wildly running around injuring his leg but without experiencing pain. Wells was successful in extracting teeth painlessly in his office using nitrous oxide. In 1845, Wells arranged to demonstrate this painless tooth extraction technique before a class of Harvard medical students at the MGH. The patient, however, was not anesthetized and screamed during the procedure. The students yelled humbug and left. Dr. Wells was devastated and left dentistry to become a salesman. It would be another 15 years before nitrous oxide became commonly used in dentistry.

Interestingly, ether had been known for almost a century before nitrous oxide was used by Davy. Ambrose Godfrey mentioned the name ether in 1730. Michael Faraday, Davy's successor, published in 1818 that ether "produced effects similar to those occasioned by nitrous oxide" (J. C. Warren 1900). It also became a common after-class enjoyment, especially by medical students who commonly referred to it as "ether frolics" (J. C. Warren 1900). In the late-eighteenth century and early nineteenth century, ether was often used to help breathing in cases of asthma and during the last stages of pulmonary tuberculosis. John Collins Warren used it for such cases in his practice. Its use began to be popular at social events; Dr. Crawford W. Long, a graduate of the Medical Department of the University of Pennsylvania, attended one such event. Long practiced in Georgia where he witnessed one of these social ether frolics. In 1842, he used ether on a patient while removing a small, half-inch in diameter cyst and later in

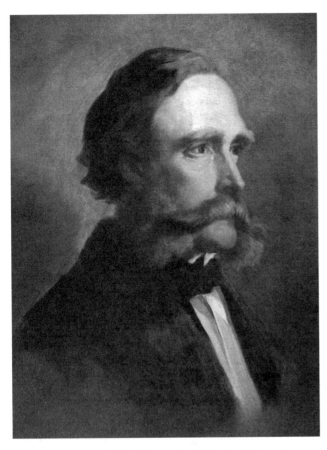

Painting of William T. G. Morton by Christian Schussele.
Massachusetts General Hospital, Archives and Special Collections.

other minor operations. The ether was successful in allowing a painless operation. However, Long did not continue to use ether in his practice. It is possible that he didn't have encouragement in his community, possibly even facing opposition by the public; or, it is possible that he found it impractical because of its short action. He did publish his results, however, in the *Southern Medical Journal* in 1849, three years after Henry J. Bigelow published the results of cases operated upon at MGH under ether anesthesia in 1846.

Meanwhile, Horace Wells and his partner William T. G. Morton opened a Boston office in 1842, where Morton practiced. About the same time that Wells was beginning to use nitrous oxide in his Hartford, Connecticut, office, Morton began to use ether as an anesthetic for tooth extraction. He had learned about the anesthetic effects of ether from Charles T. Jackson, a chemist (not related

to James Jackson, the cofounder of the MGH) and brother-in-law of Ralph Waldo Emerson. We do not know exactly how Morton learned about ether from Jackson. He may have lived in Jackson's house for a while, and he may have learned about ether while attending Jackson's chemistry lectures at Harvard. Morton was secretive about his use of ether. Jackson had experienced the effects of ether as early as 1842 when he used it to relieve respiratory problems he developed after accidentally inhaling chlorine gas. He failed to convince his students—other than possibly Morton—to experiment with ether and its effects. Morton, however, even used ether on himself. Following a successful painless tooth extraction with ether on September 30, 1846, he attracted the attention of Henry J. Bigelow (age 28) by a newspaper article the following day. Bigelow visited Morton's office to witness for himself a painless extraction under ether. After seeing the successful results, Bigelow tried to persuade John Collins Warren to operate on a patient while Morton administered ether. Jackson had convinced Morton that "tooth pulling was not a sufficient test…the crucial test lay in a public demonstration in the operating theatre of a hospital in a surgical case" (J. C. Warren 1900). After being contacted by Morton, J. Mason Warren also spoke to his father John Collins, persuading him in favor of a trial use of ether at the MGH. Since Long had not published his results using ether, word had not spread to the medical world of this outstanding discovery. Morton eventually met with John Collins, who must have been somewhat reluctant to try a painless operation again because the trial case using nitrous oxide had failed in the preceding year. To his credit, he agreed to operate on a patient under ether administered by Morton, but only after questioning Morton in detail about ether "in regard to its action and the safety of it" because the absolute composition of the substance was unknown before Morton had applied for a patent (J. C. Warren 1900). At the time, patented medicines with unknown components were referred to as nostrums. Percival's ethical guidelines in the nineteenth century stated, "No physician or surgeon should dispense a secret nostrum" (T. Percival 1859). John Collins would obviously be in a difficult position if he were to administer an unknown substance to a patient. Having always hoped for a method to end the surgical patient's suffering, however, he seized the opportunity; he did so with some risk to both his reputation and to the patient. He proceeded as no other surgeon at MGH would have been able to do.

On Friday October 16, 1846, John Collins performed the first successful use of ether as an anesthetic for a surgical operation at the MGH. Before operating, John Collins, who was age 68 and nearing retirement, spoke to those in attendance. He said:

> Since many of you have not been informed for what purpose you have been assembled here, I shall now explain it to you. There is a gentleman who claims he has discovered that the inhalation of a certain agent will produce insensibility to pain during surgical operations, with safety to the patient. I have always considered this an important desideratum in operative surgery, and after due consideration I decided to permit him to try the experiment. (J. C. Warren 1846)

He later wrote the following about the experience:

> The patient was a young man, about twenty years old, having a tumor on the left side of the neck, lying parallel to and just below the left portion of the lower jaw. This tumor, which had probably existed from his birth, seemed to be composed of tortuous, indurated veins extending from the surface quite deeply under the tongue. My plan was to expose these veins by dissection sufficiently to enable me to pass a ligature around them. The patient was arranged for the operation in a sitting posture, and everything made ready; but Dr. Morton did not appear until the lapse of nearly half an hour. I was about to proceed, when he entered hastily, excused the delay, which had been occasioned by his modifying the apparatus for the administration. The patient was then made to inhale a fluid from a tube connected with a glass globe. After four or five minutes he appeared to be asleep, and was thought by Dr. Morton to be in a condition for the operation. I made an incision between two and three inches long in the direction of the tumor, and to my great surprise without any starting, crying, or other indication of pain. The fascia was then divided, the patient still appearing wholly insensible. Then followed the insulation of the veins, during which he began to move his limbs, cry out, and utter extraordinary expressions. These phenomena led to a doubt of the success of the applications; and in truth I was not satisfied myself, until I had, soon after the operation and on various other occasions, asked the question whether he had suffered pain. To this he always replied in the negative, adding, however, that he knew the operation and comparing the stroke of the knife to that of a blunt instrument passed roughly across his neck. (quoted in R. Truax 1968)

At the end of the procedure, Warren recalled the angry words of the medical students after witnessing the failure of Well's demonstration of

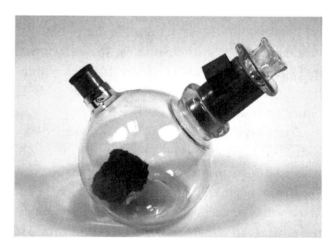

Morton's ether inhaler.
Massachusetts General Hospital, Archives and Special Collections.

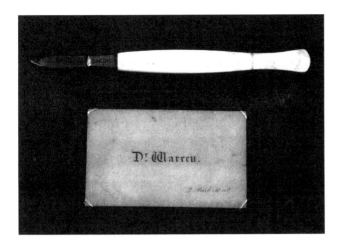

Scalpel of John Collins Warren used in first case under ether anesthesia.
Boston Medical Library in the Francis A. Countway Library of Medicine.

It is not accurately known who attended this exciting and memorable event in surgery. The scene has been preserved in a late-nineteenth century painting, and was referred to as the "First Operation Under Ether" by Robert C. Hinckley. As of 2019, the painting still hangs in the Francis A. Countway Library of Medicine, an alliance of the Boston Medical Library and Harvard Medical School. Nearly three decades after the operation, Hinckley prepared for his painting by personally investigating the names of all those in attendance in order to accurately record the event. He was not totally successful, and he used his artistic license to include some who may have been there; but he could not prove their attendance.

nitrous oxide the previous year, and he turned to the audience seated above him and said, "Gentlemen, this is no humbug." Henry J. Bigelow shouted, "I have seen something today which shall go around the world" (quoted in R. Truax 1968). Bigelow's prediction came true, starting with his father's letter about the event to his friend from Harvard, Dr. Francis Boott, in England, who informed others. Ether began to be used for surgery outside of America within one year of its successful use at the MGH.

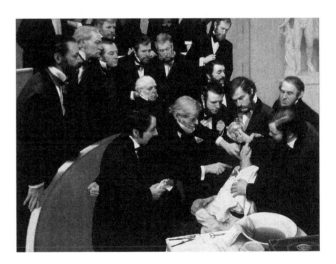

Newly commissioned painting *Ether Day 1846*, by Warren and Lucia Prosperi (2001). Many of the department chiefs and other MGH staff modeled for the artists.
Massachusetts General Hospital, Archives and Special Collections.

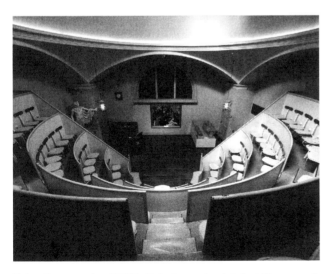

Ether Dome today (2019). Painting on back is by Warren and Lucia Prosperi.
Massachusetts General Hospital, Archives and Special Collections.

Wolfe, in his book *The First Operation Under Ether*, thoroughly analyzed the first public trial of ether. Those on the main floor included the patient Edward Gilbert Abbott; the surgeon John Collins Warren; William T. G. Morton, who administered the anesthesia; MGH surgeon Henry J. Bigelow; the patient's referring physician and cousin Dr. William Williamson Wellington; MGH senior surgeon Solomon Davis Townsend (close to Warren's age); internist and friend of Morton, Dr. Augustus

Addison Gould (who would join MGH staff later); businessman Eben H. Frost (patient of Morton), who had had a tooth removed successfully without pain while under ether, who was brought by Morton "to help reassure the patient" (R. J. Wolfe 1993). It also included members of the house staff (called house pupils or "pups"): Charles Frederick Heywood (house surgeon), Charles Bertody (house physician), and John Call Dalton Jr. (apothecary). In the seats above were possibly Jacob Bigelow, junior surgeon Samuel Parkman (not related to Dr. George Parkman), house surgeon Alfred Lambert, and numerous Harvard students. There is only some evidence that the following were in attendance: Ayer, Beckwith, Davis, Francis, Gallonpe, Hildreth, Surtleff, and Stone. Some of the students were also from the Tremont Street Medical School. J. Mason Warren was not present because he was needed for something else before the operation began. A consulting surgeon, Abel Lawrence Pierson, confirmed later that he was not present. And visiting surgeon George Hayward, who would perform the next two operations under ether at MGH, did not witness the seminal operation.

> ...
> "No hour as sweet as when hope, doubt, and fears,
> 'Mid deepening stillness, watched one eager brain,
> With Godlike will, decree the Death of Pain."
> ...
>
> "The Birth and Death of Pain" poem by
> S. Weir Mitchell, MD, LLD, October 16, 1896.
> 50th Anniversary of the public demonstration of
> surgical anesthesia. Bigelow Amphitheater
> (Grace Whiting Myers, Hx of MGH, 1872–1929. 1929)

The next day a woman was scheduled to have a lipoma removed from her arm at the MGH. After its success, it was obvious ether should continue to be used at MGH. John Collins asked Dr. George Hayward to perform the operation. It was also successful. Additional cases using ether were planned but delayed. The surgeons at MGH, including John Collins Warren, remained concerned about the chemical nature of the anesthetic. Morton had

kept it a secret, having applied for a patent. He called the substance "Letheon," hoping to make a large amount of money. Jackson and Morton publicly fought over the discovery rights of ether, forcing an investigation by both the MGH Trustees and a congressional committee. Both groups had

> expressed displeasure that Morton would try to take out a patent on a discovery that relieved suffering. No self-respecting doctor of the 1840s would have thought of patenting a breakthrough. Quack doctors regularly patented medicines and devices, but to patent such a discovery was to withhold relief from those in pain. (Bull and Bull 2011)

Morton eventually obtained his patent, but he never received the large government grant he expected because others similarly asserted they had discovered it, including Charles T. Jackson (also at Harvard); Horace Wells, of Hartford, Connecticut; and Crawford W. Long, of Jefferson, Georgia. Morton's patent was U.S. No 4848, which expired in 1860. The French government awarded a ribbon and some money to both Morton and Jackson; the MGH gave Morton $1,000 and a commemorative box.

Once John Collins and other surgeons at MGH learned the chemical nature of ether from Morton, they continued its use. The third

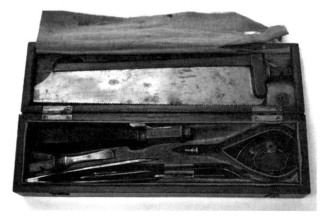

Amputation kit of George Hayward, ca. 1814.
Massachusetts General Hospital, Archives and Special Collections.

operation under ether at MGH was completed three weeks later on November 7, 1846. It was a major operation, an above-knee amputation; it was also successful and the first major musculo-skeletal operation to be completed without pain. Before beginning the operation, John Collins kept Morton in the gallery and refused to allow him in the operating space. He insisted that Morton identify the composition of his ether substance. Morton finally released information on its ingredients—sulphuric ether—so that he could continue. The amputation was performed by Hayward. The patient was a young 26-year old woman with painful probable tuberculosis of her right knee joint. She was discharged from the hospital six weeks later on December 22, 1846. On November 3, 1847—one year after ether was successfully used at the MGH—Oliver Wendell Holmes, in an introductory lecture to Harvard medical students, stated:

> In this very hour while I am speaking how many human creatures are cheated of pangs which seemed inevitable of the common doom of mortality, and lulled by the strange magic of the enchanted goblet, held for a moment to their lips, into a repose which has something of ecstasy in its dreamy slumbers. The knife is searching for disease, the pulleys are dragging back dislocated limbs, nature herself is working out the primal curse which doomed the ten-derest of her creatures to the sharpest of her trials, but the fierce extremity of suffering has been steeped in the waters of forgetfulness, and the deepest furrow in the knotted brow of agony has been smoothed forever. (quoted in A. Gawande 2012)

In the 15 months between October 16, 1846 (called Ether Day), and the start of 1848:

> 132 operations were performed at MGH using ether. On May 12, 1851, the Trustees reported that since January 1, 1848, an additional 350

operations had used some anesthetic, including 186 with sulfuric ether, 138 with chlorate ether, 25 with chloroform, and 1 with nitrous oxide gas. (Bull and Bull 2011)

A new specialty in medicine—anesthesiol-ogy—had begun.

There was some controversy in early scholar-ship on the use of ether. Henry J. Bigelow pre-sented two papers on the use of ether; the first he presented on November 3, 1846, to the Ameri-can Academy of Arts and Sciences and the second on November 9, 1846, to the Boston Society for Medical Improvement. He then published the first paper on the successful use of ether as an anesthetic. The paper was entitled "Insensibility

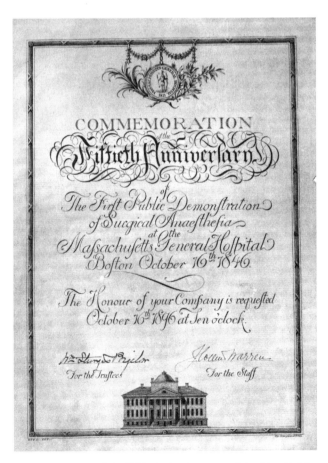

Announcement of the Fiftieth Anniversary of the First Public Demonstration of Surgical Anesthesia at the MGH, October 16, 1846. Signed by Sturgis Bigelow (H. J. Bigelow's son), Trustee and J. Collins Warren, Staff.

Massachusetts General Hospital, Archives and Special Collections.

During Surgical Operations Produced by Inhalation," published on November 18, 1846. Bigelow published his article only 33 days after the initial October 16 operation using ether and only 11 days after the third more complicated and notable operation. The third patient, Alice Mohan, was not yet even out of the hospital. The first operation had been performed by John Collins, the second and third operations by Dr. Hayward, not Bigelow. Francis Moore—in his presentation in 1996 on the 150th anniversary of the use of ether at the MGH—criticized Bigelow because his paper

described the work of Warren, Morton, and Hayward, but it didn't include them as co-authors. Bigelow was merely an observer and was junior to both Warren and Hayward. He didn't even disclose the chemical composition of the ether preparation and mentioned Warren's name only twice in the paper. He clearly attempted to usurp John Collin's moment, but it would nevertheless become known as Dr. John Collins Warren's greatest achievement. For obvious reasons, John Collins disliked Bigelow.

John Collins published his own report on his experience with it in the *Boston Medical and Surgical Journal* the following month, on December 9, 1846. In that article, he mentions 14 physicians and surgeons at MGH, but not Bigelow. He also does not refer to Bigelow's article from November 18. Other reports and publications followed by George Hayward—who had replaced John Collins as chief of surgery at MGH on November 1, 1846—as well as Abel Pierson, Samuel Parkman, and others. Parkman reported on the first use of ether to reduce a dislocated shoulder on November 18, 1846. In 1848, John Collins published a book, "*Etherization: With Surgical Remarks*," describing his experience and those of other surgeons at MGH.

The following year, he published a small book titled "*Effects of Chloroform and of Strong Chloric Ether as Narcotic Agents*," in which he documented successful cases using chloroform and cases that proved fatal. He reported that in the first year of using ether, no fatalities occurred. However, deaths were associated with the use of chloroform. He described findings at autopsies and summarized his thoughts:

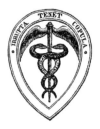

> We are therefore led to the conclusion, that the fatal result is not to be attributed to simple asphyxia, to accumulation in the heart or in the brain; but that it may be ascribed to an undiscoverable toxic action received by the lungs, and thence conveyed to the nervous centres.
> (J. C. Warren 1849)

ETHERIZATION;

WITH

SURGICAL REMARKS.

BY

JOHN C. WARREN, M. D.

Emeritus Professor of Anatomy and Surgery in the University at Cambridge; Surgeon at Massachusetts General Hospital; Honorary Member of the Medical and Chirurgical Society of London; Corresponding Member of the Royal Academy of Medicine at Paris, and of the Academies of Naples, Florence, etc.

BOSTON:
WILLIAM D. TICKNOR & COMPANY,
Corner of School and Washington Streets.
M DCCC XLVIII.

Cover, *Etherization*: With Surgical Remarks, by John Collins Warren, 1848. U.S. National Library of Medicine.

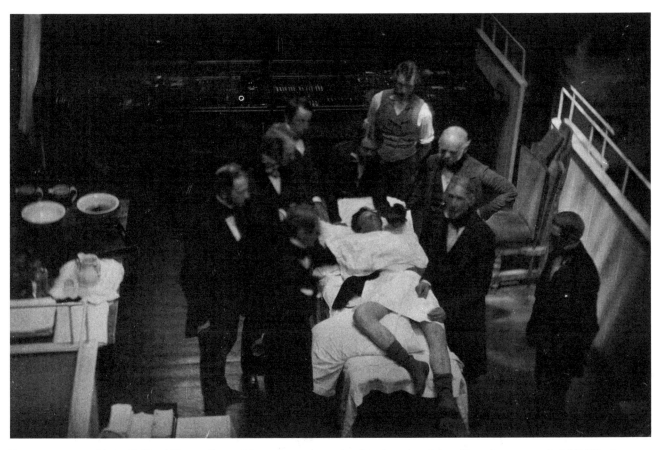

Daguerreotype of John Collins Warren (front right, next to the patient) in the ether dome. First photo record of JCW in the operating room, 1848. The J. Paul Getty Museum.

Because of the increase in deaths with the use of chloroform, John Collins warned others against its use; and because nitrous oxide was not as convenient, ether became the preferred anesthetic in America. In December 1849, Long published his article in the *Southern Medical and Surgical Journal.* It was entitled "An Account of the First Use of Sulfuric Ether by Inhalation as an Anesthetic in Surgical Operations."

J. Mason Warren was the first surgeon to use ether on a private patient at MGH. He was also the first to use ether on a child by using a new method of delivery, a sponge held over the nose and mouth replacing the glass globe used by Morton. He wrote "The domain of surgery has been enlarged by admitting into the list of justifiable operations some of whose severity would otherwise in most cases have prevented even the thought of attempting them" (J. C.

Warren 1900). J. Collins Warren agreed when he stated:

> A new era has opened to the operating surgeon. With what fresh vigor does the living surgeon, who is ready to resign the scalpel, grasp it and wish again to go through his career under the new auspices? Since the fear of pain has diminished, the number of surgical operations has remarkably increased, at least in our vicinity. (J. C. Warren 1900)

Although the number of fractures had not increased during this new era, the number of cases admitted to the hospital significantly increased. **Table 3.2** (recreated from J. C. Warren 1900) reflects the changes in surgical volume at the MGH five years before and five years after the first use of ether.

Table 3.2. Number of Surgical Cases Before and After the Introduction of Ether Number Cases (mortality %)

Total Operations	5 Years Before 184 (6.5)		5 Years After 487 (9)	
Tumors (excluding breasts)	39	(5)	122	(3)
Breast amputation	13	(8)	30	(10)
Plastic operations	6	(0)	33	(3)
Amputations	13	(15)	65	(23)
Hernia				
Strangulated	5	(60)	1	(0)
Reduced under ether	0		2	(0)
Radical cure, plastic	0		0	
Radical cure, injection iodine	0		11	(0)
Laparotomy	0		4	(75)

Data from J. C. Warren 1900.

John Collins described his interest and use of ether since he first entered practice almost a half century earlier in a small monograph:

> Many years have elapsed since I myself used ethereal inhalation to relieve the distress attending the last stage of pulmonary inflammation. So long ago as the year 1805, it was applied for this purpose, in the case of a gentleman of distinction in the city, very frequently since, and particularly in the year 1812, to a member of my family, who experienced from it great relief, and still lives, to give testimony to its effects. The manner in which it was applied was by moistening a handkerchief and placing it near the face of the patient.

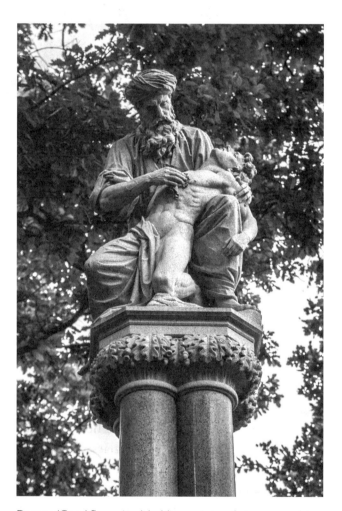

Ether Monument. Also known as The Good Samaritan. Statue and Fountain in Boston's Public Garden. Installed in 1868. Photo by the author.

Doctor (Good Samaritan) holding an injured stranger and apparently administering ether in a cloth.
Kael E. Randall/Kael Randall Images.

A new era has opened to the operating surgeon! His visitations on the most delicate parts are performed, not only without the agonizing screams he has been accustomed to hear, but sometimes with a state of perfect insensibility, and occasionally even with the expression of pleasure on the part of the patient. Who could have imagined that drawing the knife over the delicate skin of the face might produce a sensation of unmixed delight! That the turning and twisting of instruments in the most sensitive bladder might be accompanied by beautiful dream! That the contorting of anchylosed joints should co-exist with a celestial vision! If Ambrose Paré, and Louis, and Dessault, and Cheselden, and Hunter and Cooper could see what our eyes daily witness, how would they long to come among us, and perform their exploits once more! (J. C. Warren 1848)

At the time ether was first introduced, surgeons had to rely on techniques like mesmerism or hypnosis to assist patients through agonizing surgeries. Liston, well-known for performing a knee amputation within 30 seconds to alleviate patient suffering but likewise known as the only surgeon with a 300% mortality rate for a surgery performed, had exclaimed at ether's effectiveness: "This Yankee dodge beats mesmerism hollow" (A. Gawande 2012).

That Yankee was John Collins Warren.

RETIREMENT AND LEGACY

In the fall of 1846, John Collins Warren must have been thinking about his retirement. On November 1, 1846, less than a month after he performed the groundbreaking operation using ether, he stepped down as senior surgeon at the MGH. Warren was 68 years old but remained in practice. He asked Dr. George Hayward (who had also studied under Sir Astley Cooper at Guy's Hospital) to replace him as senior surgeon. Hayward had been an assistant surgeon at MGH since 1826; however, initially he and several other assistant surgeons were not allowed to operate. They probably only gave lectures to their students at MGH. Only the senior surgeon at MGH could operate, with the assistance of house pupils beginning in 1827. John Collins had not wanted this protocol to change at the time because there wasn't enough work for more than one surgeon. But in 1835, the Trustees appointed Hayward as the second surgeon; others followed until 1846 when the hospital had two surgical wards and six surgeons. Hayward assumed the responsibilities of senior surgeon and six days later performed the first major operation under ether anesthesia at MGH. Warren had temporarily turned over his responsibilities as senior surgeon

Ether Monument. At the base it states: "To commemorate that the inhaling of ether causes insensibility to pain. First proved to the world at the Mass. General Hospital in Boston, October A.D. MDCCCXLVI."

Kael E. Randall/Kael Randall Images.

to Hayward on a previous occasion when he traveled to Europe in 1837.

On December 17, 1847, John Collins informed the Harvard President of his plans to donate his anatomical museum to Harvard Medical School with a detailed history of his collection (>1,000 specimens) and a gift of $5,000 to maintain the museum, which remains a major anatomical museum as The Warren Anatomical Museum at Countway Medical Library. It contains over 15,000 specimens.

On February 15, 1847, Warren sent his resignation letter to Harvard. He gave his last lecture to the medical students on March 2, 1847. He was 69 years old. In this lecture he gave the following advice to the students (E. Warren 1860):

- to cultivate in their leisure…the higher branches of literature in their profession
- to cultivate a kind and cheerful spirit
- to evince a sympathy for their patients
- Avoid prejudice to a rival practitioner… Prosecutions for mal-practice which have become so frequent, have almost always been traced to the private hostility of a rival in the professional career
- [He wished them a] "continued zeal in the prosecution of their studies [and] abundant opportunities for relieving the poor
- an adequate reward for their labors from the rich
- [above all] a conscientious discharge of their duties through life"

The President and Fellows of Harvard accepted his resignation on February 27, 1847. He had served as the Hersey Professor of Anatomy and Surgery for 40 years; they named him professor emeritus of anatomy and surgery. He was succeeded by Oliver Wendell Holmes as professor of anatomy.

John Collins continued to see a small number of patients and operate on an occasional private patient. He continued his regular daily schedule,

spent most of his time writing, and most likely discussed cases and medical issues with colleagues and students at the MGH. He continued his interest in collecting material for his museum and his library. He walked frequently, sometimes as far as Brookline.

He officially resigned from the MGH on January 21, 1853, but continued to visit the hospital as a consultant surgeon. Captain Girdler, the hospital superintendent, was saddened by his departure. Warren, however, continued to teach and occasionally operate on private patients. He also continued to collect fossils, animal skeletons, and to write. He remained living in his home across from the Common in sight of the elm tree in the center of it, the famous tree of the Revolution (Liberty Tree) where meetings were held, effigies burned, and hangings took place.

In his early seventies, Warren began to have more physical ailments. For years he had recurrent sinus infections, and he treated himself with purging, blistering, and leeches. He was becoming short of breath after climbing stairs when visiting patients, and he had difficulty writing due to chronic inflammation of his right eye. He started to have increased episodes of light-headedness and wrote that he was becoming increasingly frail. He began to complain of increasing abdominal pain and vomiting as well as generalized aches and pains.

As aging affected his body increasingly over his last years, he remained under the care of his lifelong friend and colleague, Dr. James Jackson. In 1856, Jackson saw him almost daily. His last visit was on a Saturday, the last day Warren completed his walk to Brookline. Dr. John Collins Warren died the next morning on Sunday May 4, 1856, three months before his seventy-eighth birthday.

His funeral was the following Wednesday at St. Paul's Episcopal Church, which was filled with friends, family, and many physicians. The Massachusetts Medical Society marched in a procession to the church. The following article appeared in *The New York Times* on June 3, 1856:

The Will of the Late Dr. Warren of Boston.

The golden expectations of the numerous branches of the Warren family, which is scattered through New-England and New-York, have been disappointed by the last will and testament of JOHN COLLINS WARREN, the distinguished physician and surgeon, who recently died at Boston.

 The doctor left a property valued at about $600,000, all which, with some peculiar exceptions, he bequeathed to his surviving family, to the surprise of expectant relatives. He gave his watch guard to his brother, HENRY WARREN; a battle picture to his sister, MRS HARRIET PRINCE; $50 to the Boston Historical Society, of which he was for many years the President; and his own bones to the Medical College with which he was connected. But the bones of the celebrated mastodon he bequeathed to his own family! We presume the Medical College "wouldn't mind swapping" bones with the family, since mastodons are more scarce than men in those peculiar institutions. But as the Doctor's last will and testament does not allow this, the College will probably consider its legacy a bonne bouché, and make the most of it.

 Dr. Warren leaves two sons and three daughters, who inherit his estate. His sons are J. MASON WARREN, the distinguished surgeon, who married a daughter of Hon. B. W. Crowninshield; and SULLIVAN WARREN, who married Mrs. Elizabeth LINZEE GREEN, and lives in elegant leisure at his country seat in Brookline, one of those beautiful villages that environ Boston. One of his daughters married a son of HON. WILLIAM APPLETON, another married a son of HON. THEODORE LYMAN, and a third married a son of THOMAS DWIGHT, Esq—all "solid men of Boston."

The reference to his own bones referred to the fact that John Collins, in his will, had left his skeleton to future Harvard Medical students to be

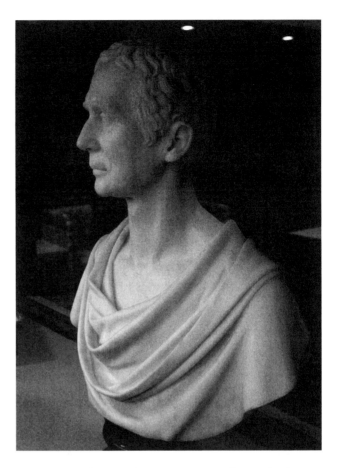

Marble bust of John Collins Warren in the Center for the History of Medicine, Countway Medical Library, Harvard Medical School. Photo by the author.

"carefully preserved, whitened, articulated, and placed in the lecture-room of the Medical College, near my bust; affording, as I hope, a lesson useful, at the same time, to morality and science" (A. M. Menting 2009). He followed the anatomists' motto of *mortui vivos docent* (the dead teach the living). His skeleton was articulated in great precision by J. B. S. Jackson, MD, professor of pathology and first curator of the Warren Museum, but it never hung publicly in the classrooms of Harvard. His wife objected and, although the restriction she sought in court was denied, Warren's skeleton was kept in a closed cabinet and never shown to the students. It remains today in the Warren Museum, and it is only viewed by and with permission of members of the Warren family. John Collins is buried with his family in the Forest Hills Cemetery in Roxbury.

Throughout his prestigious life, John Collins Warren performed operations that his father had done such as amputations, lithotomy, extirpations, and cataract removal; he was both a knowledgeable anatomist and a skilled surgeon. He was the first surgeon to reduce a strangulated hernia. He advocated early surgery for strangulated hernias because of the increase in death rates with delays in treatment. He also advocated surgery for a large variety of surgical problems; orthopaedic cases included clavicle excision, removing foreign bodies in the knees, subtrochanteric osteotomy of the femur, dislocations of the hip (he treated with pulleys and traction), amputations for compound fractures, shoulder dislocations, fractures and others.

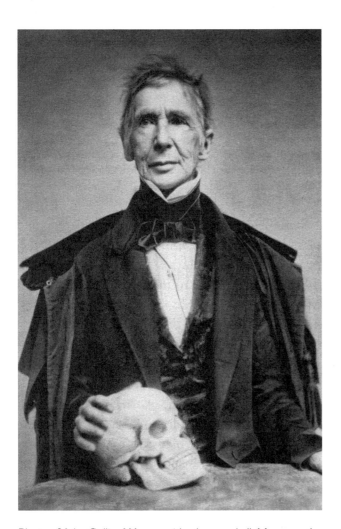

Photo of John Collins Warren with a human skull. Hangs on the wall of the first floor at the old entrance to the Bulfinch building.

Harvard Medical Library in the Francis A. Countway Library of Medicine.

John Collins never mentioned the Lowell malpractice case in his personal writings or his autobiography; he described the case in detail only in his *Pamphlet to the Massachusetts Supreme Court Justice.* He did state, "Since the use of the latter [ether] I have heard of no instance of failure in the reduction of recent dislocations...I have never failed to reduce a recent dislocation of the os femoris but would have repeatedly failed at the end of a week" (E. Warren 1860). Edward Warren writes that John Collins had seen the following types of hip dislocation: dorso-iliac, ischiatic, pubic, and thyroideal. Edward states that John Collins had successfully reduced anterior dislocations of the hip "at the end of four weeks, seven weeks and ten weeks" (E. Warren 1860). He described Warren's approach when treating a dislocated hip: the patient was bled first, then etherized, pulleys were applied to exert traction on the limb and then the leg was manipulated "according to the direction of the limb" (E. Warren 1860).

Dr. Warren had many achievements, recognitions and honors in his lifetime not already mentioned in this chapter. He was an active member of the Bunker Hill Monument Committee, which was organized to build a monument in honor of his uncle who died fighting for independence on Bunker Hill. He invested heavily and purchased three acres of land at the top of Bunker Hill; he donated and borrowed money for the monument. He petitioned and received two of the four cannons from Bunker Hill (owned by the Commonwealth of Massachusetts). The other two—and several pieces of granite which had been part of the original fortification—had been taken by the British. The two pieces of artillery were named Hancock and Adams. It took almost 20 years to complete the monument, which remains today.

John Collins was the second Hersey Professor of Anatomy and Surgery, after his father, from 1815 to 1847. He was the first dean of Harvard Medical School (1816–1817) and only one of two deans to serve on two different occasions (again in 1821–1826). He was one of two surgeons to

Box 3.2. Orthopaedic Publications of John Collins Warren

- Brown JB, Warren JC, "Two letters inscribed to John C. Warren/by John B. Brown." Var. title "Two letters on curvature of the spine." Boston: D. Clapp Jr. 1838 (republished from Boston M. & S. J., 1838).

- Brown JB, Warren JC. "Remarks on the operation for the cure of club-feet, with cases: also, letters to John C. Warren on curvature of the spine." Boston: D. Clapp Jr., 1839 (republished Boston M. & S. J., 1839).

- Haller A, Bichat X, Flagg J, Warren JC. *Anatomical description of the arteries of the human body.* Boston: Thomas B. Wait and Co., 1813.

- Warren, JC. "Removal of the Clavicle in a State of Osteo-sarcoma." *Journal of Medical Sciences*, 1833; 13.

- Warren, JC. "Physical education and the preservation of health." Boston: William D. Ticknor & Co.; 1846.

- Warren, JC. "A letter to the Hon. Issac Parker, Chief Justice of the Supreme Court of the State of Massachusetts, containing remarks on the dislocation of the hip joint, occasioned by the publication of a trial which took place at Machias, in the state of Maine, June 1824." Cambridge, MA: Hilliard and Metcalf, 1826.

Hospital Reports:
- "Case of Dislocation of the os humeri, with fracture of the Neck of the bone successfully reduced." Volume 1, ca. 1827. Warren, *The Life of John Collins Warren*, Vol. 1, 1860:238.

- Remarks by Dr. Warren on
  - fracture cases
  - hand wounds
  - compound fracture requiring amputation
- Volume 2, ca. 1827. Warren, *The Life of John Collins Warren*, Vol. 1, 1860:242.

serve as dean, the other was Edward H. Bradford, professor of orthopaedic surgery (1912–1918). There have been 23 deans of Harvard Medical School. In addition to leading in the formation of the *Boston Medical Surgical Journal*, he served as editor. He was president of the American Medical Association (1850), the Boston Society of Natural History, and other organizations. He was an honorary member of the Order of Cincinnati (an award given by George Washington to former officers for outstanding service in the Revolution), the Medico-Chirurgical Society of London, and the Parisian Medical Society to name some of his honorary memberships. He was awarded an honorary medical degree from St. Andrews University in Scotland (1802) and an honorary medical degree from Harvard in 1819. He published over 21 scientific/medical articles.

Of these, eight were some of the earliest publications about orthopaedics in the United States (see **Box 3.2**).

Oliver Wendell Holmes said that:

Dr. Warren was supreme among his fellows, and deservedly so. He performed a great number of difficult operations; always deliberate, always cool; with a grim smile in sudden emergencies, where weaker men would have looked perplexed, and wiped their foreheads. He had the stuff in him, which carried his uncle, Joseph Warren, to Bunker Hill, and left him there, slain among the last to retreat. (quoted in A. M. Sammarco 2010)

He remains one of the most influential surgeons of modern medicine.

CHAPTER 4

Warren Family

Tradition of Medical Leaders Continues into the Twentieth Century

The Warren family has made significant contributions to the profession of medicine and surgery, to Harvard Medical School (HMS), and to the Massachusetts General Hospital (MGH) throughout seven generations of physicians—beginning with Joseph and John Warren. John helped to found HMS. His son John Collins cofounded the MGH and demonstrated the first public use of ether as an anesthetic. Mason, John Collins' son, introduced plastic surgery in the United States and the use of the scientific method in evaluating patients. His son "Coll" Warren developed a research laboratory for the study of tumors at the Massachusetts General Hospital and helped to build a new Harvard Medical School at its current location in 1906. Coll's son John—great-grandson of John Collins Warren—deviated from surgery and taught anatomy at HMS. Richard Warren, nephew to John, was the next surgeon in the family. He was a general and vascular surgeon who became an expert on amputations; he led the program for amputees at the Boston Veterans Administration Hospital. Richard's nephew, H. Shaw Warren, is currently on the active staff at the Massachusetts General Hospital, leading a basic research program in adult and pediatric infectious disease.

JONATHAN MASON WARREN

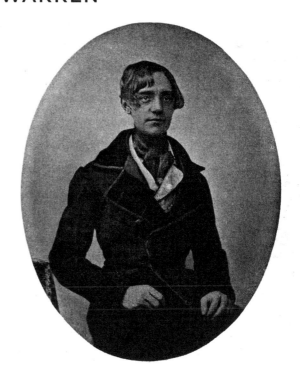

Daguerreotype of J. Mason Warren. Paris, 1844.
Collection of the Massachusetts Historical Society.

Physician snapshot

Jonathan Mason Warren

BORN: 1811

DIED: 1867

SIGNIFICANT CONTRIBUTIONS: the first plastic surgeon at the Massachusetts General Hospital; the first to use a forehead flap to reconstruct a nose in the United States; endowed the Warren Triennial Prize.

Jonathan Mason Warren, the fourth child and third son of John Collins Warren and Susan Powell Mason, would become the first plastic surgeon at MGH. He was born at home on February 5, 1811, at No. 2 Park Street. He was often referred to as J. Mason Warren or Mason. He was his mother's favorite child. Not the scholar his father was, from age nine until 14 he labored with the classes at the best school in Boston, the Latin Grammar School.

Education and Training

Throughout his youth, he was frail and sickly with frequent intestinal complaints, suggestive of recurrent gastritis or gastroesophageal reflux disease. His father was strict about his eating habits and believed it best to avoid rich foods and alcohol. John Collins exerted a domineering influence over Mason, who lost weight and was not thriving. His parents, therefore, removed him from school and arranged for him to be tutored at home. His entrance to Harvard was delayed for several additional years. Eventually, he entered as a sophomore in 1827.

With continued gastrointestinal problems and weight loss, Mason left Harvard after only three months. Although popular with many friends, he was constantly plagued by illness. His father continued to regulate and adjust Mason's diet, managing his food intake carefully, until his intake was reduced to only a small amount of plain rice with salt and sugar. Eventually his father even stopped the sugar. As was commonly prescribed for chronic illness during this period, doctors and his family recommended that Mason take a trip abroad.

When he was 17, Mason selected Cuba and traveled there with his older brother. He was so weak at the time that he had to be carried onto the ship. It wasn't long after setting sail that Mason began to feel better. He began to choose foods he liked and was soon gaining weight and strength. Most of his digestive problems disappeared. The brothers remained in Cuba for almost

six weeks. After returning to Boston with his strength restored, he eventually completed about two years of study at Harvard. In the fall of 1830, he entered the Harvard Medical School on Mason Street and began his studies under the guidance of his father, working in his father's practice at No. 2 Park Street. He was proud of his father and his family's heritage in medicine and believed that "men who thought no sacrifice too painful where great principles were at stake...upheld by a faith that knew no fatigue, no despair, no change, but, confiding in an ever-present hope, looked with assured peace to the world beyond for their reward" (H. P. Arnold 1886).

In 1832, Mason graduated from Harvard Medical School at 21 years of age. Throughout medical school, John Collins Warren advised him to avoid overeating, to avoid stimulants like wine, and to exercise regularly. He also gave him advice about his studies, emphasizing that "to obtain mechanical skill you ought daily to practice something mechanical, however, simple, even shaving or cutting sticks with a penknife, and often try your left hand" (H. P. Arnold 1886). His last category of advice was on morals, and he suggested that Mason "cultivate a high sense of religious feeling and duty" (H. P. Arnold 1886). He warned him to choose his friends carefully because he would be "known by his company" (H. P. Arnold 1886).

After graduating, Mason continued to have major weight loss, digestive complaints, loss of appetite, and fatigue. He was often depressed. Both gastrointestinal symptoms and depression remained intermittently with him for life. Another trip abroad seemed necessary. He departed on March 25, 1832, taking with him his father's advice, including a small blank book in which John Collins wrote "many rules of conduct, the dictates of his own wide observation, learning and sound judgment" (H. P. Arnold 1886). Mason landed in Liverpool, England, on May 29. He had planned to spend two years in Europe but stayed three years.

His first visit was to his father's mentor and friend, Sir Astley Cooper, who had retired except for occasional consultation and anatomical dissections. He was particularly proud of one—the thymus gland—which he sent to Mason's father. Mason spent four months in London visiting family and friends of his father, often attending rounds with Sir Charles Bell, Mr. Key at Guy's Hospital, and other leading surgeons. Mason visited the museums of hospitals and surgeons for new ideas, books, and surgical equipment and anatomical specimens, especially for his father. Mason obtained two knives from Mr. Key—one for lithotomy and a straight knife for amputation flaps—as well as newly designed vascular forceps. He also sent five casts of skulls from individuals of diverse ethnicities to his father. John Collins Warren had instructed his son to keep him informed about any new thinking, treatments, books, or instruments. In addition to visiting Cooper's home containing many anatomical specimens, he visited John Hunter's Museum.

He spent the summer touring with his friend James Jackson Jr. in Scotland. He followed Mr. Syme in his clinic, observing operations. Mason was impressed by Syme's museum, and he purchased Syme's publications on surgical excision of diseased joints. Writing to his father, Mason described Syme's use of a cautery (iron) to keep open knee and ankle joints that were infected by tuberculosis.

He arrived in Paris in late September of 1832, where he was to spend most of his three years in Europe. Many of his fellow American peers there had earned bachelor's degrees from college, and the majority of these had an upbringing among professional, business, or land-owning classes. At the time, Paris was the medical epicenter of the world and was home to hundreds of American students studying medicine. Unequaled in size and for its famous physicians and surgeons, Paris had seven major teaching hospitals: Hôtel-Dieu, Hôpital de la Pitié, Hôpital de la Charité, Hôpital des Enfants Malades, Hôpital de la Salpêtrière,

Hôpital de Bicêtre, and Hôpital Saint-Louis. During the first year of Mason's visit, the 12 hospitals in Paris treated about 65,000 patients; during this same period, MGH and McLean Hospital treated fewer than 1,000 patients.

The medical school, École de Médicine, at the University of Paris, was large. Founded during the American Revolution, it was an international leader in medical education. Medical schools in the United States were smaller, with only about six professors. The École de Médicine had 26 professors with an enrollment of about 5,000 students, which was twice the number in the United States. Classes were in French, not Latin. Only about 1% of the medical students were American. In addition to basic sciences such as anatomy, pathology and chemistry, clinical courses were given in the following surgical fields: obstetrics, clinical surgery, operative surgery, and pathologic anatomy. Orthopaedics was not a separate course. The school had a tremendous library with over 30,000 books. Harvard Medical School had few. All lectures for the American students were free.

Most of the clinicians that Mason observed—with the exception of Pierre Charles Alexander Louis—were on the faculty at École de Médicine. Louis, regarded by some as the founder of evidence-based medicine, introduced the numerical method. Mason attended many lectures at the medical school but had to visit the Hôpital de la Charité to hear Louis lecture. There, he also observed Jacque Lisfranc operate and attend patients. As a frequent visitor to Hôtel-Dieu, Mason was allowed to observe many operations performed by Baron Guillaume Dupuytren, the hospital's chief surgeon. Mason spent time in almost all, if not all, of Paris's teaching hospitals, along with some American friends: James Jackson Jr., Henry I. Bowditch, Oliver Wendell Holmes, and others. This was a joyful period of his life, and he was happy in his studies and medical experience. He had no digestive problems while enjoying his choice of French food.

At Hôtel-Dieu, Mason was impressed by the surgical skills of Dupuytren. Dupuytren's lectures were also admired by the students and "his expositions were clear and concise" (H. P. Arnold 1886). However, he was "haughty, disdainful, tyrannical and suffered no questions" (H. P. Arnold 1886). One evening while having dinner in Dupuytren's home and thinking about his own father's case, Mason asked him if he had ever seen a hip dislocation posterior and inferior. Dupuytren described two similar cases that he treated successfully with reductions accomplished soon after injury.

Without anesthesia, surgeons had to be fast. Instruments were not sterile, and surgeons rarely washed their hands before operating. Mason was surprised by the lack of concern for the patient and the emphasis on the surgeon's desire to operate rather than the patient's needs. Although an outstanding surgeon, Dupuytren was especially cruel, even becoming physically violent with patients who did not obey his orders.

Professionally, Dupuytren often publicly criticized his colleagues, which was a theme common to surgeons at the time in Paris. He focused his criticism on his competition, Jacque Lisfranc, who was head of the Hôpital de la Pitié (he also operated at Hôpital de la Charité). These two leading French surgeons quarreled often and referred to each other in their lectures as "le Brigard de la Seine" (Dupuytren, the highway robber) and "the butcher of La Pitié" (Lisfranc). Mason did not record whether he had seen Dupuytren operate on any hand deformities or perform orthopaedic operations.

Lisfranc, the powerful chief at Hôpital de la Charité, was imposing at six feet. He was quick tempered, even during his lectures where he often swore. Describing Lisfranc lecturing, Mason wrote, "I went once to hear Lisfranc thunder. He has the most powerful voice I ever heard from a lecturer. He speaks ill of everybody, and everybody of him" (H. P. Arnold 1886). Known as an excellent surgeon, Mason observed that "his amputations of fingers and toes are very neat and rapid,

and all his operations are marked by a kind of off-hand way, not premeditated" (H. P. Arnold 1886). Many patients died after surgery, from blood loss or infections. In Paris, the majority of amputees—as many as two-thirds—died after surgery.

As a bloodletter, Lisfranc had no equal, often bleeding dozens of patients at a time. Bloodletting, common in the nineteenth century, was challenged in Paris by one of Mason's favorite surgeons/teachers, Pierre Charles Alexandre Louis. Louis studied case records of 77 patients, comparing the timing of bloodletting in two groups of patients with pneumonia. Almost twice as many patients died in the group treated early:

> It is nevertheless true, that the number of patients bled on the first day, who had passed the age of fifty, was nearly twice as great as that of patients of the same age, who were bled at a later period. This must have had great influence on mortality. (P. C. A. Louis 1836)

Louis impressed Mason by using statistics and doing clinical research with cohorts of patients (what has been called the numerical method). His method of patient care included evaluating:

1. Case history
2. Symptoms and severity
3. Examination of existing and absent symptoms
4. Patient's medical record
5. Post-mortem examination if the patient died (R. Truax 1968)

This scientific approach influenced Mason, and he brought the method back to Boston along with the stethoscope, a new diagnostic tool invented by Laënnec. Holmes remarked about Laënnec's discovery, noting "Laënnec's invention of auscultation holds the next place to vaccination in the records of practical improvement during our first half century" (R. Truax 1968).

He kept a diary detailing different operations he observed. Regarding orthopaedics, he commented frequently about amputations and how unique flaps were planned, discussed cases of successful shoulder disarticulations, gunshot wounds to the extremities, fractures of all types, tuberculosis of joints, tumors, open wounds treated by hot irons, use of bandaging in treating fractures, and the use of skin grafts, which was a technique he would bring to the United States and use successfully in nose reconstruction. In one of his many letters to his son, John Collins Warren wrote:

> Practice much with tools. Get a hand-saw and saw bones daily in every direction. Saw with your left hand. Learn to shave with your left hand, and to dissect. Do all surgical operations on dead bodies methodically, carefully and frequently. This will not require much time, and you can command bodies better than here. I avail myself of every opportunity of doing the most simple operations on the dead body. (H. P. Arnold 1886)

Hip dislocations remained as one of Mason's focused attentions, namely cases of posterior and inferior dislocations into the ischiatic notch that had garnered so much adverse publicity for his father (see chapter 3). In addition to the two cases that Dupuytren stated that he had treated successfully early, Mason saw a cast of one in the museum at Leyden: "The dislocation...among them...as cast...in a case, of a dislocation behind and backwards, which showed well the formation of the new cavity for the head of the bone" (H. P. Arnold 1886). At St. Bartholomew Hospital Museum, he saw "a most perfect wet preparation of dislocation of the neck of the thigh bone, backwards and downwards" (H. P. Arnold 1886). The patient had died immediately after his accident before any treatment. It was interesting that the surgeon at St. Bartholomew had read about the trials of Mr. Lowell in Maine. Although Sir Astley Cooper had never seen such a dislocation, Mason found these four cases (two anatomic specimens and two

reported by Dupuytren) during his three years in Europe. He mentions them on six different occasions in his memoirs. Later in his publication *Surgical Observations with Cases and Operations*, he summarized hip dislocations at MGH, including 25 on the dorsum ileum, four into the foramen ovale, and 10 into the ischiatic notch. He detailed the Lowell case, including the autopsy findings of Oliver. He defends his father with these cases that he observed in Europe, reporting that Cooper later treated such cases and that he had also treated this type of hip dislocation in his own practice.

SURGICAL OBSERVATIONS,

WITH

CASES AND OPERATIONS.

BY

J. MASON WARREN, M.D.,

SURGEON TO THE MASSACHUSETTS GENERAL HOSPITAL; FELLOW OF THE
AMERICAN ACADEMY OF ARTS AND SCIENCES, ETC.

BOSTON:
TICKNOR AND FIELDS.
1867.

Cover of *Surgical Observations with Cases and Operations* by J. Mason Warren, 1867.

Warren Anatomical Museum in the Francis A. Countway Library of Medicine.

After two years in Paris, Mason returned to Great Britain, visiting London, Edinburgh, Liverpool, and Ireland for the summer. In Edinburgh, he studied with Syme and heard lectures on nerves by Sir Charles Bell. The first day he spent with Mr. Robert Liston, he observed "the reduction of the dislocated thumb of a boy, which had been some time in that state. By a cord tied around the second joint all the force was applied that could be without pulling off the thumb, and thus failing, the lateral ligament, I think was divided, and the reduction effected" (H. P. Arnold 1886). After attending the meeting of the British Association, he returned to Paris for another eight months. During the second visit, he discovered his special interest in plastic surgery, which had not yet been identified as a specialty of surgery.

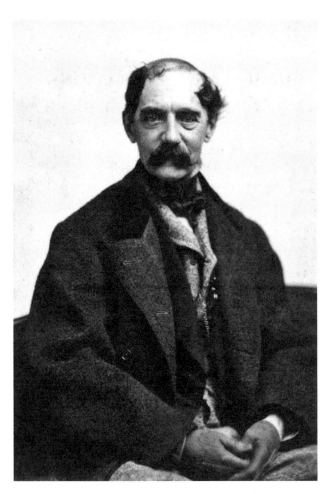

J. Mason Warren.
Harvard Medical Library in the Francis A. Countway Library of Medicine.

At the time, Professor Johann Friedrich Dieffenbach, the chief surgeon at Charité Hospital in Berlin, was visiting Paris and operating at several hospitals. He taught Mason reconstructive procedures such as V-Y advancement flaps, cleft palate repair, and use of a forehead flap to reconstruct the nose. As Mason recalls, "I had the opportunity to see Dieffenbach…exercise his skill a few days since on two noses, both of which he repaired in a very ingenious way" (H. P. Arnold 1886). Mason used this nasal flap to reconstruct a nose after returning to Boston. It was the first such case in the United States.

During his last few months in Paris and before returning to Boston, Mason took a course on bandaging by Riban. He noted that it covered "the different methods of healing fractures adopted by the French and English surgeons, and many very important things in 'La Petite Chirurgie'. This branch of Surgery I should think might be taught with more care to the rising generation at home" (H. P. Arnold 1886). This may be the first mention where a young surgeon in the nineteenth century referred to fracture care (later orthopaedic surgery) as a branch of surgery.

Medical Practice in Boston

Mason sailed from Liverpool in May, arriving in Boston the second week of June 1835. In Boston he continued to struggle with poor health, both digestive complaints and periods of depression. To recover, he would return to Europe on three more occasions before being fully prepared to resume practice in Boston again. He assumed responsibilities for his father's practice during John Collins Warren's lengthy, but deserved, vacation to Europe. Mason worked hard, grew his practice, preferred plastic reconstructive procedures, made friends easily, and married Annie Crowninshield, the daughter of a former secretary of the navy, on April 13, 1839. They began a family. Shortly thereafter, his mother died in 1840, which was especially hard on him as they were very close. Her death must have led to further bouts of depression.

In February 1846, the MGH Trustees finally appointed Mason visiting surgeon, along with five others. Holmes commented about Mason at the time: "This beloved, generous and affable man... never...lost sight of his great object to qualify himself for that...place as a surgeon which has marked for him by the name he bore" (B. P. Colcock 1972). Eight months later, his father used ether for the first time in the Bulfinch surgical theater (later called the Ether Dome). By this time, Mason was living near his father at No. 6 Park Street, with his wife and seven children. Following the first use of ether, he modified the technique of administration, using a sponge containing ether held over the patient's mouth and nose. He also performed the first operation on a private patient with ether. Mason remained in private practice, but he never had a faculty position at Harvard Medical School. He was not interested in taking time from his busy practice to teach.

Like his grandfather, Mason repaired hair lips. He was described by many as an excellent surgeon; he introduced the broad field of plastic surgery—not yet named as such—to the United States. Some of his most significant contributions include restoring the roof of the mouth (hard palate) in hair lip deformities by suturing the periosteum over the defect, nose restoration with a forehead flap, use of other flaps (arm flap), and skin grafts in reconstruction of defects caused by cancer, trauma, and infection (in cases of tuberculosis).

Norwalk, Connecticut, Train Wreck

A near-death experience occurred to Mason, his wife, his son Collins (Coll), and a nephew. On April 30, 1853, while returning by train from an American Medical Convention in New York City, a terrible train accident happened in Norwalk, Connecticut. The train was speeding as it approached the bridge in Norwalk, and the drawbridge was opened at the time for a passing steam ship. The engine, along with the first two cars and half of the third car plunged into the river. Over 60 among the 200 passengers died; many were injured. Some physicians were also lost. Mason and his family were in the third car; their seats faced only wreckage in front as they and passengers behind them teetered on the edge of the bridge. They escaped without physical injury, but psychologically Mason was permanently affected by the experience. He and others worked tirelessly to rescue and treat the injured. First reports in the press headlined "Frightful and Fatal Railroad Accidents! The cars thrown off the bridge at Norwalk...Dr. Warren and others from Boston safe" (H. P. Arnold 1886). It wasn't long after this traumatic experience that Mason, his wife, and Collins returned to Europe for a family vacation while Mason also visited medical museums and hospitals.

Mason's health remained problematic, including digestive complaints and symptoms of depression. During a later trip to Rome, Mason and Annie rented an apartment at the Piazza de Spagna. Mason also experienced what sounds like sciatica, forcing them to return home. The trip was long; during which his father died. Mason arrived back in Boston on July 3, 1856, two months after John Collins Warren's death. Before they moved

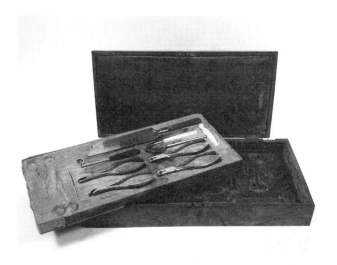

J. Mason Warren's instrument case. Courtesy Massachusetts General Hospital.

Massachusetts General Hospital, Archives and Special Collections.

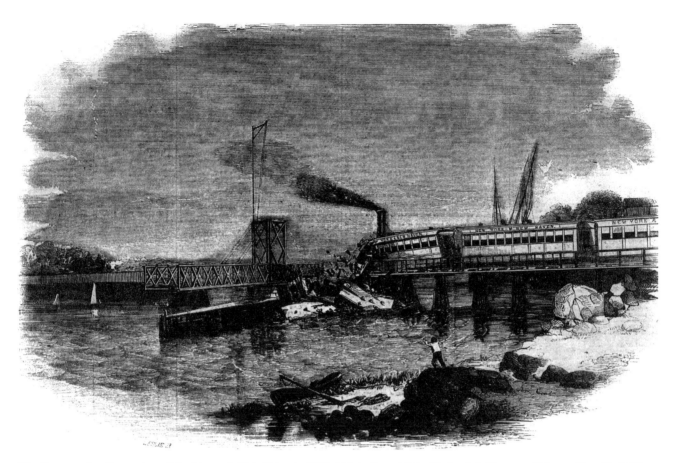

The Catastrophe. Illustration of the Norwalk Train Wreck, 1853. Originally published in Leslie's Illustrated News, May 21, 1853. The Connecticut Historical Society.

into his father's house at No. 2 Park Street, Annie first insisted all manner of medical memorabilia and phenomenon—including skeletons and pickled specimens—be removed.

Legacy

Despite his own health struggles, Mason remained happy and continued to work hard in his surgical practice. He published about 25 articles, lectures, and books, including four on orthopaedic topics such as treating wry neck with division of the sternocleidomastoid muscle and hip disarticulation for osteosarcoma of the femur. Mason included 400 cases—many orthopaedic—in the second edition of his book, *Surgical Observations with Cases and Operations*, which his son Collins (Coll) described as the definitive voice on surgery at the time. Most likely, Mason eventually developed intestinal cancer.

He died on August 19, 1867, at 56 years of age. His 25-year-old son, Coll, summoned home from Europe, arrived three days before his father died.

In honor of his father's memory, Mason left an endowment to MGH in his will, which was used to establish the Warren Triennial Prize in 1871. The prize is awarded every three years to scientists for "the best dissertation on some subject in physiology, surgery, or pathologic anatomy" (F. A. Washburn 1909); its modern day focus includes "fields relating to medicine and includes a cash award of

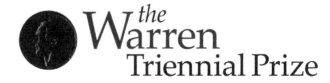

The Warren Triennial Prize and Medal.
Massachusetts General Hospital, Archives and Special Collections.

$50,000" (MassGeneral.org, n.d.) plus a handsome medal. In 2011, it was awarded to two scientists who discovered a method to convert adult stem cells into cells like embryonic stem cells and the use of those stem cells in animal models of disease. In the 141 years of its existence, 22 of the honorees have also received the Nobel Prize in Medicine.

JOHN COLLINS "COLL" WARREN

Physician snapshot

John Collins "Coll" Warren

BORN: 1842

DIED: 1927

SIGNIFICANT CONTRIBUTIONS: Fundraiser for Harvard Medical School and the Cancer Research Laboratory in Collis P. Huntington Memorial Hospital; introduced Lister's antisepsis concept to MGH surgeons; tumor surgeon

The second John Collins Warren was commonly called Coll or Col and signed his name as J. Collins Warren. He did so to differentiate himself from his famous grandfather, John Collins Warren. He was born on May 4, 1842, as the second child and only son of Mason and Annie. Growing up, he always planned to follow his family's tradition in medicine; this dream was reinforced by many trips abroad meeting famous physicians/surgeons, often waiting in the garden along the Charles River while his father made rounds, or at other times watching his father operate.

Education and Training

After graduating from Boston Latin School, he enrolled at Harvard. By his second year, he had committed himself to a career in surgery, but then the Civil War erupted (April 12, 1861) the same year. Coll considered enlisting in the army, but his parents were opposed. The family reached a consensus, deciding that Coll would begin his medical studies while an undergraduate. He attended lectures at the medical school on North Grove Street, next to the MGH. The Battle of Gettysburg (July 1–3, 1863) erupted immediately after he finished his coursework, and he and his classmates found themselves establishing their careers right at the heart of the tension of the Civil War.

Having finished two years of lectures, but without any apprentice time, he did join the army and was assigned to a hospital in Philadelphia as an acting medical cadet where he dressed wounds. There were few patients in his hospital, allowing him to continue his medical studies at Jefferson Medical School. He was given a great opportunity to study under Joseph Pancoast and Samuel D. Gross. He often had the opportunity to assist Gross at surgery. But in early 1864, the number of wounded increased with General Grant's campaign. Coll, a volunteer, was advanced to an acting

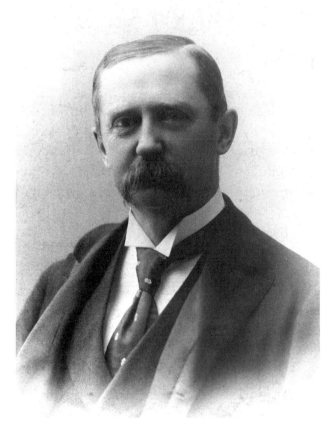

Photo: J. Collins (Coll) Warren.
Boston Medical Library in the Francis A. Countway Library of Medicine.

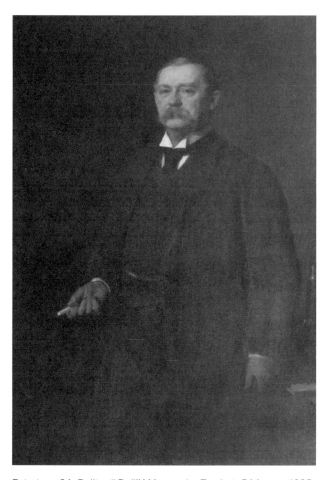

Painting of J. Collins "Coll" Warren, by Frederic P. Vinton, 1905.
Massachusetts General Hospital, Archives and Special Collections.

England. The term *pup* eventually was used to identify interns and later junior residents at the MGH; it disappeared in the early 1970s. At the time Coll was a house pupil, the surgical staff consisted of six surgeons, including his father, Mason; three surgeons assigned to an east service and three to a west service. In 1866, Coll took and passed his final exams at Harvard Medical School. He spoke fondly of his father's influence on his education as a mentor and guide.

House pupils on the surgical service treated wounds; removed foreign bodies, including bone fragments; and applied dressings. Each surgical house pupil was equipped with scissors, dressing and artery forceps, a probe and director, a *porte-caustique*, and a knife, but they were not yet familiar with sterility issues at the time. They assisted in operations, including washing the instruments after an operation and preparing the ether dome for the surgeon. Patients were monitored postoperatively by their pulse, general status, breathing, temperature of the skin, and the state of the wound.

House pupils assisted surgeons in treating fractures on the ward. Femur fractures were treated in Buck's traction, which was a popular method. They also used fracture boxes to treat fractures of the leg. The fracture box, while unreliable, allowed surgeons to drain compound fractures, replace

assistant surgeon. Placed in charge of two hospital tents near Richmond, Virginia, he was responsible for about 50 patients. Wounds were severe, and Coll found himself dressing wounds and giving morphine injections to ease the soldiers' pain. He expressed that "the syringe was a novelty at the time…this little instrument became by far the most valuable part of my equipment" (R. Truax 1968). It was a difficult time for Coll because there were no trained surgeons to care for his patients. He must have felt very inadequate, and he became increasingly determined to complete his surgical education.

After the Civil War ended in 1865, he began one year as a house pupil, or pup, at the MGH. Since 1811, the term *house pupil* had been used for medical students making hospital rounds at the Almshouse. The term probably dates back to

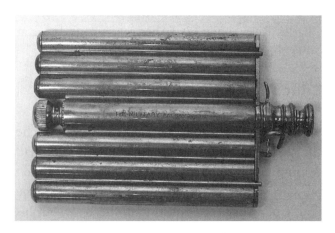

Military metal syringes with cylinders of morphine, atropine and Digitalin.
Massachusetts General Hospital, Archives and Special Collections.

dressings and apply pads to keep the bone fragments aligned and secure. It was not uncommon for the house pupils and the surgeons to contract an infection from their patients' wounds.

Coll also experienced the advent of new operations, including orthopaedic cases, with the use of ether anesthesia. Infected joints were resected instead of amputated. Attempts to save a limb by removing bone or joint, in the cases of infections and tuberculosis, increased at the MGH. Coll's father, Mason Warren, successfully excised the knee joint three times.

After his year of training at MGH and the completion of his studies at Harvard Medical School, Coll, like his father and grandfather, went to Europe to further his education. He chose to also visit Berlin and Vienna after being influenced by his older colleagues. In Germany, the hospitals were owned by the government. The staff consisted of university faculty where the professor dictated in a department. As such, the hospitals' primary purpose was for education and research. After arriving by ship first in England, Coll visited several famous surgeons at the request of his father. At St. Bartholomew's, he observed James Paget's successful knee joint resections without gangrene development. At the University College Hospital, he saw a Pirogoff amputation by Mr. Erichsen. He was impressed by many of the surgeons he visited, including Timothy Holmes at St. George's Hospital, who wrote the surgical authoritative textbook of the day, Holmes's *System of Surgery* (six volumes). After almost two months in England, Coll traveled to Germany.

After learning German in Dresden, Coll worked at the famous Allgemeines Krankenhaus, which had opened in Vienna in 1697. He began his studies in medicine before concentrating on surgery, and he learned the important tools of auscultation and percussion. Later, in another visit to Europe, Coll studied with Lister, learning his principles of antisepsis. We do not know whether Coll knew of Ignaz Semmelweis's landmark studies on hand washing, which dramatically reduced deaths from puerperal fever. The studies were completed on the obstetrical service at the Allgemeines Krankenhaus almost 20 years (1847) before Coll's arrival, eight years after Semmelweis published his research and 12 years before Pasteur's germ theory (1878). Coll doesn't mention Semmelweis in his *Reminiscences*.

After two semesters in Vienna, Coll was notified that his father was severely ill. The telegram he received stated, "Come home first steamer…" (R. Truax 1968). He sailed home on July 31, 1867, arriving August 16, 1867. His father died three days later. He was faced with a dilemma of either returning to Europe to complete his studies or taking over his father's practice. Ultimately, he followed O. W. Holmes's advice to complete his surgical education. Returning to Vienna, he focused his education on surgery. The university department had a new chairman, Professor Theodor Billroth, who was an innovative and leading voice on surgical training.

Coll became well educated in surgery and surgical pathology studying with Billroth in Vienna. He studied Billroth's recently published classic book on surgical pathology and treatment, and he observed many of Billroth's operations and frequent autopsies, which were caused primarily by infection. For example, Billroth's mortality rate from infection after goiter removal was 36%. Later, Halsted visited Billroth (1879). Amazed by Billroth's surgical expertise, he stated, "Slowly it dawned upon us that we in America were novices in the art as well as the science of surgery" (W. Halsted 1924). Coll observed that the devastation of infection after surgery increased with the increased rate of operations following the successful use of ether by his grandfather 20 years before he studied in Vienna.

Except for trephining for skull fractures, the abdomen and thorax remained off limits for surgeons until four years later when Billroth operated in both the thorax and the abdomen, becoming the founding father of abdominal surgery. Coll was extremely fortunate to learn about the surgical treatment of tumors with his experience working under Billroth, the recent publication of Virchow on tumors, and a private course he arranged with another new professor in Vienna, Alfred Biesiadecki, assistant under Professor Karl Rokitanasky in the Institute of Pathological Anatomy. Biesiadecki introduced him to laboratory techniques of tissue sectioning, staining and microscopic analysis. He was convinced to focus his career on the diagnosis and treatment of tumors; he published his first paper on keloid development in the *Proceedings of the Imperial Academy of Science* (1868).

After spending a total of two years in Vienna—one in medicine and one in surgery—Coll traveled to Berlin, the epicenter of scientific medicine and its advancements. Continuing with his focus on surgery and pathologic anatomy, he studied under Bernard von Langerbeck, the leading surgeon in Germany; Rudof Virchow, the father of modern pathology; and his successor, Julius Cohnheim.

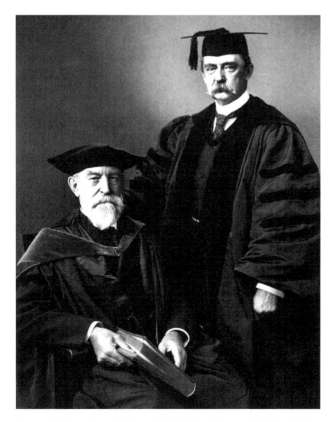

Henry P. Bowditch (left) and J. Collins Warren (right), 1906.
Harvard Medical Library in the Francis A. Countway Library of Medicine

Virchow not only classified tumors, but first described the pathophysiology of pulmonary thromboembolism.

In his private course with Professor Langerbeck, Coll observed many orthopaedic operations, including joint excisions for gunshot wounds (following the Prussian-Austrian War) for the elbow, hip, knee, and ankle. According to Coll, Langerbeck stressed preservation of the periosteum in these cases to avoid ankylosis. Coll was able to practice many of these operations on cadavers under Langerbeck's supervision.

Following the spring and summer of 1868 in Berlin, Coll went to Paris for a brief visit with plans to return to Berlin. There, in the laboratory of Claude Bernard, he met Henry Pickering Bowditch, the elder brother of Charles Pickering Bowditch who had graduated with Coll at Harvard College. Postponing his plans to return to Boston, Coll became close friends with Bowditch, a friendship that continued after they returned to Boston. Their friendship was largely responsible for the later success of the new medical school at Longwood Avenue. He decided to study for a while in the laboratory of Louis Antoine Ranvier at the Collège de France, already famous for his studies on nerve fiber anatomy. The opportunities for observation by students were difficult at the time, which was a change for the worse since his father had studied in Paris. Students had to obtain tickets for simple visits to hospitals, and tickets were difficult to obtain. Coll did manage to continue some limited studies in surgery with Jacques Maisonneuve at Hôtel-Dieu and Auguste Nélaton, originator of Nélaton's line, at Hôpital St. Louis. It was while in Paris that Coll first heard of the surgeon Joseph Lister, who successfully used carbolic acid to prevent wound infections in Glasgow. He also heard about Louis Pasteur. Anesthesia was also increasingly being used in operations, although not fully embraced by all surgeons. Coll recalled only seeing chloroform used in Europe and England. He only saw ether used once when he administered it for Liebreich in Paris. In his

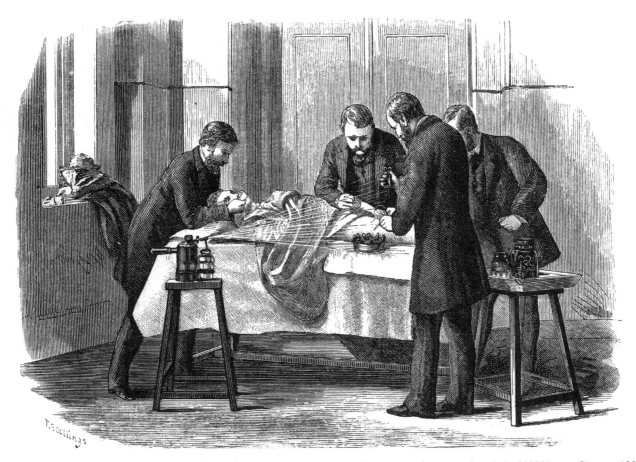

Lister's Carbolic acid spraying treatment. From *Antiseptic surgery: its principles, practice, history and results* by W. Watson Cheyne, 1882. Wellcome Library/Wikimedia Commons.

Remembrances, he noted "I do not remember having seen ether given during my three years in Europe…one exception…when I gave ether for Liebreich in Paris" (quoted in E. D. Churchill 1958). He had stayed in Paris for most of the academic year.

With only a few months left before returning to Boston, he limited his studies to surgery and went to England with plans to eventually visit Lister in Glasgow, which he would consider the most important facet of his experience as a student. In London he visited Timothy Holmes at St. George's Hospital. It was Holmes who first demonstrated antiseptic treatment of wounds to Coll. Holmes' early attempts included having the instruments as well as the surgeon's hands washed in carbolic acid. Coll wrote, "I do not remember any preliminary cleansing of the hands" (quoted in E. D. Churchill 1958). At Guy's Hospital, he

attended lectures and clinics of Thomas Bryant, whose textbooks on surgery were used by Harvard medical students. Coll was first introduced to a specialty hospital while visiting England. He was impressed by Bernard Edward Brodhurst's proposal that orthopaedics be a separate specialty and his promotion of his specialty at the Orthopaedic Hospital. In his *Remembrances*, Coll wrote:

> Mr. Brodhurst's work at the Orthopaedic Hospital seemed to me to be of an advanced character and an improvement on what I have seen at home, although at this time Louis Sayre in New York, whom I had heard lecture on one occasion in Gross's clinic in Philadelphia, had already placed this branch of surgery on a substantial basis and Buckminster Brown in Boston was beginning to develop orthopaedic surgery as a specialty. (E. D. Churchill 1958)

Upon traveling to Glasgow, he met Sir James Simpson, Mr. Joseph Bell, and Mr. James Syme (Lister's father-in-law), but the highlight of his visit was seeing Lister's successful technique of treating compound fractures, surgical wounds, and abscesses. He recalls Lister being self-aware that he was on the vanguard of surgical advancement, realizing his techniques would be accepted and adapted in the future. His tenure under Lister left a lasting impression upon him and influenced his own scientific approach to medicine and surgery; in addition to his learning, he brought back samples of plaster from Lister with him on his voyage home.

Lister had been Professor at the Royal Infirmary in Glasgow for about eight years. He had been developing his concepts on antisepsis for about three years after learning of Pasteur's research. During the year prior to Coll's visit, he had published his first papers in the *Lancet*, "On Compound Fractures and Preliminary Notice on Abscess" and "On the Antiseptic Principle in the Practice of Surgery." He had received his medical degree at the University of London where he studied with William Sharpey (of Sharpey's fibers). As a student, he observed the first use of ether by Robert Liston in England on December 21, 1846, two months after its public use by John Collins Warren. Liston prided himself on being able to complete an above-knee amputation in 30 seconds, but he also has an infamous record as the only surgeon to have a 300% mortality rate for an operation. While amputating one patient's leg, he also inadvertently amputated the index finger of his assistant. Both the patient and the assistant later died from postoperative infections. Simultaneously, Liston severed the coattails of a close observer, who died of a probable heart attack at the time. Nevertheless, overall Liston had a very low mortality-rate of postoperative infection, only 15%, compared to the average rate, which was greater than 50%. It was his habit to wash his hands and change to a clean apron before each operation long before Semmelweiss published his landmark study on postpartum fever prevention from hand washing. Joseph Lister, after graduation from medical school, was recommended to James Syme, professor of surgery at Edinburgh, by Sharpey. He remained as Syme's assistant until assuming the chair in Glasgow.

Medical and Surgical Practice

On September 6, 1869, Coll Warren began his practice as a physician and surgeon, as his father and grandfather had done before him, at No. 2 Park Street. He was appointed physician to outpatients at the Massachusetts General Hospital. In 1872, he received an appointment as surgeon to outpatients and in 1876 was appointed visiting surgeon. During his three-year stay in Europe, the Ether Dome was no longer used for surgery. A new surgical wing had been added to the hospital that included a new surgical amphitheater, later named the Henry J. Bigelow Operating Theater in 1890 (see chapter 29). Dr. Henry J. Bigelow was the senior surgeon and an influential surgeon of the time.

With the new tools to fight infection given to him by Lister, Coll expected his colleagues to

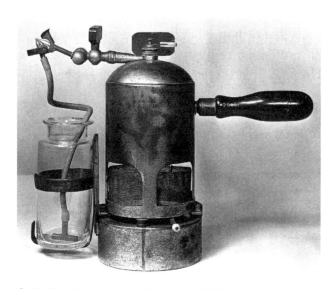

Carbolic acid sprayer used by Lister (1866). Wellcome Library.

eagerly accept Lister's technique to improve their patients' safety. Unfortunately, that did not happen. Henry J. Bigelow had tried the Lister technique of antisepsis before Coll returned to the MGH but remained unconvinced about its effectiveness. Coll found that surgeons could not be easily persuaded to change their techniques, and he was forced to watch them continue to practice surgery while not following asepsis technique.

In his enthusiasm to advance Lister's principles, Coll published an excellent explanation of his principles of antisepsis in a letter to the *Boston Medical and Surgical Journal*. He also used Lister's technique successfully with a dressing given to him by Lister in a patient he had operated on for breast cancer. But the old guard under Bigelow's leadership prevented Coll from bringing this new important discovery into the practice of surgeons in the United States. Bigelow did not accept the protocol until seven years later in 1876. Acceptance by established surgeons was slow but, as Lister had predicted, the next generation of surgeons were convinced of the usefulness of antisepsis techniques. The surgeons at MGH had brought two major advances to surgery in the United States following the use of ligatures to control bleeding: the first public use of ether (general anesthesia) and the use of Lister's antisepsis carbolic acid dressings (preventing wound infections, the most frequent cause of death after compound fractures, amputations, and surgery).

As his practice grew, Coll worked in his laboratory at home and at the medical school on North Grove Street, having received an appointment as instructor in surgery at Harvard in 1871. He studied tumors. In 1872, he received the Boylston Prize for discovering that the rodent ulcer was a type of cancer. Just six months before the great fire of Boston on November 7, 1872—which destroyed Trinity Church and 65 acres in downtown Boston (including 776 buildings) and just spared the Warren's homes at No. 2 and No. 6 Park Street—Coll (age 31) married Amy Shaw (age 21). Her father (deceased) was a member of the Parkman family.

They lived at No. 2 Park Street until 1874 when they moved into a house at 58 Beacon Street, which was given to them by Amy's mother. In 1874 they also had their first son, John, and a year later their second, Joseph, was born. Amy was left a partial invalid after Joseph's birth. Coll's practice was large, but for over 30 years he devoted himself to improvements and growth of the facilities of Harvard Medical School, first the Boylston Street campus and then the present Longwood campus (see section on Harvard Medical School).

Coll was personally well liked and very successful as a surgeon. He taught medical students surgical oncology and established a ledger of tumors at MGH entitled "Microsurgical Examinations of Tumors." He continued to pursue the incorporation of Lister's principles into surgical practice at MGH, witnessing the transition to

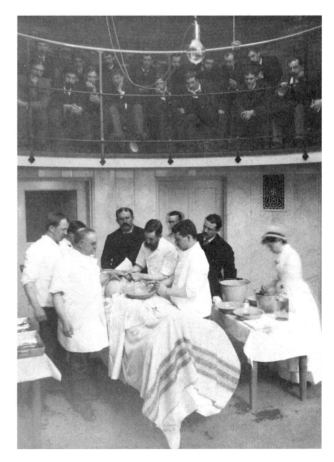

J. Collins "Coll" Warren doing first operation in Ward E, 1888.
Massachusetts General Hospital, Archives and Special Collections.

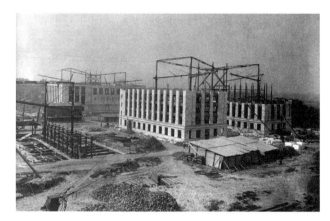

Construction of the new HMS buildings on Longwood Avenue (1904).
Harvard Medical Library in the Francis A. Countway Library of Medicine.

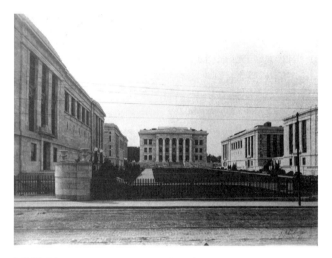

HMS. New construction completed. Photo by Elmer Chickering.
Harvard Medical Library in the Francis A. Countway Library of Medicine.

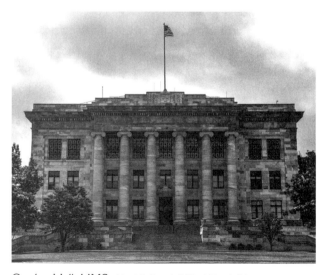

Gordon Hall, HMS. *Kael E. Randall/Kael Randall Images.*

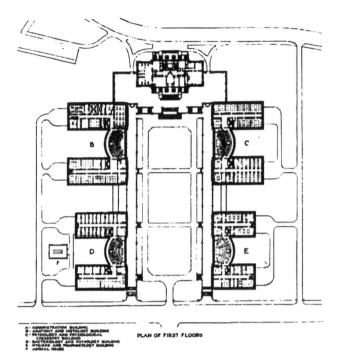

HMS. First floor plans (1906).
Harvard Medical Library in the Francis A. Countway Library of Medicine.

asepsis and the use of sterilization. Medical students were soon graduating who were unfamiliar with the stink and grime of the past. After Bigelow resigned in 1886, surgeons began to operate in the abdomen. Coll Warren did a successful hysterectomy for the first time at MGH in the Bradlee Ward.

In spite of his outgoing, warm personality and his athletic skills as an ice skater and mountain climber, Coll had his troubles, too. As head of the family, he cared for his invalid wife, was responsible for his mother, sisters, his uncle who remained a patient in McLean Hospital for years, and two of his father's spinster cousins (Abby and Rebecca Brown). Illness also struck Coll in 1917, and he has the distinction of being the first patient admitted to and having surgery in the newly built Phillips House at the Massachusetts General Hospital. Phillips House was the answer to his grandfather's dream that MGH would ensure that wealthier patients would have the comforts of home in a hospital.

Fundraising Endeavors and Other Contributions

It was remarkable that he had the time and energy to plan and raise enormous amounts of money needed for the new campus of Harvard Medical School. Although he had many successes, Coll Warren was most proud of an honor bestowed upon him by the Trustees of MGH. He had raised the money for a laboratory in the Collis P. Huntington Memorial Hospital for Cancer Research, completed in 1922. The Trustees renamed it the J. Collins Warren Laboratory. He felt it was his greatest contribution.

From 1873 to 1881 he was editor of the *Boston Medical and Surgical Journal*. Dr. J. Collins Warren had become a full professor of surgery at Harvard Medical School in 1893, and this professorship later became the Moseley Professorship of Surgery in 1899. In 1896, he was elected president of the American Surgical Association. The title of his presidential address was "The Influence of Anesthesia on the Surgery of the Nineteenth Century." His publications (n=46; four on orthopaedic topics) included "Surgical Pathology and Therapeutics," "The Anatomy and Development of Rodent Ulcer," "The Healing of Arteries after Ligature in Men and Animals," and "A Case of Laminectomy for Depressed Fracture of the Spine," an interesting orthopaedic case report. In 1900, he edited the *International Textbook of Surgery*. That same year, he was one of four American surgeons to be given an honorary fellowship in the Royal College of Surgeons of England, along with Drs. Halsted, Weir, and Keen. Coll retired from MGH in 1905, and he became professor emeritus in 1907. He remained a member of the Board of Overseers of Harvard University.

With the dedication of the new medical school buildings in 1906, Harvard awarded Dr. Warren the degree of doctor of laws:

> John Collins Warren, Instructor and Professor of Surgery in Harvard University for thirty-five years; author, and eminent practitioner in surgery; the enthusiastic, winning and indefatigable promoter of the great undertaking of the Medical School, who knew how to inspire others with his own well-grounded hopefulness and ardor. (E. D. Churchill 1958)

He also received a doctor of laws degree from Jefferson Medical School (1905), an honorary degree of LLD from McGill University (1911), and honorary membership in the American College of Surgeons (1913). His wife, Amy Warren, died in 1923, just before her seventy-third birthday. Coll's health declined; with him becoming increasingly frail, sick, and almost blind. He died at age 85 on November 3, 1927. He died having performed a critical role in transforming surgical technique in the United States in contributing to the enduring legacy of Harvard Medical School.

JOHN WARREN

The eldest son of J. Collins Warren, John Warren, was born on September 6, 1874. He had no middle name. His brother, Joseph, did not follow the family tradition into medicine; he became a lawyer. However, John did enter medicine and received an AB from Harvard in 1896 and his medical degree from Harvard in 1900 at the age of 26. Harvard Medical School had evolved to become four years in length.

Education and Training

Although shy, John Warren was very popular, did well in school, and enjoyed tennis. During medical school, he lived with his parents. He became fascinated with anatomy and planned a career in surgery like his father, grandfather, great-grandfather, and John and Joseph Warren (the original physicians in the family). His father's cousin was Thomas Dwight, the head of the Anatomy Department and the Parkman Professor of Anatomy. He

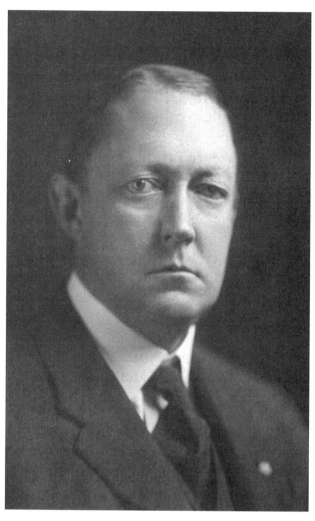

John Warren (Anatomist), 1921.
Harvard Medical Library in the Francis A. Countway Library of Medicine.

Physician snapshot

John Warren
BORN: 1874
DIED: 1928
SIGNIFICANT CONTRIBUTIONS: Anatomist, *Warren's Atlas of Anatomy*

had replaced Dr. Oliver Wendell Holmes. Dwight was also a surgeon but stopped practicing and developed his career to teach anatomy, which was possibly the model for John Warren. He was an expert on comparative osteology. John loved gross anatomy and followed Dwight into a career in teaching anatomy; he never practiced surgery.

Academia

After graduation, having decided not to pursue a career in surgery, he was appointed assistant in Anatomy. He was promoted to demonstrator in anatomy in 1901, assistant professor in 1908, and associate professor of anatomy in 1915. He was both an anatomist and a teacher, teaching anatomy to medical students in 1915. He had the wonderful opportunity to study some of the great books on anatomy that his great grandfather had collected: *De Humani Corporis Fabrica* by Versalius, *Opera Chirugica* by Ambrose Paré, *The Anatomy of the Human Body* by John Bell, *Anatomia Reformata* by Thomas Bertolinus, as well as his own collection. John enjoyed collecting books.

But WWI broke out, interrupting almost two years of his academic career. He enlisted, entering the first officer-training camp at Plattsburgh, graduating as a major. He spent his short army career training medical officers at Camp Greenleaf, Georgia. Remaining unmarried, John returned to live again (at age 45) with his parents on Beacon Street and resumed his career as a teacher of anatomy at Harvard Medical School. He walked daily to his office at the medical school on Longwood Avenue from 58 Beacon Street, frequently walking back home to have lunch with his aging father and then returning to his classes before walking back home in the evening. He did this long walk four times daily.

Accurate and careful dissection of the human body was essential in his mind. He admonished students to not take for granted their experience with dissecting a human body. He also saw a great need for a detailed dissection manual. With his assistant, Dr. Alexander S. Begg, he completed a modern dissection guide (300-pages long) in 1924, *An Outline of Practical Anatomy*. He had also been working for almost four years on an anatomical atlas for surgeons, an atlas that he would not finish.

Working frequently on his anatomical atlas, John did his own meticulous dissections and supervised the drawings of his dissections. Following his father's death, he went to Europe for a vacation

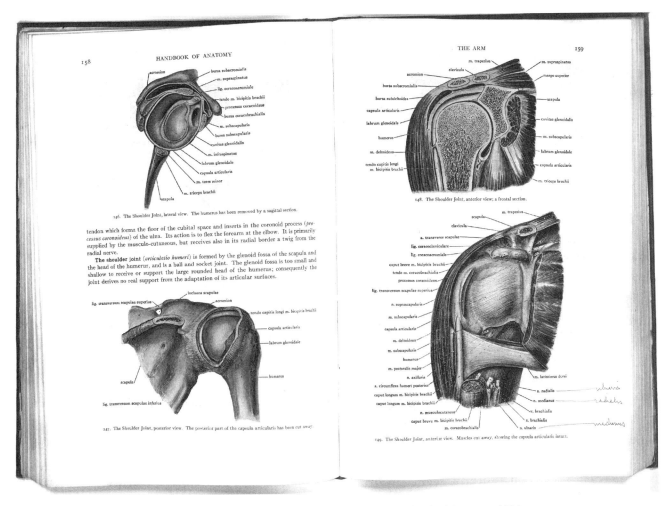

Example; H.F. Aitken's detailed drawings from Warren's dissections in his *Handbook of Anatomy*, 1930.

Harvard Medical Library in the Francis A. Countway Library of Medicine.

and to add to his book collection. Injuring his knee in Italy, probably a patellar tendon rupture, he returned to Boston. Dr. Philip D. Wilson Sr. operated on him in the Phillips House on July 1, 1928. Dr. Wilson was an expert on orthopaedic problems; later becoming the chief at the New York Hospital for the Ruptured and Crippled (Hospital for Special Surgery). The operation was successful. As was the custom at the time, John remained in the hospital for over two weeks. On the morning of July 16, 1928, he was found dead as a result of coronary occlusion. It was only eight months after his father's death. He was 53. For the first time in five generations of physicians/surgeons, Boston was without a Warren physician/surgeon.

Legacy

John Warren had been working on his anatomical atlas for eight years, and it remained unfinished at the time of his death. He left the atlas to the anatomy department. Members of the department completed his book and published it in 1930 as the *Handbook of Anatomy Adapted for Dissecting and Clinical References from Original Dissections* by John Warren, commonly called "Warren's Atlas." The text was by Robert M. Green, MD. Also included in his will was his large collection of 2000 books dating as early as the fifteenth century, which he left to Harvard University where they remain today.

RICHARD WARREN

Physician snapshot

Richard Warren
BORN: 1907
DIED: 1999
SIGNIFICANT CONTRIBUTIONS: Vascular surgeon;
amputee expert; leader in the Veterans Administration;
listed nine sacrifices required of surgeons

Known as Rich by his friends and colleagues, Richard Warren was the son of Joseph and Constance Warren. His father, the brother of John Warren (anatomist), was a distinguished lawyer in Cambridge and a professor at Harvard Law School. After graduation from Harvard College and Harvard Medical School in 1934, he interned in surgery at MGH and completed a surgical residency at the Peter Bent Brigham Hospital. After a fellowship with Dr. Jonathan Rhodes at the University of Pennsylvania, he returned to Boston to practice surgery but was interrupted by World War II.

He entered the Medical Corps as a captain, became chief of a hospital surgical service in Britain (as a major) for almost four years, and received a battlefield promotion to lieutenant colonel by the surgeon general because of his outstanding work. While in England, his father died. None of his three siblings entered medicine. They included Mary; Joseph, who died at a young age; and Howland, who followed his father's footsteps planning a career in law. His older brother married Dr. Francis D. Moore's daughter.

After the war, Rich returned to Boston as chief of the surgical service at the Veterans Administration Hospital in West Roxbury and surgeon at the Peter Bent Brigham Hospital. He remained as chief at the VA for 14 years. He served as a consultant on the surgical service at MGH. Committed to teaching, Harvard appointed him a clinical professor of surgery. He focused much of his career on vascular and cardiovascular surgery; starting an open-heart surgery program at the VA Hospital. For a brief period, he also served as director of

the Department of Surgery at Cambridge Hospital. As an author of many publications and books, he co-authored a book entitled *Lower Extremity Amputations for Arterial Insufficiency* with Eugene Record, MD, a colleague in orthopaedic surgery at the MGH. He also wrote a review in the *Archives of Surgery* on another textbook, *Amputees and their Prostheses* by Mohinder Mital and Donald Pierce, orthopaedic surgeons at MGH. He edited a major textbook, *Surgery*, in 1963.

In recognition of his academic and writing accomplishments, he was selected as chief editor of the *Archives of Surgery*, a position he held for seven years. Introducing new parts of the journal while guiding the journal through the difficult financial period in the 1970s, he was responsible for ensuring its stable future. Dr. Arthur Baue of Yale wrote that "His disarming integrity and wonderful Yankee individualism provided for the *Archives* a uniqueness that we hope can be continued" (A. E. Baue 1977).

Richard Warren was president of the New England Surgical Society in 1969. In his presidential address, he described "a balanced list of justifiable demands and sacrifices...whereby the surgeon may travel the golden middle road to his own happiness...to the best care of...patients needing surgical help" (R. Warren 1970). Written over 40 years ago, he listed nine justifiable sacrifices that he advised surgeons to consider. They remain a list of admirable recommendations today:

To live near the hospital.

To strive for shortened hospital stays.

To work on committees.

To take time to teach nurses and other nonmedical hospital personnel.

To be selective in demands on resources. A useful slogan for house staff to learn is "Think of it, but don't do it."

To take time to teach younger surgeons, but not 'unload' responsibility by removing oneself from the patient.

To make home visits when indicated and to make one's home phone number freely available.

To standardize fees, respect the public till, and help young men along by sharing practice.

To keep within one's physical ability and time.

(R. Warren 1970)

Richard Warren died from Parkinson's disease on September 23, 1999. He was an excellent and dedicated teacher, a deep-water sailor, and was largely responsible for elevating the Veterans Administration hospitals as major teaching centers for medical schools.

H. SHAW WARREN

Physician snapshot

Howland Shaw Warren Jr.

BORN: 1951

DIED: N/A

SIGNIFICANT CONTRIBUTIONS: Physician-scientist; specialist in infectious diseases

Shaw Warren, the nephew of Richard Warren, was one of Howland Warren's three children; he was born on May 16, 1951. His father Howland was Richard's brother. Shaw has continued the tradition of a Warren practicing medicine. After graduating from Harvard College and Harvard Medical School, he interned in medicine at Chapel Hill, completed a medical residency at Beth Israel Hospital in Boston followed by a fellowship in infectious disease at Beth Israel Hospital. Interested in a career in clinical medicine and research, he completed research fellowships at the Dana Farber Cancer Institute and the Institute Pasteur in Paris.

He is an associate professor of pediatrics at Harvard Medical School, with hospital appointments at the Boston Shriners Hospital for Children, Massachusetts General Hospital, and Spaulding Rehabilitation Hospital. He is clinically active in the adult and pediatric infectious disease units, and is a lead investigator in a laboratory at the MGH Charlestown Navy Yard research facility where he focuses on sepsis, or "the interactions of the bacterial cell wall with the host and its secondary inflammatory consequences" (H. Shaw Warren 2019). As principal investigator of many grants, Shaw leads an active laboratory and is a frequent contributor to scientific literature.

Orthopaedics Emerges *as a* Focus *of* Clinical Care

"Boston: The Cradle of Orthopaedics"

—**Thornton Brown, MD**, ca. 1983, unpublished Osgood Lecture (MGH HCORP Archives)

"The People of the United States are under great obligation to that small northeastern corner of the country which is called New England. The men and institutions of New England have had an immeasurable influence on thought and progress in this land. In the field of medical education [including orthopaedics] the contributions have been large."

—**J. G. K. (John G. Kuhns)**, "Dr. Robert B. Osgood," *Archives of Surgery*, 1943; 45:589.

"Orthopaedics—a specialty which may be considered to have obtained its adolescence, if it did not actually have its birth, here in Boston."

—Obituary of **Robert William Lovett**, 1859–1924, *Boston Medical and Surgical Journal*, 1925; 192:374.

CHAPTER 5

John Ball Brown
The First American Orthopaedic Surgeon

John Ball Brown became the first surgeon in the United States to limit his practice to orthopaedics. He also went on to open the first orthopaedic specialty hospital in the country. He was born to Dr. Jabez Brown and Anna Ball Brown, who had already lost a son of the same name in 1777 at six years old. John Ball Brown inherited the name from his brother when he was born on October 20, 1784, in Wilmington, Massachusetts. Brown's father was also a physician and his second cousin was Dr. Aaron Dexter, the first professor of chemistry and materia medica at Harvard Medical School. After attending Phillips Academy (Dover) and several other schools, he entered Brown University in 1802. At age 22, he graduated with a bachelor's degree in 1806.

EDUCATION

Following in his father's footsteps, John Ball began his study of medicine in Salem, Massachusetts, with a friend and colleague of his father, Augustus Holyoke, MD. Holyoke was highly respected and experienced; he was 84 years old when John Ball became his apprentice. After one-and-a-half years, Holyoke advised him to apprentice with Dr. Moses Little, also in Salem. Finishing his studies in the early summer of 1809, Brown began to practice medicine in Dorchester. Although busy in the summer caring for 16 cases of typhoid fever, his practice never grew.

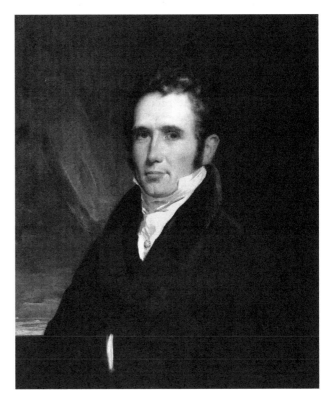

Chester Harding, American, 1792–1866. Dr. John Ball Brown, about 1826. Oil on canvas. 76.49 x 63.82 cm (30 ⅛ x 25 ⅛ in.). Museum of Fine Arts, Boston. Bequest of Buckminster Brown, M.D., 14.424. Photograph © 2021 Museum of Fine Arts, Boston.

Physician Snapshot

John Ball Brown

BORN: 1784

DIED: 1862

SIGNIFICANT CONTRIBUTIONS: First surgeon in the United States to limit his practice to orthopaedics and to open the first orthopaedic specialty hospital; initiated a prototype of telemedicine

In January 1810, he moved to Boston. He states in his autobiography that "when I first came to Boston it was a bold push. I knew nobody who could be of much service to me in any way" (J. B. Brown 1852). He took and passed his examination for a license to practice medicine by the Censors of the Massachusetts Medical Society. During his first year practicing in Boston, he collected $450 of his $600 in charges. During this time, he also attended classes at Harvard Medical School in Cambridge. Brown lived and practiced in several different locations in Boston over three or four years, first on Court Street near the Revere House and then at the corner of Providence and School streets, opposite City Hall. Next, he switched to West Row Court. He also lived for many years on Montgomery Place. He records in his autobiography that he completed his Harvard examinations and received a medical degree in 1813. He was 29 years old. He continued to attend classes and studied anatomy and surgery under John Warren and chemistry under Aaron Dexter, his second cousin, at Holden Chapel in Cambridge.

FAMILY LIFE

In 1814, he married John Warren's daughter, Rebecca Warren (1789–1855), who was also the sister of John Collins Warren, the leading physician/surgeon in Boston at the time. General Joseph Warren became his uncle by marriage. Shortly thereafter, Rebecca and some of her family followed many other Bostonians in moving out of the city because of the threat of an attack by the British in the War of 1812. John Ball remained to continue his practice at West Row Court. Upon Rebecca's return, they purchased a home at Montgomery Place. Five of his six children were born in this house, including Buckminster Brown. Rebecca Warren Brown, in order to earn additional money for the family, became a distinguished and prolific writer, including writing many books for children.

SURGICAL APPOINTMENTS

John Ball Brown went on to establish orthopaedics as a surgical specialty. In 1817, he was "appointed Surgeon and Physician to the Boston Alms House" (J. B. Brown 1852). Little is known about his involvement in patient care and operative procedures at the Almshouse. At the time he was appointed, the Almshouse was located on Leverett Street. It was later replaced by the Leverett Street Jail. Appointments were for one year and were made by the Board of Overseers of the poor. During his first year, a major outbreak of typhus hit the Almshouse. "My post was rather a dangerous one and certainly a very responsible and laborious one" (J. B. Brown 1852). A future superintendent of the MGH, Gamaliel Bradford, almost died. Brown recorded that "some of my pupils were taken down with it" (J. B. Brown 1852). Rewarding his outstanding service, the Board of Overseers made the unusual decision to reappoint him for a second year. He was also given a bonus of $100 in addition to his salary. Dr. Brown was deeply honored and wrote:

> It was the handsomest compliment I ever had. The having charge of the Institution was of service to me in my profession. It gave me much experience, enabled me to take pupils and made me more known. (J. B. Brown 1852)

Other than Boston Dispensary (where Brown oversaw one district), the Almshouse was the only other hospital in Boston. The Massachusetts General Hospital (MGH) was not built yet at the time. While at the Almshouse and in charge of one of the three districts of the Boston Dispensary, John Ball Brown instructed many students. There were few other clinical-practice opportunities for medical studies in Boston. He lists several in his autobiography: Dr. Charles A. Cheever (Portsmouth, NH), Dr. Charles Wild (Brookline, MA), Gamaliel Bradford (became superintendent of MGH),

Mr. Keeting (son of a rich Boston merchant), Dr. J. V. C. Smith (mayor of Boston in 1854), Dr. Hildreth (South End in Boston), and several others whom he could not recall as he was writing his autobiography some 35 years later.

After the opening of the MGH in 1822, Brown was appointed junior surgeon in 1823 under John Collins Warren, his brother-in-law. He resigned three years later in 1826, but he remained as consulting surgeon (1829–1836). He continued in private practice between 1826 and 1829, but we do not know whether he continued in a role at MGH during this time. His name does not appear as surgeon in any of the early surgical logs of the MGH. In a letter from Dr. J. C. Warren to Brown in 1822, he listed Dr. Brown's responsibilities: "visit hospital daily…carry out the directions of the chief surgeon…be present for all operations…watch over the apothecary… and do such other duties as may be required by the attending surgeon" (quoted in L. K. Eaton 1957). Before beginning these responsibilities, Brown asked to make rounds with Dr. Warren in order to obtain respect from patients and medical students. We do not know why Brown later resigned as associate surgeon, but another assistant resigned after eight months because the pay was not high enough and the position lacked prestige. There is no record of Dr. Brown having held a Harvard faculty position.

SPECIALIZATION IN ORTHOPAEDICS

In 1838, one year after moving his family into their new home at 8 Joy Street (several blocks from MGH), he had already begun to focus on treating spine deformities. However, the pivotal factor in his developing specialty was when two of his sons contracted Pott's disease. His first son, John Warren Brown, died at age 14. Buckminster, his other living son, developed a severe kyphoscoliosis. He recorded in his autobiography that "My

mind was drawn to the study of spinal complaints" (J. B. Brown 1852). He wrote:

> Having lost my eldest son (as you well know) by inflammation of the great spinal cord, and having now my second son confined to his bed by a lateral curvature of the spine, my attention has been forcibly drawn to the study and treatment of spinal disease generally, and to the correction of other deformities of the human body, such as distortion of the limbs, club feet, etc., etc. (J. B. Brown 1838)

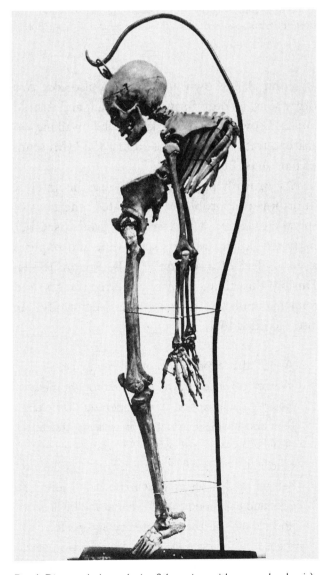

Pott's Disease (tuberculosis of the spine with severe kyphosis). Warren Anatomical Museum in the Francis A. Countway Library of Medicine.

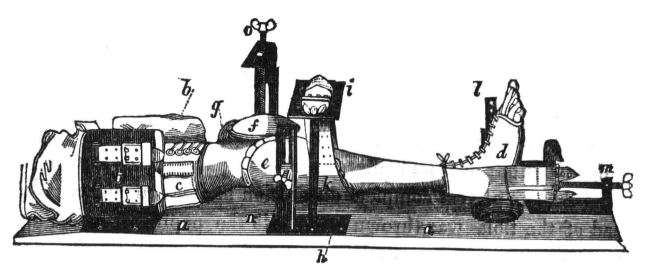

Apparatus used by Brown to correct a chronic knee contracture. Published in Brown & Brown, *Reports of Cases Treated at the Boston Orthopedic Institution*, Boston: Cabinet Office, 1850. Collection of the Massachusetts Historical Society. Photo by the author.

John Ball Brown and Rebecca also lost two other sons, George Brown as an infant and Arnold Welles Brown, "who was killed while walking on railroad tracks at the age of 25 in 1852" (Museum of Fine Arts, Boston, n.d.).

As Brown's practice grew so had his interest in orthopaedic problems. He treated nine cases of spinal curvatures. There were not many cases, but he noted "each case lasts some time and requires a good deal of attention" (J. B. Brown 1852). During this time, Brown preferred braces and joint manipulation to treat skeletal deformity. He also recorded that:

> About this time my brother-in-law Dr. J. C. Warren returned from Paris and brought me M. Bouvier's description of the operation for club-feet and process of nature in splicing the tendons. This was in French. My daughter Abby read it to me…After she finished I requested her to read it again which she did. I jumped up…and explained that is rational and I will do it and soon I had the opportunity and performed the operation on a little girl. I never had heard of the operation before and it was entirely unknown here. This case was quite successful… (J. B. Brown 1852) (see Case Report 7.1, chapter 7).

Dr. J. C. Warren also gave Dr. Brown a club-foot apparatus from Paris. Brown recorded he "had especially altered and improved [the apparatus], so much so that Dr. Jules Guerin told my son (Buckminster) that they had nothing so good for the purpose…Dr. Wm. J. Little of London told him the same thing" (J. B. Brown 1852).

After almost a decade of interest in orthopaedics, including foot and spine deformities, at age 54, Brown limited his practice to orthopaedics and

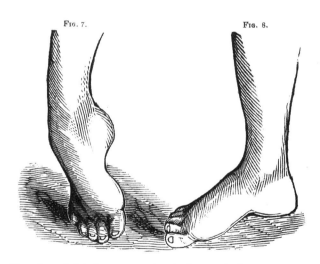

Drawing of club foot correction; before and after treatment. Published in Brown & Brown, *Reports of Cases Treated at the Boston Orthopedic Institution*, Boston: Cabinet Office, 1850. Wellcome Library.

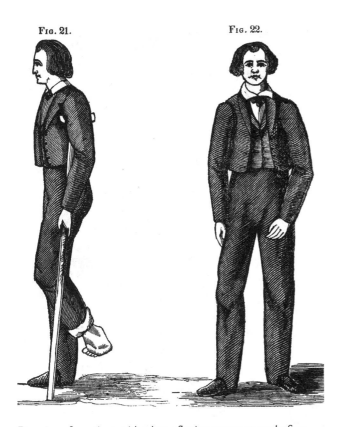

Fig. 21.   Fig. 22.

Drawing of a patient with a knee flexion contracture; before and after treatment (Buckminster Brown and J. B. Brown 1850). Published in Brown & Brown, *Reports of Cases Treated at the Boston Orthopedic Institution*, Boston: Cabinet Office, 1850. Wellcome Library.

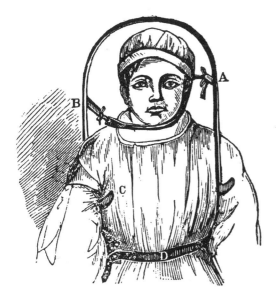

Torticollis brace used by John Ball Brown. Published in Brown, *Report of Cases in the Boston Orthopedic Institution*, Boston: David Clapp & Son, 1844.

Collection of the Massachusetts Historical Society. Photo by the author.

opened the first orthopaedic specialty hospital in the United States (see chapter 7). Buckminster, who would later join him, was 19 at the time. At the time, specialization was not valued. In fact, according to Shands (1970), specialization was still despised as late as 1846. Brown did not seem to share this viewpoint and believed strongly in specialization. He wrote, "It is natural to suppose that an individual who gives exclusive attention to any one subject, will make greater progress in it than one who devotes his attention promiscuously to a variety of subjects" (J. B. Brown 1840). His practice continued to grow, and his orthopaedic hospital—at about 60 beds—was very busy. In his obituary, the Massachusetts Medical Society (1866) offered the following description:

> His reputation for the treatment of clubfoot, wry neck, affections of the spine and other disorders of the human frame became very great…patients not only from various neighboring states and from the south but from the far West and even the Sandwich Islands (Hawaii) journeyed to Boston for the sole purpose of being placed under his care. He was not only skillful in performing the operations necessary for the cure of these annoying and perplexing cases but more difficult to accomplish, he followed them up by mechanical means with patience and energy until he had attained a successful result. He was possessed of a great mechanical ingenuity in the invention and application of special surgical apparatus.

His hospital attracted the most experienced in the profession in Boston. There were 23 consulting surgeons at the orthopaedic hospital, including John Collins Warren. In addition to his surgical and mechanical skills, John Ball Brown displayed remarkable marketing skills and diagnostic innovations, both additionally responsible for his successful growing practice. He essentially was the first physician to use a form of telemedicine. Very early in his practice at the Boston Orthopedique

Infirmary he would ask people from Canada and other states requesting his advice about foot deformities to send him daguerreotypes (first commercially successful photographs) of the affected foot. He would provide them with a diagnosis and a plan of treatment. Many would then travel to Boston and his Orthopedique Infirmary. Further, Brown would request daguerreotypes of patients he had treated from their local physicians. By doing so, he could manage patients postoperatively from a distance, advise local care and see his results.

In 1839, one year after specializing, Brown published the first American orthopaedic book, *Remarks on the Operation for the Cure of Club Feet with Cases*. Brown viewed this operation as one of the most influential advancements in surgery at the time. The book was 27 pages in length and included letters about curvature of the spine to John Collins Warren. He discussed cases and reported their clinical results after tenotomy of the Achilles tendon, which were the first reports of this operation in the United States by an American-trained surgeon. In addition to cutting the Achilles tendon, Dr. Brown also divided the anterior tibial tendon and occasionally divided the flexor and extensor tendons of the great toe in patients with clubfeet. Although receiving little attention, Brown was a strong advocate (as was Sayre later on) that the clubfoot deformity be diagnosed at birth and treated early with manipulations and corrective shoes to prevent later surgery. Probably his second most common operation was for spine deformities, including scoliosis and wry neck. He divided the sternocleidomastoid off the sternum, occasionally off the clavicle, in patients with torticollis. In spine deformities, such as scoliosis and tuberculosis, the common releases were of the trapezius, longissimus dorsi and the sacrolumbalis muscles. Following these surgical releases, Brown would apply an apparatus he designed for clubfeet and another he designed for torticollis. He did not usually use any apparatus to correct spine deformities but instead preferred

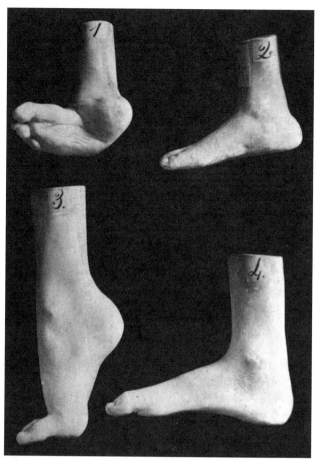

Daguerreotypes of corrections of club feet in two patients. Published in *Cases of Orthopaedic Surgery, with Photographic Illustrations of the Cases Presented* by Buckminster Brown, Boston: D. Clapp & Son, 1868. Read before the Massachusetts Medical Society at its annual meeting.
University of California Libraries/Internet Archive.

strengthening exercises. In one patient with probable arthrogryposis, he described releasing tendons in the patient's feet as well as the palmaris longus for the hand/wrist. Likewise, Brown also understood tenotomy was a method to prepare for physical therapy (strengthening exercises and massage), the preferred treatment.

There is some debate over whether Brown or William Ludwig Detmold was the first orthopaedic surgeon in the United States. Detmold, a surgeon from Hanover, Germany, also practiced orthopaedics in New York at the time. In 1838, the year Brown opened his orthopaedic hospital in Boston, Detmold published case reports of his technique

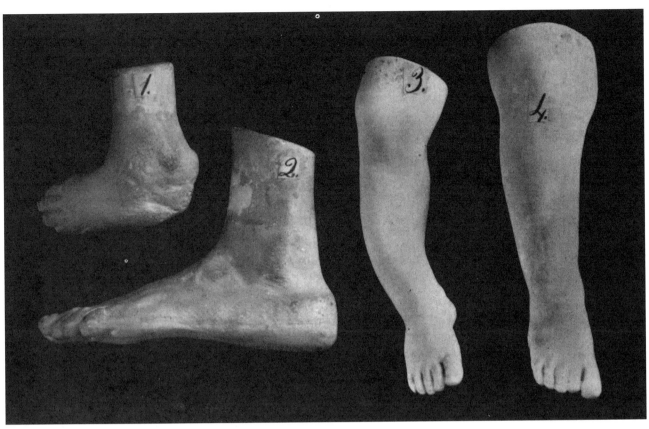

Daguerreotypes of correction of a clubfoot (left) and a bowleg Deformity (right). Published in *Cases of Orthopaedic Surgery, with Photographic Illustrations of the Cases Presented* by Buckminster Brown, Boston: D. Clapp & Son, 1868. Read before the Massachusetts Medical Society at its annual meeting. University of California Libraries/Internet Archive.

for subcutaneous Achilles tenotomy; two years later he reported on the treatment of 167 patients with clubfoot deformity. According to Edgar M. Bick (1976), "the operation was not generally accepted until Brown's reports appeared." Detmold was an immigrant from Germany to New York City in 1837, after studying with Stromeyer in Hanover. He did not specialize in just orthopaedic surgery; he also ran a school called "Dr. Detmold's Practical School of Medicine and Surgery." Graduates were trained in medicine, surgery, and obstetrics. In 1841, he began a clinic for crippled children at the College of Physicians and Surgeons. He continued there until 1861.

With continued advancement of specialization, surgeons at this time were evolving into orthopaedic surgeons. Brown recognized the importance of this new surgical armamentarium to the practice of orthopaedics. He correctly noted that:

It [orthopedics] was practiced a hundred years ago—in the eighteenth century—but the discovery (of recent date) that tendons could be divided with impunity gave new life to this most useful, but which had become obsolete, art…From time immemorial, no age has been exempt from pretenders to cure club-feet, spinal disorders, etc. etc. These pretenders have mostly consisted of quacks and machine-makers, who knew nothing of anatomy and physiology. Regular surgeons, finding the uncertainty, difficulty and frequent impossibility, of curing these deformities had relinquished the practice of orthopedy to these ignorant men, who applied such means as their cupidity and stupidity might suggest. The practice of orthopedy is a distinct branch of surgery, as much as dentistry, or the profession of the oculist or aurist, and should be practiced exclusively. It certainly requires all of one man's mind to treat these deformities judiciously. It would be better for the profession and for the public at large, if the duties of the profession were divided and subdivided…It is reasonable to suppose that an individual who gives his exclusive attention to any one subject, will make greater progress in it than one who devotes his attention promiscuously to a variety of subjects. (J. B. Brown 1844)

LEGACY OF JOHN BALL BROWN

In addition to his advocating for specialty hospitals, his marketing skills and diagnostic innovations, Brown also advocated for public reporting. He said a "recent introduction of the practice of orthopedy on a scientific basis…and an account of their success which has been the result of their treatment should be taken from the case-book and presented to the public" (Buckminster Brown and J. B. Brown 1860). He received public accolades

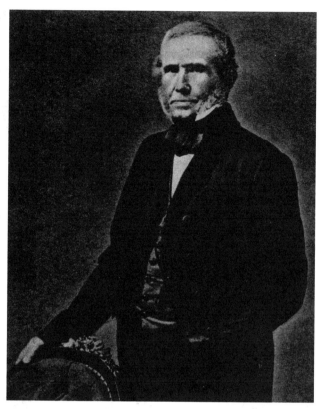

John Ball Brown. Published in *Bulletin of the Warren Anatomical Museum, Harvard Medical School, No. 1: Pathological Anatomy*, 1910.

Warren Anatomical Museum in the Francis A. Countway Library of Medicine.

Box 5.1. Publications of John Ball Brown

"Curvature of the spine." *The Boston Medical and Surgical Journal*, 18:139–142, 1838.

"Remarks on the operation for the cure of club-feet, with cases." Boston: D. Clapp Jr., 1839.

"Remarks on the operation for the cure of clubfeet, with cases." *The Boston Medical and Surgical Journal*. 21:153–159, 1839.

"Report of cases in the Orthopedic Infirmary of the City of Boston." Boston, D. Clapp Jr., 1840.

"Reports of cases in the Boston Orthopedic Institution." Boston: D. Clapp Jr., 1844.

"Reports of cases in the Boston Orthopedic Institution: with some preliminary observations on spinal curvature, distortion of the chest, and spinal irritation." Boston: D. Clapp Jr., 1845.

"Reports of cases, treated at the Boston Orthopedic Institution: or Hospital for the Cure of Deformities of the Human Frame: with some preliminary observations on the present state of the institution, and on club foot, spinal curvature, distortions of the chest, stiff joint, and spinal irritation." Boston: John Wilson and Son, 1850. (co-author Buckminster Brown).

"The Daguerraean art in medicine and surgery." *The Boston Medical and Surgical Journal*. 57 (19): 386. Dec. 10, 1857.

"Observations on lateral & angular curvature of the spine, wry-neck, club-foot, and other orthopedic affections: with report of cases." Boston: John Wilson and Son, 1860. (co-author Buckminster Brown).

John Ball Brown's signature. Harvard Medical Library in the Francis A. Countway Library of Medicine.

for his care. For example, Reverend Chauncey Eddy of Saratoga, New York, wrote:

> I have seen patients of four surgeons of three different cities and none of them except Dr. Brown's had apparatus at all suited for the purpose. Any surgeon can separate the cords well enough; but the cure depends more upon the machinery that is afterwards used, then all things else. I have reason to presume that there is none in the country to be compared with that invented and used by Dr. Brown. (C. Eddy 1842)

Most of John Ball Brown's few publications were limited to orthopaedic surgery (see **Box 5.1** for a complete list).

John Ball Brown died on May 14, 1862 at age 78. At the time, he was

> still in the enjoyment of an uncommon share of health and freshness of appearance for a man at his period of life. He was suddenly seized with his last illness and at once calmly recognized that death was making its approaches with mathematical certainty. Having expressed his last wishes, he quietly awaited the termination *sans peur et sans reproche* [without fear and without reproach]. (C. Eddy 1842)

He was a giant in the advancement of orthopaedics in the United States with a legacy that continues to this day.

CHAPTER 6

Buckminster Brown

Founder of the John Ball & Buckminster Brown Chair

Buckminster Brown was the only son of John Ball and Rebecca Brown to follow in his father's footsteps as a surgeon. He was born in Boston on July 13, 1819. We know very little about his early life except that as a teenager he developed Pott's disease, which left him with a severe kyphoscoliosis. He was treated with bed rest for almost eight years; the continued isolation he experienced throughout his life from his condition may have influenced his dedication and commitment to his profession.

EDUCATION AND TRAINING

After four years at Harvard Medical School, he graduated at 25 years old with a medical degree in 1844. He had attended classes at the school on Mason Street, which remained open until 1846. Buckminster went to England and Europe to continue his studies in medicine and surgery. He was probably influenced in this decision by his uncle, John Collins Warren, and his cousin, Mason Warren, both of whom studied in Europe. Buckminster focused his additional training on orthopaedics, studying under Little in London, Guérin and Bouvier in Paris, and Stromeyer in Germany. According to Siffert (1958), Buckminster hoped his diversity of training would allow him to introduce a variety of surgical instruments and apparatus in the United States. While studying at the

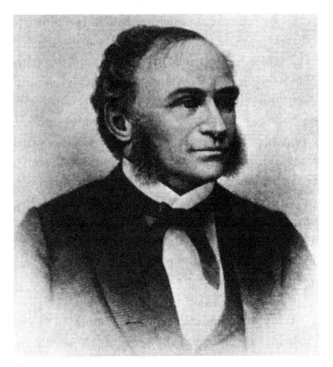

Buckminster Brown. Published in *Biographical Encyclopaedia of Massachusetts of the Nineteenth Century*, New York: Metropolitan Pub. And Engraving Co., 1879.
Boston Public Library/Internet Archive.

Physician Snapshot

Buckminster Brown

BORN: 1819

DIED: 1891

SIGNIFICANT CONTRIBUTIONS: Educator and mentor of the next generation of orthopaedic surgeons; established John Ball & Buckminster Brown Chair at Harvard Medical School; implemented new method of continuous traction to treat congenital dislocated hips and Pott's disease

Royal Orthopaedic Hospital in London under Dr. William J. Little and Mr. Lawrence, he observed that their treatment of tuberculosis of the spine was prolonged bed rest in the prone position. Little, who had contracted polio at four years of age, developed a severe equinus deformity of his left leg. He was never happy wearing a brace and sought a surgical correction. He was aware of the early work in 1823 of the French surgeon, Jacques-Mathieu Delpech, who reported his results with tendon releases in clubfeet. Delpech, however, stopped operating on clubfeet, influenced by the severe criticism of his surgical methods. About eight years later, his methods were used by Stromeyer in Germany. In 1836, Little went to Hanover, Germany, seeking Stromeyer's opinion about his equinus deformity. Other consultants he had seen had all advised him against surgery. Upon observing Stromeyer operate with positive results, Little underwent an Achilles tenotomy. He had excellent results from the procedure even without anesthesia or any form of antisepsis. Little brought the procedure back with him and was the first to complete it in London in February 1837. The operation became popular, and Little subsequently published his "Treatise on the Nature of Club Foot" in 1839.

When Buckminster arrived in London in 1844, Little had already opened his specialty hospital, the first in Britain focused on orthopaedics, four years earlier. This hospital eventually became the Royal National Orthopaedic Hospital, and Peltier (1993) considers Little to be the father of orthopaedics in Britain. Buckminster may also have visited St. George's Hospital where Bernard E. Brodhurst, another expert in the surgical treatment of clubfoot, and Sir Benjamin Collins Brodie worked.

Upon leaving London, Buckminster traveled to Paris. He visited Jules Guérin, who had established an orthopaedic hospital for patients with skeletal deformities in 1834, and Sauveur-Henri Victor Bouvier. Another American surgeon (Valentine Mott) had also visited Guérin and wrote, "In one operation, some half of a hundred nearly (in the case I refer to, forty-three muscles and tendons were divided) of these ropes of the human body were cut asunder, and the patient stretched out upon the table in his natural shape" (quoted in Peltier 1993). At the time, Guérin had been also appointed as chief of the orthopaedic service at Hôpital des Enfants Malades in 1839. In addition to tenotomies for clubfeet, Buckminster observed Guérin's methods for treating congenital dislocation of the hip as well as his special devices (as well as Little's) to maintain correction of deformities after tenotomy.

Back in the United States, John Ball had designed his own device to treat foot deformities after surgical releases. Buckminster had brought a model of this device with him and later wrote that it was "considered by Little, Guérin and others as one of the most perfect they have seen" (Buckminster Brown 1846). Buckminster was especially impressed with Guérin's method of treating congenital dislocated hips and Pott's disease. He later writes in an article on orthopaedic treatments in Europe stating: "The treatment of clubfeet is a subject which is now so thoroughly understood on both sides of the water than I need scarcely refer to it here. The chief difference consists of in the form of apparatus employed" (Buckminster Brown 1846).

After spending the winter of 1844–1845 in Paris, Buckminster traveled to Hanover, Germany, to visit Louis Stromeyer. He also visited Dr. Zuick's orthopaedic hospital in Vienna to learn about new treatments for scoliosis. He traveled to a specialized institution, which at the time was called the Institution for Cretins and Idiots, in the Swiss Alps. Impressed with the results of treatment in these unfortunate patients, he said, "In some future communications I shall take occasion to refer to a novel and effectual method now pursued for straightening the best limbs of rickery children, for the diagnoses and cure of stammering in those cases which admit of a cure, and also for the treatment of some of the varieties of scrofulous (tuberculosis of the cervical lymph nodes) diseases and of nervous debility" (Buckminster Brown 1846).

SPECIALIZATION IN ORTHOPAEDICS

Buckminster returned to Boston in 1846, almost two years after setting sail for London. At the time, "orthopaedic surgery was then in its infancy in New England" and in the United States (C. Foster 1893). Buckminster joined his father's practice at the Boston Orthopedic Institution, initially as a general practitioner/surgeon, but he soon devoted most of his focus to orthopaedic problems. The Boston Orthopedic Institution functioned without ether for its first eight years. After its introduction at Massachusetts General Hospital (MGH) in October 1846, however, both John Ball Brown and Buckminster soon began to work with it as well. Buckminster worked very hard "in spite of constant suffering and physical weakness that obliged him to economize every ounce of strength for his work" (C. Foster 1893). Others described him as an "inquiring student and a forceful teacher" (R. S. Siffert 1958).

Because of his own health condition, Buckminster had a special affinity and commitment to the rehabilitation of children's orthopaedic health conditions. He became a strong advocate for disabled children with cerebral palsy and other serious diseases that impaired function. In his writings, Buckminster discussed how these children were able to thrive and even learn to communicate and learn a trade after treatment. In 1863, he was appointed surgeon at the Good Samaritan Hospital, a position he held until 1880.

FAMILY LIFE

The year following his appointment, Buckminster (age 45) married Sarah Alvord Newcomb (age 31). They were second cousins once removed; Sarah was the granddaughter of General Joseph Warren, and Buckminster was the grandson of John Warren and nephew of John Collins Warren.

FORWARD-THINKING TREATMENT

Known as a skillful orthopaedic surgeon, "his sense of touch was also very keen, and he learned much through the ends of his fingers. To watch him as he manipulated a contracted tendon, or a carious spine was an object lesson" (C. Foster 1893). Buckminster emphasized total care of the patient's orthopaedic problem: nonoperative, operative, and, importantly, postoperative care. He also emphasized early treatment as preventive of future complications. Buckminster was a frequent user of mechanical devices, including traction, to correct without surgery or improve a deformity after surgery. He even designed his own devices (called apparatus) for clubfeet, hip deformity, and contracture (including congenital dislocation), deformed knees, bowlegs, torticollis (in addition to his father's brace) and the spine. His back brace for spinal deformity was similar to that of C. F. Taylor's in New York, and he used a Sayre jacket for selected cases. According to L. Mayer (1950), "he was an orthopaedist in the best and broadest sense of the word, using all means—operative, mechanical and medicinal. His mechanical ability was great, and his surgical dexterity was equally remarkable."

Buckminster was critical of applying common and often inadequate methods and devices to all patients with certain conditions. He advocated for tailoring treatment to the individual patient, emphasizing further reevaluation and adjustment at each stage of treatment. He was especially critical of treatments that immobilized the patient, including taping, plaster and static splints, and other apparatus. He probably learned to value manipulation and mobilization from the French and his German mentors as well as his own experience. As a patient himself with a severe spine deformity, he had been on the receiving end of treatment through immobilization. Years of bed rest obviously influenced his thinking regarding rest versus activity.

In addition to his widely recognized skill in correcting clubfoot deformities, Buckminster was known for his treatment of congenital dislocation of the hip. He abandoned the belt and spring method used at the time, designing a new method

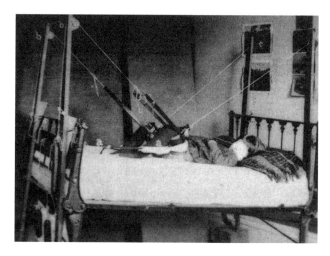

Four-year-old child with bilateral dislocated hips; treatment in traction (Buckminster Brown 1885).
Boston Medical and Surgical Journal, 1885; 62: 541–546.

of continuous traction. In 1885, he reported its successful use in a four-year old child with bilateral dislocated hips (see chapter 8). The patient was treated in traction for 13 months. Bradford and Lovett (1890) referred to this case in their book, *A Treatise on Orthopaedic Surgery*, when they wrote "To Dr. Buckminster Brown of Boston belongs the honor of first having secured a cure by this method of continuous traction."

Spinal tuberculosis was common in children, and both Buckminster and his father had tremendous experience in treating Pott's disease. Between them, they treated over 500 cases. Buckminster advanced new methods and defied current practices of "rest, sunshine, cod-liver oil, stimulants and lactophosphate of lime" (R. S. Siffert 1958). He believed these accepted practices furthered deformity, and he instead advocated for traction "with a pad under the gibbus to correct the deformity" (R. S. Siffert 1958). Buckminster (1858) wrote, "In caries of the vertebrae, the true

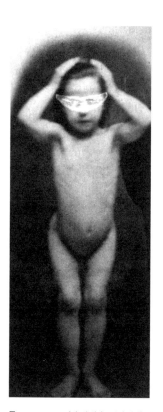
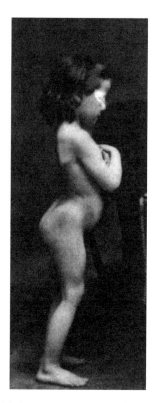
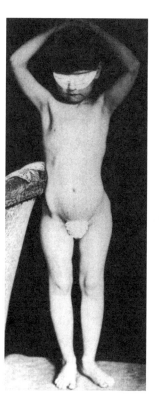
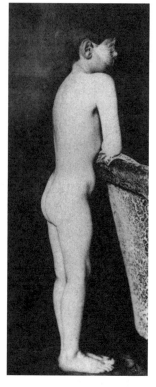

Four-year-old child with bilateral dislocated hips; before treatment (Buckminster Brown 1885).
Boston Medical and Surgical Journal, 1885; 62: 541–546.

Results of treatment in traction for more than one year (Buckminster Brown 1885).
Boston Medical and Surgical Journal, 1885; 62: 541–546.

principle, bearing in mind the state of the bones, is undoubtedly to treat the disease as a fracture, so far as this is possible consistent with the health of the patient."

Many of these patients died and Buckminster performed their autopsies. He described the location of the lesions in terms of body versus posterior elements. Although he did not have access to any imaging technologies, he nevertheless classified the types of lesions as:

- slow absorbing
- ulceration with caseation or pus
- caries sèche (dry caries) (R. S. Siffert 1958)

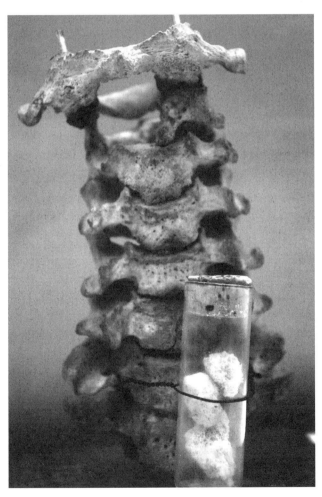

Tuberculosis of the upper cervical spine with sudden death after fracture of the odontoid process. Autopsy performed by Buckminster Brown.

Warren Anatomical Museum in the Francis A. Countway Library of Medicine.

Buckminster also used his own designed brace (like C. F. Taylor's) to treat children with scoliosis not associated with Pott's disease. Buckminster wrote, "The Treatment of this affection [scoliosis] by the same dressing (plaster of Paris jacket) as that which is applied in vertebral disease [Pott's Disease], is advocated. On this point we [Buckminster Brown] feel obliged to differ in toto from our author [Sayre]" (Buckminster Brown 1878). Brown strongly believed the etiology of scoliosis was multifactorial. He thought poor posture, constitutional debility, and genetics were all influential factors (R. S. Siffert 1958). He believed that children who were active out-of-doors did not develop scoliosis. He also observed that early mild cases of scoliosis were relatively easy to correct. His interest in the development and treatment of scoliosis was so great that he had begun to write a book on lateral curvature of the spine and its treatment, which remained unfinished at his death.

Careful application of surgery and thorough follow-up care was very important to Buckminster. He stressed personal attention throughout the full process. According to Charles C. Foster, who was a student and assistant to Buckminster for 10 years:

Thoroughness and patience characterized all of Dr. Brown's work...Treatment, once begun, was carried out in every detail, and continued as long as might be necessary. He never gave up, no matter how discouraging and intractable a case might be but preserved until it resulted as he had expected it to do...As a surgeon, his patients trusted him implicitly; as a man, they loved him and never forgot him. Some of his old patients corresponded with him for years. At the time of his death, several of them came long distances to attend his funeral, and many others sent letters of condolence. (C. Foster 1893)

Box 6.1. Publications of Buckminster Brown

"Orthopaedic surgery in Europe." *The Boston Medical and Surgical Journal*, 34:429–433, 1846.

"On the pathological and physiological effects of ethereal inhalation, with an appendix containing an additional case and experiments." Boston: D. Clapp, 1847.

"The treatment and cure of cretins and idiots: with an account of a visit to the institution on the Abendberg, Canton of Berne, Switzerland, during the summer of 1846." Boston: W.D. Ticknor & Co., 1847.

"The treatment and cure of cretins and idiots." *American Journal of Medical Sciences*, 14:109–117, 1847.

"Reports of cases, treated at the Boston Orthopedic Institution: or Hospital for the Cure of Deformities of the Human Frame: with some preliminary observations on the present state of the institution, and on club foot, spinal curvature, distortions of the chest, stiff joint, and spinal irritation." Boston: Cabinet office, 1850 (co-author John B. Brown).

"A case of extensive disease of the cervical vertebrae: with clinical observations on this and some other form of caries of the spine: also, a report of an operation for neuralgia." Boston: J. Wilson & Son, 1853. Repr. from: *American Journal of Medicine and Science*, Philadelphia, 25:120–131, 1853.

"Hints on the diagnosis and treatment of clubfoot." *The Boston Medical and Surgical Journal*, 21:715–726, 1879.

"Spinal caries, or angular curvature." *The Boston Medical and Surgical Journal*, 58:176–181, 1858.

"Cases of talipes, or club-foot." Boston, D. Clapp, 1858. Repr. from: *The Boston Medical and Surgical Journal*, 58: 209–213, 1858.

"Observations on lateral & angular curvature of the spine, wry-neck, club-foot and other orthopaedic affections: with report of cases" Boston: John Wilson & Son, 1860 (co-author John Ball Brown).

"Clubfoot, Spine Curvatures and Analogous Affections." Boston: John Wilson & Son, 1860.

"Memoir of John Warren, M.D., first professor of anatomy and surgery in Harvard Medical College." In Gross, S., Editor: *Lives of eminent American physicians and surgeons of the nineteenth century*. Philadelphia, 1861, Lindsay and Blakiston, pp. 86–115.

"Femoral aneurism treated by immediate compression." *The Boston Medical and Surgical Journal*, 74:129–132, 1866.

"Cases of orthopedic surgery, with photographic illustrations of the cases presented." Read before the Massachusetts Medical Society at its annual meeting. Boston: D. Clapp & Son, 1868.

"Cases in Clubfoot Read Before the Massachusetts Medical Society at its Annual Meeting," June 3, 1868.

"Femoral aneurism cured by direct compression, while the patient was taking active exercise; death from peritonitis six years afterwards; with an account of the post-mortem appearances by Henry H.A. Beach." Cambridge: Riverside Press. Repr. from: *The Boston Medical and Surgical Journal*, 93: 461–469. 1875 (co-author: Henry H.A. Beach).

"Spinal disease and spinal curvature. Their treatment by suspension and by the use of the plaster of Paris bandage. A review." Cambridge: Riverside Press, 1878. Repr. from *The Boston Medical and Surgical Journal*, 98: 18–21, 1878.

"Review of Sayre, Lewis A., Spinal disease and spinal curvature." (London, 1877, Smith Elder & Co.), *The Boston Medical and Surgical Journal*, 98:18–21, 1878.

"Hints on the diagnosis and treatment of club-foot." *The Boston Medical and Surgical Journal*, 101:715–726, 1879.

"The Influence of the prevailing methods of education on the production of deformity in young persons of both sexes." Cambridge: Riverside Press, 1879.

"False anchylosis of the hip joint." Rec. *Boston Society for Medical Improvement*. 8:127–129, 1880–1882.

"Description of an apparatus for the treatment of contracture and false anchylosis of the hip joint." *The Boston Medical and Surgical Journal*, 104:514–515, 1881.

"Extension in the treatment of diseased vertebrae." Cambridge: Riverside Press, 1884. Repr. from: *The Boston Medical and Surgical Journal*, 111:1–3, 1884.

"Double congenital displacement of the hip. Description of a case with treatment resulting in a cure." Boston: Cupples, Upham & Co., Repr. from: *The Boston Medical and Surgical Journal*, 112:541–546, 1885.

ADVANCEMENT OF HARVARD MEDICAL SCHOOL

Buckminster was a charter member of the American Orthopaedic Association (1887) and a member of the Massachusetts Medical Society; he served as secretary and treasurer of the Boston Medical Association and as librarian of the Boston Society for Medical Improvement. He was also a member of the Massachusetts Medical Benevolent Society. He published numerous articles and case reports on specific orthopaedic disease and deformities (see **Box 6.1**).

He died December 24, 1891, at the age of 72. In his will, he left his collection of photographs and casts to Harvard Medical School and established an endowment for a professorship in orthopaedic surgery, which was later called the John Ball and Buckminster Brown Chair of Orthopaedic Surgery. He left $40,000, and, with another $10,000 donated by his sister Rebecca, the endowment for the chair in 1891 totaled $50,000 (accepted by Harvard in 1895). This amount equaled $1,220,538 in 2008 dollars. Edward Hickling Bradford, Buckminster's most famous student, continued to further his work in establishing Boston as a city on the forefront of orthopaedics. These two accomplishments of Dr. Brown were pivotal in putting orthopaedics on the map at Harvard Medical School.

His qualities as a physician, as a surgeon, and as a human being are detailed in his obituary, written by C. Foster in 1893:

> Dr. Brown was an orthopedist in the best and broadest sense of the word, using all means—operative, mechanical and medicinal. Conservative by nature, he was ready yet to adopt any new method as soon as its value was clearly proved…Confident in his own skill, in his long experience, and his well tried methods, he quietly watched various procedures taken up by the profession with enthusiasm and gradually allowed to pass into oblivion…His favorite quotation was, "Genius is the talent for taking pains." (C. Foster 1893)

CHAPTER 7

The Boston Orthopedic Institution
America's First Orthopaedic Hospital

The first orthopaedic specialty hospital in the United States opened in Boston in 1838. It was originally named the Orthopedique Infirmary and later referred to as the Boston Orthopedic Institution. It was opened and operated privately by John Ball Brown when he was 54. He called it the Hospital for the Treatment of Deformities of the Human Frame. At the time, he had already begun to limit his practice to orthopaedics, which he did entirely within the span of opening his new hospital. Both Drs. Brown agreed that "This institution is the first and only one conducted on scientific principles in the United States" (J. B. Brown and Buckminster Brown 1850).

Interestingly, for some unexplained reasons, the Boston Orthopedic Institution has received little

Advertisement for the "Boston Orthopedic Infirmary for the Treatment of Spinal Distortions, Club Feet, etc."
Boston Medical and Surgical Journal, January 1839; 19: 420.

recognition in the history books, possibly because it was privately owned and not a general hospital. The lengthiest descriptions of the Institution are contained in Shands's *The Early Orthopaedic Surgeons of America*, in Bicks's "American Orthopedic Surgery: The First 200 Years," and Cohen's "The Boston Orthopaedic Institution." Other references are brief at best. Leo Mayer's classic history "Orthopaedic Surgery in the United States of America" begins with the formation of the American Orthopaedic Association in 1887 and doesn't mention the Boston Orthopedic Institution. It is also not covered in Sir Harry Platt's "The Special

Orthopedic Hospital–Past and Present," published in 1964. Platt describes many orthopaedic specialty hospitals in England and Europe but only two in America in the nineteenth century, both in New York. He mentions the Society for the Relief of the Ruptured and Crippled and the New York Orthopaedic Hospital and Infirmary.

ORIGINS AND GROWTH

Brown modeled his Institution after Dr. Guérin's Orthopaedic Institution of Paris. He originally

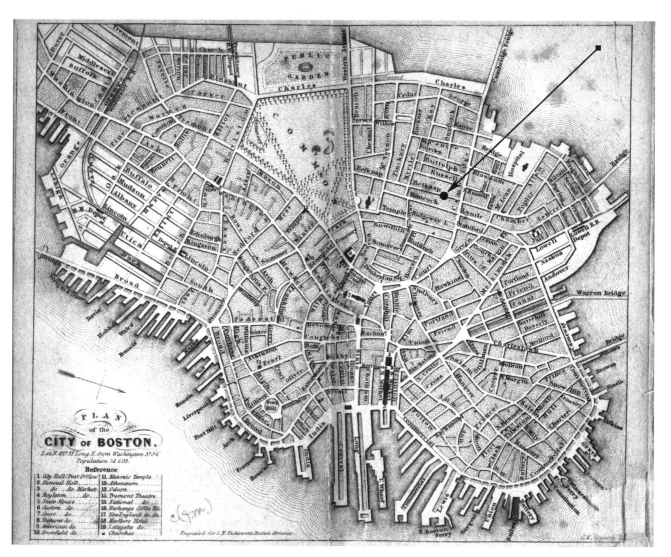

Plan of the city of Boston, engraved by George W. Boynton for Samuel N. Dickinson's *Boston Almanac*, 1840. MGH is in the upper right and the Boston Orthopedic Institution is located at the dot on the map.
Norman B. Leventhal Map & Education Center/Boston Public Library.

opened the hospital within his home where he, his wife, and their children (including Buckminster) lived. It was located at 65 Belknap Street, now re-named Joy Street. As of 2019, the building remains. The original announcement for the Institution listed 22 physicians/surgeons who endorsed the hospital's focus on scientific principles. It appeared in the *Boston Medical and Surgical Journal* in 1839 and stated:

Orthopedique Infirmary

For the treatment of spinal distortions, club feet, etc. 65 Belknap Street, Boston. Patients from a distance can be accommodated with board in the immediate neighborhood.
    John B. Brown, MD, Surgeon

We the subscribers approve of Dr. John B. Brown's plan of an infirmary for the treatment of Spinal Affections, Club Feet and other Distortions of the human body, and will aid him by our advice whenever called upon. John C. Warren, George Hayward, Edward Reynolds, Jno. Randall, J. Mason Warren, John Jeffries, John Homans, M.S. Perry, W. Channing, George C. Shattuck, H.J. Bigelow, Enoch Hale, W. Strong, George Parkman, D. Humphreys Storer, George W. Otis, Jr., Winslow Lewis, Jr., J.H. Lane, Edw. Warren, Geo. B. Doane, John Ware, George Partlett, John Flint.
    Boston, August 1, 1838 (*Boston Medical and Surgical Journal 1839b*)

Brown also named five consulting surgeons who "render their advice and aid gratuitously whenever it is desired...John C. Warren, M.D., Professor of Anatomy in Harvard University. George Hayward, M.D., Professor of the Principles of Surgery and Clinical Surgery in Harvard University. J. Mason Warren, M.D., S.D. Townsend, M.D. and Winslow Lewis, Jr., M.D" (J. B. Brown 1845).

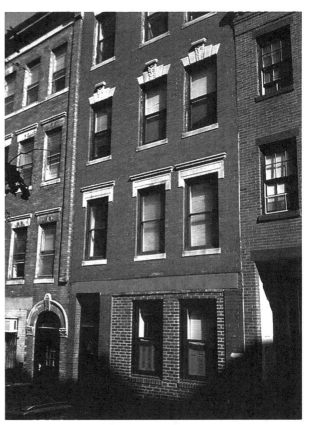

Joy Street location of the building that housed the Boston Orthopedic Institution, 2016. Photo by the author.

Brown's practice continued to grow rapidly as word spread of the specialized center. Patients arrived from across diverse locations in the United States, and he was unable to accommodate all his patients in his home. First, he rented part of a house across the street, and later he rented a whole house on Pinckney Street. An additional announcement in the *Boston Medical and Surgical Journal* stated:

An institution is now in successful operation, in Boston, for the cure of spinal distortions, club-feet, etc...Under these favorable auspices, there is every reason for believing that the infirmary will prove a useful institution, that it will be judiciously and scientifically managed. In Paris, the Orthopaedique Institution has been appreciated by the benevolent, there being a large capital invested in apparatus adapted to the various distortions and deformities of the body—particularly in children and young persons of both sexes. Dr. Brown has recently received a minute report from the two surgeons who control it, which presents a detailed account of the principles and modes of treatment. Spinal affections are continually increasing amongst us, as an accompaniment of civilization, and it is important, therefore, that the best mode of correcting and preventing them, should be based upon true anatomical and psychological principles. Until within a few years, comparatively, their complaints, even in Europe, were left to the management of quacks and machine-makers; and much unnecessary suffering and derangement of health has been the unfortunate result.

Much has been said, of late, of the effects produced on the general condition of the body by compressing the whole trunk in such a manner as to impede the functions of the vital organs. A mode of practice is at this moment in vogue of casing up the patient in a metallic corselet, which is not justified by any discoveries in anatomy…We view Dr. Brown's plan of operations for restoring distorted limbs and spinal curvatures, as unexceptionable, because they are sustained by the acknowledged principles of anatomy and physiology. To long professional experience, this gentleman unites a mechanical ingenuity and skill, without which no success can be expected in this peculiar department of surgery. In view of the great and good object he proposes, we cordially

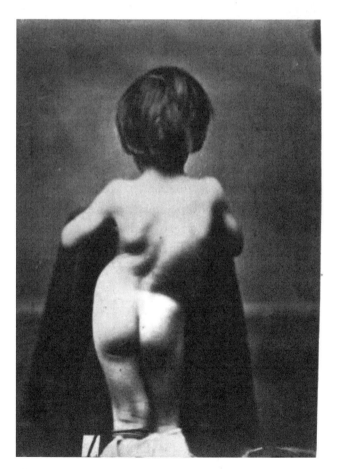 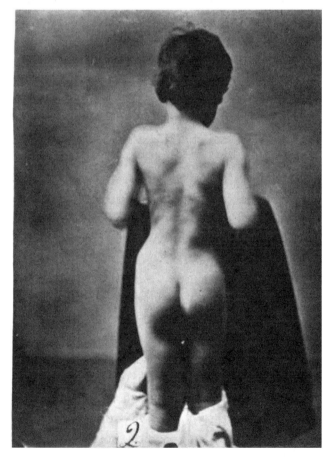

Photo of patient with scoliosis; before and after treatment (Buckminster Brown 1868). Published in *Cases of Orthopaedic Surgery, with Photographic Illustrations of the Cases Presented* by Buckminster Brown, Boston: D. Clapp & Son, 1868. Read before the Massachusetts Medical Society at its annual meeting. University of California Libraries/Internet Archive.

wish the infirmary success, and freely express a hope that the community will appreciate the advantages of having it located in this city—under the direction of one who manifests a determination to exert every power to sustain it with increasing reputation. Although comparatively in its infancy, we are assured that the applicants are numerous, and it is much to be deplored that many calls are from that class of worthy, industrious poor, who are wholly unable to pay for the necessary apparatus. In spinal distortions, particularly, the success of Dr. Brown is extremely encouraging, and will have a tendency to prevent patients from going on expensive journeys for medical advice which can be obtained at home…a little girl, three years of age, both of whose feet were turned in (vari), together with…the bones of the legs being so curved that the fibula rested on the anterior part of the tibia, after having been six months a subject of the infirmary, could stand in an erect position…the most difficult and unpromising subject that could have been selected. She was placed under Dr. Brown's care, we understand, by the recommendation of the President of the Massachusetts Medical Society. On the whole, we are gratified with the progress which he is making in this benevolently devised institution, which only requires to be extensively known to be upheld by the strong arm of an intelligent community. (Boston Medical and Surgical Journal 1839a)

By 1845, he needed even more space and moved his Boston Orthopedic Institution to 49 Chambers Street, which no longer exists. In 1845,

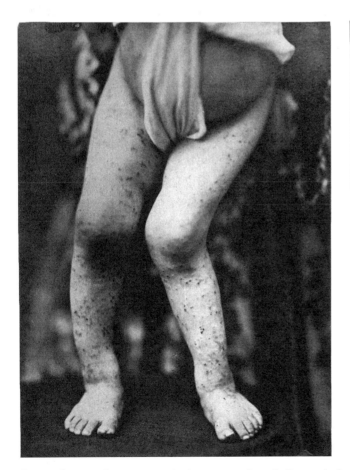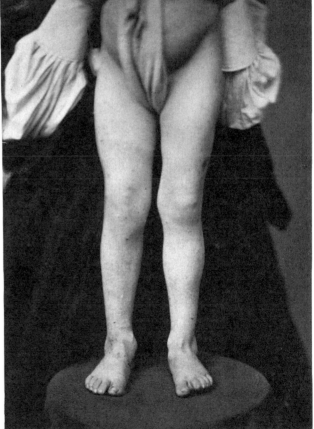

Genu valgum and genu varum in the same patient; before and after treatment. Donated by Buckminster Brown.
Warren Anatomical Museum in the Francis A. Countway Library of Medicine.

however, Chambers Street was an extension of Joy Street on the opposite side of Cambridge Street, which was very close to his home. Conveniently located near Beacon Hill, it was only a few blocks from the Massachusetts General Hospital. It contained about 60 beds and a large outpatient infirmary; most beds were filled with spinal or club-feet cases. It was stated to be:

> A large and commodious house…[it] contains large halls for orthopedic exercises, and private apartments for lodging and board. It is under the surveillance of an experienced matron, who resides in the house, and a respectable widow woman takes care of the house, and furnishes board to patients, either at the common table or in their private rooms, as may be necessary… There is a Library in the Institution, for the benefit of patients, and from which they are at liberty to take books free of charge. (J. B. Brown 1840)

By the time Buckminster joined his father in practice in 1846, the Boston Orthopedic Institution had been opened for eight years. Having visited the orthopaedic specialty hospitals in London (Royal National Orthopaedic Hospital founded by Little), Paris (hospital founded by Jules Guérin), Hanover (Stroymeyer's orthopedic institute), and Vienna (Zurick's orthopedic hospital and the Institution for Cretins and Idiots), Buckminster brought back to his father and the Boston Orthopedic Institution new ideas for treatment, new types of mechanical devices, different approaches and types of tenotomies as well as organizational and operational ideas to improve his father's institute. Shortly after he returned, ether became available. It must have been a tremendous gift and opportunity for both John Ball and Buckminster to suddenly be able to operate on patients in the Institution without causing pain during surgery. They could begin to slow their technique and concentrate on details of the surgical anatomy and desired correction. Of course, sepsis remained a significant problem for another 20 years, until Lister's antisepsis techniques became commonly used in the United States.

TREATMENT ADVANCES

Operations were performed without anesthesia for about eight years before ether was successfully used as an anesthetic at the Massachusetts General Hospital in 1846. Thereafter, both Drs. Brown used ether as an anesthetic for operations performed at the Institution. On February 13, 1839, senior Brown was among the first to use Stromeyer's subcutaneous tenotomy for clubfoot and was also an early performer of Guérin's tenotomy for scoliosis and torticollis. He always considered these procedures as supplementary to the primary treatment of mechanotherapy. Brown reported his first case of tenotomy in a patient with a clubfoot in 1839; he eventually began to perform over 100 tenotomies (both for foot and spinal deformities) over the course of two years. Patients sought out his expertise for the procedure.

Case Report 7.1. Stromeyer's Subcutaneous Tenotomy For Clubfoot

"February 13, 1839.—J. A. G., of Milton, Mass., came under my care with two club-feet. She is 3 ½ years old; never has walked. February 21st, at 3 o'clock, P.M., divided the tendo-Achilles in both feet. The ends separated about an inch. The feet came round very well; brought the heels immediately down, agreeable to M. Bauvier's direction. The child appeared to suffer little or nothing from the operation. There was not a drop of blood from the left foot, and only four or five from the right. Drs. J.M. Warren and J.W. Gorham were present; also Mr. J.W. Phelps, machinist. Saw her at 5 o'clock, two hours after the operation. She was sitting quietly upon the sofa, eating her bread and milk. Saw her again at 7 the same evening…and 7 the next morning…child has…suffered no inconvenience…She stood erect on the soles of her feet on the 18th, and began to walk on the 36th day after the operation" (J. B. Brown 1839).

After Brown surgically treated the clubfoot in this three-and-a-half-year-old patient, the child's physician in Milton (Dr. Jonathan Ware) wrote to him on August 30, 1839 and said, "The little girl actually unable to stand…is now…able…to walk about the house. The operation and applications by which you have been successful in relieving her, I would earnestly and confidently recommend to…all persons having children similarly afflicted" (J. B. Brown 1839). His uncle, Dr. John Collins Warren, wrote: "Dr. Brown. . . In compliance with your request, I can state that I have seen a number of such cases of club-foot operated on by you, which appeared to be much improved and in a fair way to be cured" (J. B. Brown 1839).

ADVOCACY FOR SPECIALIZATION

John Ball Brown was a strong advocate for the specialty of orthopaedic surgery as well as his specialty hospital. He wrote in his "Reports of Cases in the Boston Orthopedic Institution, or Hospital for the Cure of Deformity of the Human Frame" that:

> Deformities of the human frame cannot be conveniently and judiciously treated except in a hospital or institution expressly devoted to this object. It is not for the interest of any general practitioner of medicine and surgery to be at the expense of furnishing himself with the variety of apparatus (some of which is very expensive) required in treating these deformities. (J. B. Brown 1844)

Further, in reference to a general hospital such as the MGH treating orthopaedic patients, he stated:

> There would be an impropriety in patients of this description being mingled with patients who usually resort to that useful institution suffering all kinds of diseases…they have not the accommodations as it regards room…furnished with every variety of apparatus for correcting every variety of physical deformity; and then a skillful surgeon should be hired to give his whole attention to this business, with two or three mechanics under his direction…It requires a peculiar combination of talents to practice this branch of business with success…and do the most good in the community. (J. B. Brown 1844)

Brown—along with Lewis Sayre—was a strong advocate for the early diagnosis (at birth) of clubfoot and early treatment with manipulation and corrective shoes. Both men promoted evaluating all newborns for clubfoot (Bick 1976). Even Dr. John Collins Warren, a generalist in surgery and medicine, agreed with Dr. Brown's opinion about the importance and need of specialty care. He said:

> Dr. Warren remarked that he had been in a position to see a great number of the cases operated upon by Dr. Brown, and also after treatment, and that he had truly been surprised at the perfection of the cures and the great care and unwearied attention by which this favorable result was accomplished. He thought it very important that all of this class of cases should be placed in the hands of some one or two of the profession who had given great attention to the subject, and who had the necessary variety of apparatus by which alone a successful issue could be obtained. He said that various cases were brought to the Hospital [MGH]—poor patients—upon whom they felt obliged to operate, and that in a short time sores would appear upon the feet, and various other drawbacks would occur, and before the patients left the institution the surgeons were heartedly sick of the cases. (Buckminster Brown 1858)

Drs. Brown also referred to an observation of Dr. Little in briefly describing a case at the MGH. Dr. Little, in his observations on club feet, stated: "Indeed, it will often be found that the amount

REPORT OF CASES

IN THE

ORTHOPEDIC INFIRMARY

OF THE

CITY OF BOSTON.

BY JOHN B. BROWN, M.D.

SURGEON OF THE INFIRMARY.

Republished from the "Boston Medical and Surgical Journal."

Cover of the first *Report of Cases in the Orthopedic Infirmary of the City of Boston* by John Ball Brown, Boston: D. Clapp, Jr., 1840.
Collection of the Massachusetts Historical Society. Photo by the author.

REPORTS OF CASES

TREATED AT THE

BOSTON ORTHOPEDIC INSTITUTION,

OR

HOSPITAL FOR THE CURE OF DEFORMITIES OF THE HUMAN FRAME;

WITH SOME

PRELIMINARY OBSERVATIONS ON THE PRESENT STATE OF THE INSTITUTION,

AND ON

CLUB FOOT, SPINAL CURVATURE, DISTORTIONS OF THE CHEST, STIFF JOINT, AND SPINAL IRRITATION.

BY

JOHN B. BROWN, M.D.
Fellow of the Mass. Medical Society; formerly Surgeon, and afterwards Consulting Surgeon, at the Mass. General Hospital.

AND

BUCKMINSTER BROWN, M.D.
Fellow of the Mass. Medical Society, Member of the American Medical Association, and of the Boston Society for Medical Improvement.

BOSTON:
CABINET OFFICE, 128, WASHINGTON STREET.
1850.

Cover of *Reports of Cases Treated at the Boston Orthopedic Institution*, by John Ball Brown and Buckminster Brown, Boston: Cabinet Office, 1850.
Collection of the Massachusetts Historical Society. Photo by the author.

of pain and fatigue is greater in cases of talipes, than in those where the deformity has reached its highest grade" (Buckminster Brown and J. B. Brown 1850). Drs. Brown commented: "A striking instance of this has lately been brought under our notice, at the MGH…a young and beautiful girl, seventeen…obliged to have her foot amputated, on account of a [painful] sore" (J. B. Brown and Buckminster Brown 1850). She had developed osteomyelitis of the metatarsals and phalanges following a chronic ulcer that developed when she was one year of age. Dr. J. Mason Warren performed an amputation while she was under ether anesthesia.

John Ball Brown wrote three books on reports of cases that he had treated at the Infirmary

(1840, 1844, and 1845) before his son Buckminster joined him in his practice. He was a strong believer in reporting his treatment results to all physicians as well as to the public. Later, he and Buckminster would write two more reports on cases treated at the Institution, one in 1850 and a final one in 1860. Even though the Hospital for the Ruptured and Crippled "claimed that [it] was the first institution to be organized within the United States for the treatment of orthopaedic conditions" (F. Beekman 1939), according to its seventy-fifth anniversary volume (1939), it did not open its doors to patients until May 1, 1863, which was 25 years after the Boston Orthopedic Institution opened (1838).

THE CLOSING OF THE BOSTON ORTHOPEDIC INSTITUTION

The Boston Orthopedic Institution eventually closed, but the exact date is unknown as there is no information available after 1851. Buckminster and his father had been in practice together for at least five years before it closed. John Ball Brown was 67 years of age; Buckminster was only 32. Jonathan Cohen (1958) suggested that John Ball probably retired, although he was healthy until just before his death at age 72 in 1862. Buckminster, however, was in the early years of his practice, and he didn't assume his position at the House of the Good Samaritan until 1861. His health couldn't have resulted in his leaving the Boston Orthopedic Institution because he led the orthopaedic service at the House of the Good Samaritan for 19 years (until 1880), and he was in charge of 24 beds dedicated to the treatment of musculoskeletal deformities in children. Also, both John Ball and especially Buckminster continued to publish cases between the years 1851 and 1861. Where did they operate during this period? Surely Buckminster continued to practice and operate, but here the trail runs cold.

Some of the confusion about the closure of the Boston Orthopedic Institution is because it was no longer listed in the Boston Directory after 1851. In 1852, Brown's wife noted that a large laundry and two homes belonging to her husband were destroyed by fire. Since Dr. John Ball Brown and his family continued to live at 8 Joy Street, these burned buildings most likely included the facility at 49 Chambers Street. We do not know whether this catastrophe was responsible for the absence of the listing of the Boston Orthopedic Institution in the Boston Directory after 1851. The July 1851 Boston Directory clearly lists Dr. J. B. Brown as surgeon at two locations—Orthopedic Institution at 49 Chambers and his house at 8 Joy. Dr. Buckminster Brown is listed as a physician with an office at 2 Bowdoin (near Bowdoin Square, a few blocks from his father's house). In 1852, J. B. Brown's house remained at 8 Joy; Buckminster's office was listed at 1 Bowdoin in 1852. The 1854 Business Directory's listing of physicians listed J.B. Brown at 8 Joy and Buckminster Brown at 26 Beacon (on the opposite side of Beacon Hill from his former office). One possibility is that both Browns continued to care for patients at 8 Joy Street where the Orthopedic Institution had begun. Other possibilities are that they both worked at 8 Joy Street and at Buckminster's office on Bowdoin Street (later 26 Beacon Street) or each worked at their own office. The patients most likely were housed around the city as Dr. J. B. Brown had started when the Institution was located on Chambers Street.

It is difficult to determine the dates of surgery and the location of treatment for many of their published cases because they often presented the same case in different publications, and they commonly don't state where the patient was treated and rarely reported the year of surgery. However, in their 1860 publication "Observations on Lateral and Angular Curvature of the Spine, Wry-Neck, Club-Foot, and Other Orthopedic Affections with Report of Cases," J. B. Brown and Buckminster Brown gave dates of surgery in two cases after 1851. The first was June 1853:

> F. P., aged sixteen years, had an injury of the right foot and ankle some three years since… the foot turns out…he walks on the inner edge…The muscles on the outer side of the leg, ankle, and foot, and the flexor of the toes, are contracted. These muscles were all divided, and the foot placed in an apparatus. In six weeks, this patient went home with a perfectly straight foot…In the fall of 1859, F. P. visited Boston…His foot is in all respects perfect both in form and in usefulness. (J. B. Brown and Buckminster Brown 1860)

The second case included a surgery on September 8, 1859:

The subject was a lad, eighteen years of age. When eleven years old…caught his pantaloons (in a rapidly turning shaft), and he was whirled around with the shaft…on examination…a great portion of the gastronomii muscles of the left leg had been torn off…The surgeons brought together the jagged fragments as well as they could by stitches and adhesive plaster; but…the heel stood five inches from the ground when we first saw the young man; and he walked entirely on his toes…from the time of the accident, seven years previous. The operation was on the 8th of September, 1859; and in three weeks the foot had acquired its normal position…the young man did not return home until about six weeks from the time he came, as we thought it best to continue the application of the apparatus. (J. B. Brown and Buckminster Brown 1860)

John Ball Brown had resigned from his consultant position at the MGH (1836), Buckminster Brown was never on the staff of MGH, and the House of the Good Samaritan didn't open until 1861, so it is most likely both Drs. Brown completed these published surgical cases and others at their offices and the Boston Orthopedic Institution. Dr. John Ball Brown died in 1862, the same year that Dr. Buckminster Brown joined the staff at the recently opened House of the Good Samaritan. Buckminster went on to continue to influence the development of the specialty of orthopaedic surgery there (see chapter 8). Although the Boston Orthopedic Institution has been largely invisible in the chronicles of history, the Drs. Brown led the way for important advances in orthopaedic history at the institution.

House of the Good Samaritan
America's First Orthopaedic Ward

Anne Smith Robbins established the House of the Good Samaritan in Boston in 1861 "for women with advanced consumption who were without means of support" (S. A. Knopf 1922). Robbins did not grow up poor herself, but after living in various boarding houses when she became unexpectedly penniless, she became intimately familiar with the experiences of poor women with incurable or chronic illnesses. Such women were not admitted to hospitals at that time, and, after Robbins received an inheritance, it became her goal to change their circumstances. The House of the Good Samaritan was incorporated on June 11, 1860, and the first patient was admitted on January 7, 1861, two months before Abraham Lincoln's inauguration on March 4 and eight years before the founding of Boston Children's Hospital.

The House of the Good Samaritan would eventually become the first hospital in the United States to create an orthopaedic ward; in particular, it treated disabled children with severe spinal deformities. At its founding, it was located at 6 McLean Street, close to Massachusetts General Hospital (MGH) as well as the Boston Lying-in-Hospital at 24 McLean Street, which was temporarily closed. It was very near to where the Boston Shriner's Hospital is located in 2019. Robbins wrote about her dreams for the hospital:

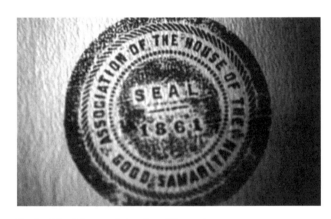

Seal of the House of the Good Samaritan.
Boston Children's Hospital Archives, Boston, Massachusetts. Photo by the author.

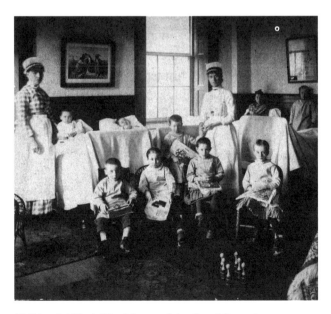

Children's Ward, The House of the Good Samaritan Hospital. 1863.
Images of America. Children's Hospital Boston. Charleston, SC: Arcadia Publishing, 2005. Boston Children's Hospital Archives, Boston, Massachusetts.

It being well known that there is a great want in the city not sufficiently met by any of the hospitals and institutions now existing. It is hoped that a subscription may be raised to meet this difficulty in a degree. (House of the Good Samaritan Records)

Anne Smith Robbins' plan was supported by many of Boston's leading physicians, including J. Mason Warren, James Jackson and Henry J. Bigelow. Robbins wrote:

There is a class of women, many of them Americans, who being either patients discharged from the MGH as incurable, or who have been refused admission there on that account are forced to seek for shelter in very poor boarding houses or in the almshouse, where they are made to suffer for want of the comforts and quiet as requisite to lessen the miseries of prolonged illness. [The House of the Good Samaritan is] for those disabled by long and lingering illness, who cannot be received into, or kept in, the MGH. (House of the Good Samaritan Records)

According to its original bylaws, a Board of Managers elected visiting physicians and nurses. All admissions were "under the advice and consent of the visiting physicians and a committee [the secretary and one of the female managers]" (House of the Good Samaritan Records). The records indicate that "all patients appropriate for admission, owing to illness and poverty, will be received without regard to religious faith, but Americans decidedly have preference" (House of the Good Samaritan Records). For almost two years, the small building housed only women with tuberculosis, but it gradually expanded to include "phthisis, scrofula, Brights disease, typhoid fever, dyspepsia, anemia, paralysis and dropsy, debility, hysteria, heart disease, destitution and spinal disease" (House of the Good Samaritan Records).

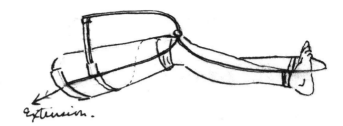

Drawing of a leg brace to correct a knee flexion contracture.
The House of the Good Samaritan Records 1860–1966. Archival Collection—AC4. Box 16, Volume 24, p. 81. Surgical Records, Nov. 1879–Aug. 1889. Boston Children's Hospital Archives, Boston, Massachusetts.

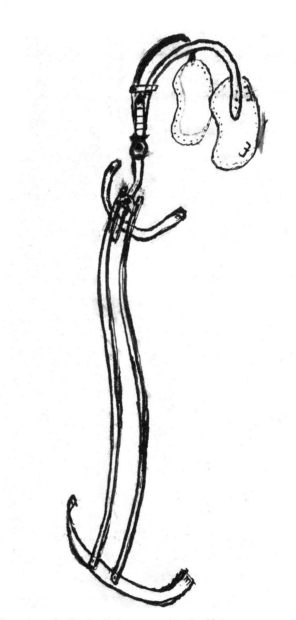

Drawing of a Torticollis brace used in the 19th century.
The House of the Good Samaritan Records 1860–1966. Archival Collection—AC4. Box 16, Volume 24, p. 213. Surgical Records, Nov. 1879–Aug. 1889. Boston Children's Hospital Archives, Boston, Massachusetts.

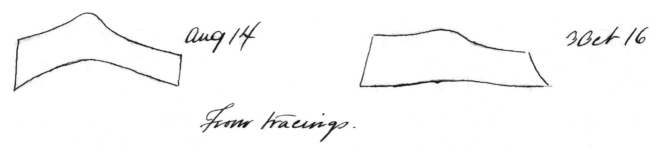

Tracings of a knee flexion contracture before treatment (August 14) and after treatment (October 16).
The House of the Good Samaritan Records 1860-1966. Archival Collection—AC4. Box 16, Volume 24, pg. 82. Surgical Records, Nov. 1879–Aug. 1889. Boston Children's Hospital Archives, Boston, Massachusetts.

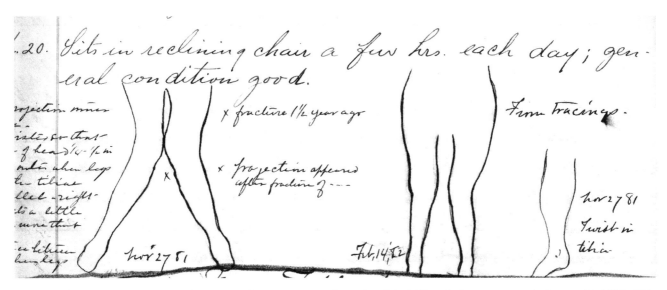

Tracings of Bilateral knee valgus deformities before treatment (November 27, 1881) and after treatment (February 14, 1882). This method of documenting a patient's improvement was common before the discovery of x-ray.
The House of the Good Samaritan Records 1860-1966. Archival Collection—AC4. Box 16, Volume 24, pg. 52. Surgical Records, Nov. 1879–Aug. 1889. Boston Children's Hospital Archives, Boston, Massachusetts.)

OPENING THE ORTHOPAEDIC WARD

The House of the Good Samaritan opened its orthopaedic ward in May 1862. A superintendent wrote that the orthopaedic ward was opened "due to the Founder [A. S. Robbins] finding a child of four, suffering from tuberculosis of both hips, tied to the leg of a chair while his mother went out to work" (House of the Good Samaritan Records). Buckminster Brown was placed in charge of the orthopaedic ward and remained so for almost 20 years until 1880. At age 62, he became Consulting Surgeon, and he "only resigned his place

because he felt himself unable longer to attend to…patients…He remained as Consulting Surgeon until his death" (House of the Good Samaritan Records).

Just as his father, John Ball Brown, had attracted patients from the United States and abroad to the Boston Orthopedic Institution, so did Buckminster Brown receive patients "coming from all parts of the United States and the British Provinces" at the House of the Good Samaritan (C. C. Foster 1893). With the increasing demand of orthopaedic patients, two new wards opened in 1862 providing orthopaedics with a total of 24 beds. The expansion resulted in a

Case Report 8.1. Treatment for Bilateral Hip Displacement

[Excerpted from Buckminster Brown's 1885 "Double Congenital Displacement of the Hip; Description of a Case with Treatment Resulting in a Cure," *Boston Medical and Surgery Journal*.]

On the fourth of April, 1882, a little girl four years of age was brought to me to be treated for what was thought to be an unusual example of spinal curvature. On examination I found a double hip displacement…The condition of the hips at this time was as follows: No trace of a cotyloid cavity could be discovered. When the patient was recumbent…traction on the legs would readily bring the heads of the femur into their normal position…they would slip upward by the natural contraction of the muscles…There was no action of a muscle or group of muscles as would demand or warrant the use of the knife…The walk was the extreme of that sideward movement which is expressed by the term waddle…The great trochanter is…a rounded prominence high up on the ileum, bordering the crest… The excessive lordosis is conspicuous…the consequent prominent, overhanging abdomen and compensatory bend of the knees are well seen…

The child was brought to Boston…on the thirtieth day of December, 1882, she was placed upon the bed…my treatment must be divided into distinct stages. First, it

was requisite to relax and extend the large mass of glutei and other pelvic muscles…I commenced with warm poultices…enveloped the pelvis and hips…renewed twice a day for one week…a firm leather belt three inches wide, padded…was buckled around the hips (1/6/1883)… four long straps were attached…from the ilium…each side…front and back….were buckled to the rail at the head of the iron bedstead. Two perineal straps were fastened…lower edge of this belt…gave firm, unyielding counter-extension.

Direct extension was made by…stiff leather bands… encircling the legs above the knees and above the ankles. A cord to which weights were suspended passed over… pulleys at the foot…the use of the bands alternated: sometimes above the knees, and sometimes above the ankles… knee-bands were preferable…extension…directly upon the pelvic muscles…weights…three pounds were used at first…afterward increased…the head of the bedstead… raised by…wooden blocks…eight inches high…

About the middle of February…the femoral heads now being in normal position, the thighs were flexed to nearly right angles with the body and then spread…knees tied to the edge of the bedstead on each side and the feet secured to the opposite side…This position was painful and could

"very considerable increase in…annual expenditure, particularly as a larger portion of the cases admitted into these wards…[were] of a surgical nature, requiring various expensive appliances for relief" (House of the Good Samaritan Records). The wards filled immediately while hundreds continued to wait on admission.

Siffert (1958) described Buckminster Brown as especially committed to pediatric orthopaedics because of his own experience with childhood disability and rehabilitation. Buckminster treated many patients with hip and spine disease in the new specialty ward. In doing so, he documented patients' outcomes as recovered, relieved, not relieved, or died. In 1865, he treated a young boy with tuberculosis of the knee. The child's knee was

flexed more than 90 degrees, and he was unable to walk or stand. Robbins (1865) wrote:

In April we admitted a little boy of six years to be treated for contraction of the knee…arising from scrofulous of the knee joint…(his) lower leg was fixed at more than a right angle to the thigh…In the early part of June an operation was decided upon…(risk): joint disorganization by disease… result: was so successful that the child is now the happy possessor of two available legs of equal length. (House of the Good Samaritan Records)

At that time, ether had only been recently introduced and they were just beginning to operate on severe deformities. Successfully reducing be borne but two or three hours...of the day...After...the legs were weighted as before...the rest of the twenty-four hours...At no time were the limbs allowed...without extension...Graduated compresses were placed across the dorsum ilii...above the trochanter...An attendant...drew the small weight downward...the knee was raised toward the abdomen...Four hours a day this passive exercise was continued, two hours for each limb. This may properly be termed the stage of excavation...The course was pursued...until July 20, 1883.

The hips remained in position...last time either had been displaced was on March 28, 1883.

June 2, 1883. The patient was removed to the seaside to a hotel in the neighborhood of my summer residence. July 20, 1883. The first test was made to test the strength of the tissues by which the heads of the femurs were retained in their sockets. I pushed the limbs upward...and backward, with considerable force. There was firm resistance in each direction...this experiment was frequently renewed...until finally the body was moved by pushing against the rim of the acetabulum, which was now unquestionably formed... The patient now used active movements of the limbs...

The fourteenth day of January, 1884, the little girl sat up in bed, for the first time for thirteen months...A cart was constructed...the patient sat...only to allow...the toes to touch the floor...At first she only imitated walking, but soon was able to propel herself through two large rooms and a hall with ease. The Hip joints worked perfectly... In April the patient bore her own weight...May 14th she began to walk in her carriage...

June 11th. Walked by herself without support a distance of three feet. Did this six times...

June 28th. Commenced to use canes, which gave her confidence in walking. On the thirtieth of June, 1884, the patient left Boston for her home in the southern part of the State...

January 20, 1885. The child walks well without canes...

February 18, 1885. The walk has much improved...some degree of muscular atrophy between the trochanter and the crest of the ilium, on each side...

March 28, 1885. The lateral movement of the shoulders disappeared some weeks since...Nélaton's line, passing over the summits of the trochanters, indicates that the heads of the femurs are in their normal position...

May 25, 1885. The child's walk is normal.

Buckminster Brown, 1885

See photos, Chapter 6

---

the contracture was a significant accomplishment. Buckminster also published his own case reports, which included notes recording the first case of reduction of dislocated hips in the United States. See **Case Report 8.1** for details.

EXPANSION AND TRAINING OF FUTURE ORTHOPAEDIC SURGEONS

Few of the annual reports remain from the House of the Good Samaritan. A report from January 1, 1872, noted that "We beg here to renew our grateful acknowledgement—to those gentlemen to whom we have so long been indebted for the

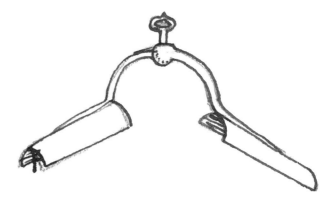

Drawing of a hip abduction splint used at The House of the Good Samaritan. The House of the Good Samaritan, 1860-1966. Archival Collection—AC4. Box 16, Volume 24, p. 87. Surgical Records. Nov. 1879–Aug 1889. Boston Children's Hospital Archives, Boston, Massachusetts.

good gift of our medical care and surgical service...to Dr. Thomas Dwight who took temporary charge of the surgical patients during the absence

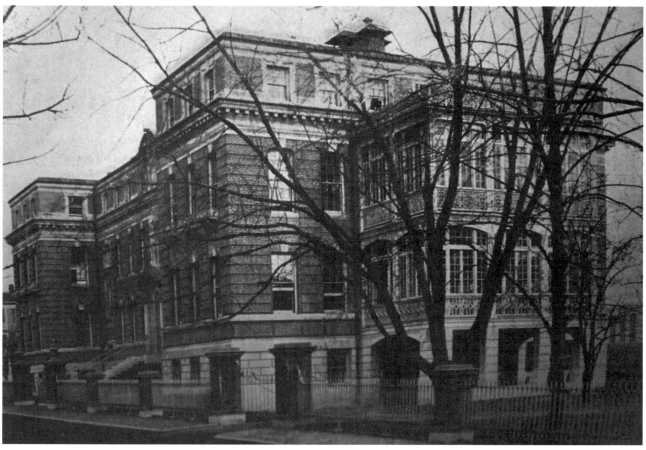

The House of the Good Samaritan. 25 Binney Street (ca. 1906).
Images of America. Children's Hospital Boston. Charleston, SC: Arcadia Publishing, 2005. Boston Children's Hospital Archives, Boston, Massachusetts.

of Dr. Brown" (House of the Good Samaritan Records). We do not know why Buckminster was absent or for how long. However, the January 1, 1892, annual report recognized his contributions:

> There is another that deserves the honorable mention we so gladly accord to it, that is of Dr. Buckminster Brown. Dr. Brown was elected surgeon in 1864 and retained his office until 1880. During those years his devotion to this house was unflagging, to his skill and care we owe some remarkable and interesting results. Never possessed of vigorous health, he continued his work with wonderful persistence, and only resigned his place because he felt himself unable to attend to our patients. He always retained his cordial regard for our welfare, and came from time to time to congratulate us on our success. His name remained as Consulting Surgeon until his death. (House of the Good Samaritan Records)

Dr. Edward H. Bradford, who had been mentored by Buckminster, was employed at the House of the Good Samaritan in 1876, and later, in 1880, followed him as chief orthopaedist. Bradford had started his practice in Boston in 1876 after graduating from Harvard Medical School and spending two years studying in European orthopaedic centers. He had observed and admired Buckminster's orthopaedic contributions and continued additional orthopaedic studies with Taylor at the New York Orthopaedic Hospital. In the annual report from January 1, 1891, Bradford emphasized the importance of the cases of hip disease treated at the House of the Good Samaritan:

The number of cases of hip disease which… have been treated in the last eight years at the hospital, is of value…within comparatively short time hip disease was considered one of the most incurable of disorders…in our small ward fifty cases have been thoroughly treated in the last eight years. Many of these cases were of the most severe type of the disease, and a careful investigation of their present condition gives most gratifying results…of the cases heard from—twenty-nine,—all were well with the exception of four. Of these four, three had died of some intercurrent disease, and only one had died of hip disease. Those results are rarely obtained, even in excellent hospitals, and give evidence of thoroughness in nursing and care which cannot be too highly praised. (House of the Good Samaritan Records)

Because of an increasing demand for more beds, the House of the Good Samaritan moved to Binney Street at Francis Street in 1905. Its inpatient capacity increased to 40 beds. In 1914, an additional ward of 20 beds was added for the care of women with inoperable cancer. The orthopaedic service remained active under Bradford's leadership.

The House of the Good Samaritan also had an important role in the training of future orthopaedic surgeons, and it provided certificates to trainees (residents) between 1905 and 1923. In the May 21, 1946, annual report, Mrs. Henry B. Chapin wrote that Dr. Bradford, Dr. Goldthwait, and other major figures in orthopaedics had had their early training there.

CLOSURE OF THE ORTHOPAEDIC WARDS

Competing demands for beds (especially with a plea by the medical staff for more beds to treat rheumatic heart disease) and the large expense of caring for orthopaedic patients (including adults at the time), eventually led the board of managers to plan the closure of the orthopaedic wards after 60 years. Letters from the medical staff included arguments that although orthopaedic beds were needed in Boston, their costs were high. Space demands, including a large elevator, an x-ray facility and an occupational therapy room equipped with looms, were too much for the House of the Good Samaritan to continue to support. They also argued that orthopaedic beds were no longer required for the chronic care of patients with rickets. Pressure even came from the Boston Association of Cardiac Clinics who supported the change.

Dr. Robert Soutter's letter to Miss Catherine A. Codman, Chairman of the Board of Managers, House of the Good Samaritan. November 18, 1924.

The House of the Good Samaritan, 1860–1966. Archival Collection—AC4. Patient Records. Boston Children's Hospital Archives, Boston, Massachusetts. Photo by the author.

At this point in time, other hospitals in Boston had now established orthopaedic wards and the House of the Good Samaritan was no longer the only available service for orthopaedic patients. On November 5, 1924, the chairman of the board of managers wrote to Dr. Robert Soutter, associate of Dr. E. H. Bradford, and informed him that a decision had been made to close the orthopaedic wards. He replied to Miss Codman on November 18, 1924, saying, "I cannot say that it is without much regret that it seems necessary to close the orthopedic wards for children" (House of the Good Samaritan Records). He accepted staying on as a consulting surgeon.

By 1930, the House of the Good Samaritan had 74 beds; 54 occupied by children with rheumatic heart disease. It was the largest center for the treatment of rheumatic heart disease in children in the United States. On December 9, 1946, it merged into Children's Hospital (see chapter 14) when new treatment options using penicillin and steroids had left its beds increasingly empty. With physician support and generous donations, the House of the Good Samaritan remained open and independent for 65 years. On March 15, 1967, the House of the Good Samaritan became legally incorporated into the Boston's Children Hospital Medical Center. The House of the Good Samaritan had had a pivotal role in the influence of the creation of orthopaedic specialty wards and in the training of future generations of orthopaedic surgeons.

Section 3

Harvard Medical School

The ignorance and general incompetency of the average graduate of American Medical Schools, at the time he receives the degree which turn him loose upon the community, is something horrible to contemplate, considering the nature of a physician's functions and responsibilities. The mistake of our ignorant or student young physician or surgeon means poisoning, maiming and killing; or, at the best, they mean failure to save life and health which might have been saved, and to prevent suffering which may be have prevented. The Harvard Medical School has successfully begun a revolution in this period.

—**Dr. Charles W. Eliot**, President's Report 1871–1872 (Deans Files, Harvard Medical School)

Harvard wanted a medical school…not only to train men learned and skillful in what is now known and applied, but expectant of progress, and desirous to contribute to new discovery…men whose chief interest lies in medical and surgical progress rather than in the cautious application of what is now supposed to be known.

—**Dr. Charles W. Eliot**, President of Harvard, Letter H. L. Higginson, 1907
(Deans Files, Harvard Medical School)

Half of what we have taught you is wrong. Unfortunately we do not know which half.

—**C. Sidney Burwell**, Dean of Harvard Medical School 1935–1949,
statement to a graduating class (Deans Files, Harvard Medical School)

CHAPTER 9

Orthopaedic Curriculum

Harvard University began discussing the establishment of a medical school as early as 1764. However, that same year the library building was destroyed by fire. It contained a complete male and a complete female skeleton as well as a collection of medical books. These were the same books and skeletons Joseph Warren studied as an undergraduate at Harvard. In 1770, Ezekiel Hersey donated €1,000 to Harvard for a professorship of anatomy and surgery. The next year a group of Harvard undergraduates interested in anatomy formed "The Anatomical Society" and later, the "Spunkers"—a secret society of students

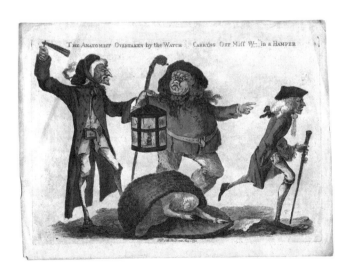

Cartoon of William Hunter, who introduced the use of cadavers in Medical education, being chased off by a night watchman. Painting by William Austin, 1773.

Carl H. Pforzheimer Collection of Shelley and His Circle, New York Public Library.

who robbed bodies from graves, possessed skeletons and anatomic books, and dissected animals and human cadavers. During the 1780s, John Warren successfully gave lectures and demonstrated anatomical dissections at a military hospital for students and any interested persons from the public

By 1782, there was overwhelming support among Harvard students for the establishment of a medical professorship, and President Willard and members of the Harvard Corporation charged a committee to report to the board on the topic. The committee reported on September 19, 1782, that the university's library should collect books on anatomy, surgery, physic, and chemistry; obtain complete anatomical and surgical equipment; and raise sufficient funds for professors of anatomy and surgery, physic (art or practice of medicine), materia medica (pharmacology), and chemistry. They recommended that every student who passed examinations should receive a certificate from the university and be allowed to practice medicine, also that the university apply to the General Assembly of the Commonwealth for a law allowing bodies of criminals and those who died by suicide to be given to the professor of anatomy for purposes of teaching anatomy and surgical operations by dissection. Finally, the committee suggested that, since the college lacked funds to pay these new professors: "the Corporation...[should] elect [to] those Professorships some gentlemen of public spirit and distinguished ability who would undertake the business for the present for the fees that may be obtained from those who would readily attend their lectures" (T. F. Harrington 1905a). On November 22, 1782, the Corporation voted:

> That there be three Professors chosen as soon as circumstances will permit, and that Anatomy and Surgery be assigned to one; the Theory and Practice of Physic to another, and Chemistry and Materia Medica to a third.
>
> Written votes being brought in for a Professor of Anatomy and Surgery, it appeared that Dr. John Warren of Boston was chosen.
>
> That the filling of the Professorship of the Theory and Practice of Physic and of Chemistry and the Materia Medica be for the future consideration of the Corporation.
>
> That the President and Professor Wigglesworth be a committee to form an article for the Medical Institution on the subject of conferring medical degrees, and to compose an introduction for ushering it into the public view, together with such remarks as they may think expedient, and to make a report to this Board at some future meeting.
>
> Voted, that the gentlemen who shall be first elected a Professor superintend all the branches as far as may be consistent with the prosecution of his own particular branch till another is chosen.
>
> The question being put whether the Corporation will now proceed to the choice of a Professor of Anatomy and Surgery, it was voted in the affirmative.
>
> That the filling of the Professorship of the Theory and Practice of Physic and of Chemistry and the Materia Medica be for the future consideration of the Corporation.
>
> That the President and Professor Wigglesworth be a committee to form an article for the Medical Institution on the subject of conferring medical degrees, and to compose

> an introduction for ushering it into the public view, together with such remarks as they may think expedient, and to make a report to this Board at some future meeting. (T. F. Harrington 1905a)

The committee's recommendations were accepted, and the Corporation asked John Warren to develop plans for a course of medical studies at Harvard in Cambridge. This included instruction plans for anatomy, physiology, and surgical operations.

EARLY MEDICAL INSTRUCTION

The first medical school lectures were given in the basement of Harvard Hall, but in less than one year they were moved to Holden Chapel, where all lectures were given for about 25 years. In 1810, they moved to a new Boston location at 49 Marlborough Street. See **Table 9.1** for additional details.

Table 9.1. Locations of Harvard Medical School

1782	Harvard Hall, Cambridge
1783	Holden Chapel, Cambridge
1810	49 Marlborough Street, Boston (now 400 Washington Street)
1816	Mason Street, Boston
1847	North Grove Street
1883	688 Boylston Street
1906	Longwood Avenue, Boston

Data from T. F. Harrington 1905.

The content of Warren's lectures indicate he prioritized the teaching of anatomy over that of surgery. Although not named, orthopaedics was a large focus of these early lectures. Both intact skeletons and skeletal parts from amputated limbs were studied in detail. Warren's yearly course always began with his lecture on osteology, which he often delivered in Latin (see chapter 2). Warren's first course included a week of lectures and

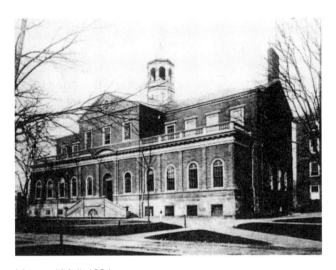

Harvard Hall, 1906.

Harvard Medical Library in the Francis A. Countway Library of Medicine.

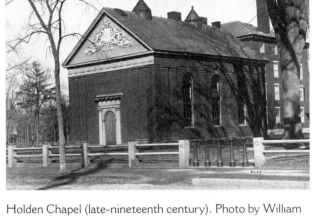

Holden Chapel (late-nineteenth century). Photo by William Notman and Son (Montreal Canada), 1874.

Roosevelt 560.12-022 (olvwork416445), Houghton Library, Harvard University.

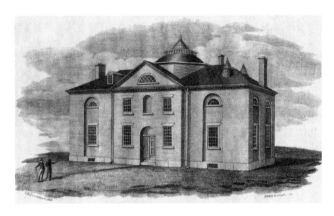

Massachusetts Medical College at Harvard University on Mason Street, 1816–1846.

Harvard Medical Library in the Francis A. Countway Library of Medicine.

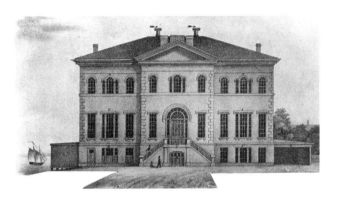

Massachusetts Medical College on North Grove Street, 1846–1883. Published in *The Harvard Medical School. A History, Narrative and Documentary, 1782-1905*, Vol. II, by T.F. Harrington, 1905. Internet Archive.

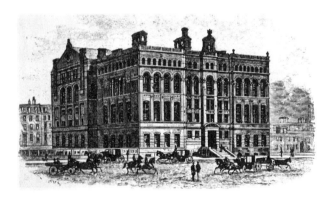

Harvard Medical School; Boylston and Exeter Streets, 1883–1906. Published in *The Harvard Medical School. A History, Narrative and Documentary, 1782-1905*, Vol. III, by T.F. Harrington, 1905. Internet Archive.

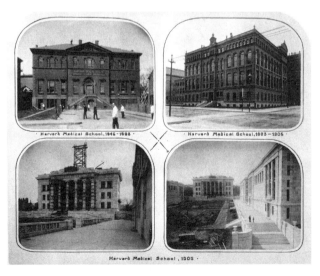

Photos of Harvard Medical School in three different locations, 1846–1906.

Harvard Medical Library in the Francis A. Countway Library of Medicine.

Mortui Vivos Docent
(The dead teach the living)

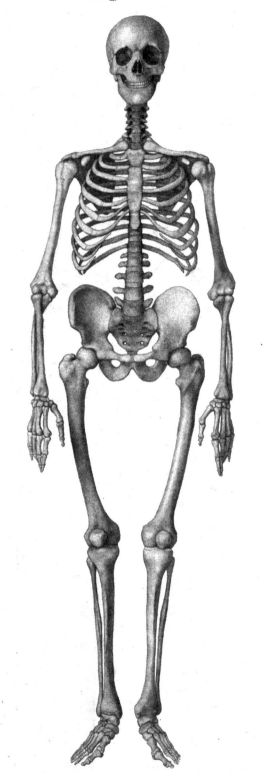

Human Skeleton. Etching by George Stubbs, from *A comparative anatomical exposition of the human body with that of a tiger and common fowl*, London 1804–06.

© Photo: Royal Academy of Arts, London. Photographer: John Hammond.

demonstrations of each of the following topics over the course of six weeks:

   I. Osteology, or a definition of the bones
  II. Myology, of the muscles
 III. Splanchnology, of the viscera contained in the large cavities
 IV. Angeiology, of the blood vessels and Lymphatics
  V. Neurology, of the Nerves
 VI. Adenology, of the Glands (T. F. Harrington 1905a)

Lectures began October 6 and ended November 17. By 1790, his lectures expanded to include the brain and the thoracic and abdominal cavities along with dissections.

After Warren's death, lectures on bones, joints, and muscles were continued by his son John Collins Warren (see chapter 3), who was fascinated by all skeletons (human, animal, and fish). For more than 25 years, MGH had the following schedule for lectures:

Hospital, Medical Visit [9-11 AM] …; Surgery, Saturday at 12; Dr. Jackson Monday and Thursday 3 P.M., other days 11 to 12; Dr. Channing, Friday afternoon at 3. Tuesday and Saturday 9 A.M.; Dr. Bigelow, Tuesday 3 P.M., Wednesday and Friday 9 to 10; Dr. Warren daily at 12… time allotted to the examination of each candidate for a degree was fixed at forty minutes; ten minutes for surgery and anatomy; and from five to eight minutes at least for other branches.
(T. F. Harrington 1905b)

There was no examination in orthopaedics. Examinations were given in anatomy, physiology, chemistry, materia medica, pharmacy, midwifery, surgery and the theory and practice of medicine. In 1831, lectures for medical students were

delivered at the Massachusetts Medical College in Boston [Harvard Medical School]…

Students attending the Lectures of the Professor of Anatomy and Surgery are admitted to see the Surgical Practice in the Massachusetts General Hospital…On January 15, 1835, the Corporation voted to establish a professorship on the Principles of Surgery and of Clinical Surgery…"to give Elementary Lectures on the Principles of Surgery, and Clinical Lectures on the surgical cases in the Massachusetts General Hospital." (T. F. Harrington 1905b)

Each student was charged an attendance fee of $10 for the surgical lectures. Dr. John Collins Warren presented the anatomy and operative surgery lectures; Dr. George Hayward provided the principles of surgery and clinical surgery lectures.

After Dr. Hayward's resignation in 1849, Dr. Henry J. Bigelow was appointed professor of

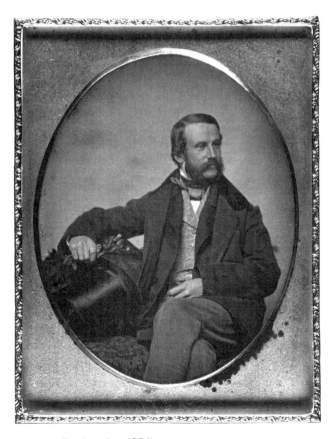

Henry J. Bigelow (ca. 1854).

Harvard Art Museums/Fogg Museum, Loan from the Massachusetts General Hospital Archives and Special Collections. Photo © President and Fellows of Harvard College.

surgery. Bigelow, along with six other professors, wrote an article in 1850 titled "Practical Views on Medical Education," which argued that:

In Surgery, of which several subordinate specialties constitute distinct living professions; it is not to be admitted that the means or time of any course of lectures, can furnish full and complete instruction. Certainly, it must be difficult to arrange a course of lectures on any of the extensive sciences which now constitute medicine, if it be indeed true, that "the teachers are not justifiable in suppressing any portion." It is the business of lecturers in medical schools to condense and abridge the sciences which they respectively teach, to distinguish their essential and elementary principles, to sift carefully the useful from the superfluous, and to confine…their teachings…to what is true and profitable, and likely to be remembered and used by their hearers…to teach him well what he can and should master, and briefly to point out to him the sources, fortunately abundant, from which he may obtain the rest…Lectures are chiefly wanted to impress by demonstration the practical branches of science, and are most effective in places where the facilities for such demonstrations can be commanded. Anatomy requires extensive exhibitions by the teacher, and personal dissection by the student…Surgery is acquired by witnessing numerous operations, surgical diseases, illustrated explanations, and by personal practice on the dead body… The exacted evidence of three years of well conducted study, is better than the exhibited ticket of a six months course…The things to be avoided by medical teachers are technicalities which are unintelligible to beginners…excessive minuteness in regards to subjects, which are intricate and but little used, and therefore destined to be speedily forgotten. (J. Bigelow et al. 1850)

This seminal article on surgical pedagogy was important because there were no entrance requirements yet for medical school and medical curriculum was still in the very early stages of development. At the time, some students could not even read, and examinations were oral to accommodate this fact. Examinations were also rushed and not sufficiently evaluated.

During this time frame of early pedagogical determinations, HMS also debated which students it permitted to apply for admission. The issue of when and what studies minorities were permitted to pursue or which they were excluded from at Harvard is complex and poorly documented, including for the orthopaedic program; the topic is worthy of a book in itself. See **Box 9.1** for an overview.

Box 9.1. Minority Admissions to Harvard Medical School

- **1847**: Harriet K. Hunt, a white woman from Boston, was granted permission to attend lectures, but that permission was withdrawn in 1850.

- **1850**: Three black men were admitted to study medicine. However, they were later (exact date unknown) expelled in response to protests by faculty and students.

- **1860**: HMS admitted the first black male student in 1860.

- **1936**: Fe del Mundo, a female Filipino physician, was allowed to attend lectures, but women were not permitted to apply for admission to the school.

- **1945**: Women were officially allowed admission to HMS.

Harvard began publishing a "Catalog of Officers and Students of Harvard College" in 1850. In addition to listing the professors and students of Harvard Medical School, it also listed the courses consisting of daily lectures, demonstrations, operations, and examinations. From 1850 to 1860, anatomy and surgery were listed as courses and orthopaedic surgery was not mentioned. In 1865,

the first clinical instruction was given in a sub-specialty of surgery, ophthalmology. Over time, Harvard "fulfilled its early ambition of teaching medicine as a clinical endeavor...although it never had direct control over any of the five Boston hospitals whose facilities it used; close relationships, Faculty and staff overlap, and material advantages had combined to produce an abundance of teaching opportunities" (M. F. Nigro 1966).

There is something very solemn and depressing about the first entrance upon the study of medicine. The white faces of the sick that fill the long row of beds in the hospital wards saddened me and produced a feeling of awe-stricken sympathy. The dreadful scenes in the operating theatre—for this was before the days of ether—were a great shock to my sensibilities, though I didn't faint, as students occasionally do. When I first entered the room where medical students were seated at a table with a skeleton hanging over it, and bones lying about, I was deeply impressed, and more disposed to moralize upon mortality than to take up the task in osteology which lay before. It took but a short time to wear off this earliest impression. I had my way in the world to make, and meant to follow it faithfully. I soon found an interest in matters which at the outset seemed uninviting and repulsive, and, after the first difficulties and repugnance were overcome, I began to enjoy my new acquisition of knowledge.

—Oliver Wendell Holmes
(quoted in T. F. Harrington 1905)

In the early and mid-nineteenth century, rival medical schools had begun to appear in New England and in Boston. One such school was the Boylston Medical School, located on the corner of Essex and Washington Streets and founded by Harvard graduates. The first and only course in orthopaedic surgery in New England, taught by Henry W. Williams, was introduced at the Boylston Medical School in 1847. This new medical school and others eventually failed, however, because Harvard recruited the best teachers and modified its courses.

EDUCATIONAL REFORM

In 1869, Charles W. Eliot, a professor of chemistry at MIT and former assistant professor of mathematics and chemistry at Harvard, was elected as president of Harvard. Earlier that same year he published "The New Education: Its Organization" in the *Atlantic Monthly*. In his essay, he persuaded his readers of a need for a new type of distinctly American university, one in which universities combined the best aspects of liberal arts and more technical education; his essay ultimately persuaded the Harvard trustees to select him as president. Under Eliot's leadership, Harvard Medical School issued reforms to bring order to the curriculum.

Immediately upon assuming his presidency, Eliot was confronted by Henry J. Bigelow, who "defended the status quo with vehemence and dedication. He firmly believed that the school was successful and Eliot's visions of the school 'were unrealistic and unfair'" (M. F. Nigro 1966). Eliot firmly believed: "all medical progress hinges on scientific discovery" (M. F. Nigro 1966) and new research should be the guiding force behind all activity at HMS. Initially, Oliver W. Holmes was a staunch ally of Bigelow, but Holmes later accepted Eliot's vision for medical education and the role of HMS. Even though Bigelow had made many important clinical discoveries, he objected to expanding the curriculum in non-clinical areas. He thought "the average community required only an average doctor and that the average doctor needed only an average knowledge...most eminent men are in a large degree self-made" (M. F. Nigro 1966). Bigelow also believed that advances occurred because of "haphazard growth...stemming from his own career...[and he] was understandably unsympathetic and even hostile to science and research generally, and to their invitation into the practical art of medicine...[He felt that] science was fickle, worthless, wasteful, cruel, and most important useless to the practitioner" (M. F. Nigro 1966). In contrast to Bigelow, Eliot believed that "science needed no justification on

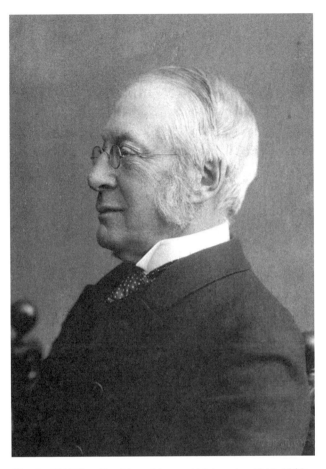

Charles W. Eliot, President, Harvard University, 1869–1909. HUP Eliot, Charles W. (38a), olvwork361310. Harvard University Archives.

any grounds, but [that in] the search for truth... Truth and right are above utility in all realms of thought and actions" (M. F. Nigro 1966). Eliot instituted the majority of his reforms at HMS within a single year.

The transition led by Eliot began in November 1869 and lasted until October 1871. His aim was "to correct the flaws...excessive autonomy of the school within the University [not under the university's control]...and failure to treat medicine as a scientific and academic as well as a clinical endeavor [it lacked a devotion to research]" (M. F. Nigro 1966). In a powerful symbolic step, Eliot attended a faculty meeting of Harvard Medical School in November 1869 and sat in the chair's position, a first for a Harvard president and clearly demonstrating "a new chief was in town" (M. F. Nigro 1966). Eliot's reforms are outlined in **Box 9.2**. HMS was typical of the other better medical schools and "indeed many of the points of contention which troubled Harvard Medical School in 1871 still confront American Medical Schools...maximum utilization of a given period of study; appropriate emphasis on medical, clinical, scientific or other training; the best teaching methods for various disciplines; and the most suitable kind of student for medicine" (M. F. Nigro 1966).

Box 9.2. President Charles W. Eliot's Reforms at HMS

1) *Calendar*. The Harvard Medical School calendar was changed to match that of the university with classes held between September and June. Before 1869, the medical school calendar included daily lectures during the winter and personal instruction or recitations in the summer. Both were now combined between September and June.

2) *Financial structure*. Harvard's "Corporation assumed control of the receipts and expenditures of the school...[and] salaries of faculty [were] drawn up" (M. F. Nigro 1966). Previously, Harvard Medical School was financially independent and the students purchased tickets for specific classes.

3) *Education*. Education changes included increased entrance requirements, and the development of a standard curriculum for all students, including required examinations. Eliot had found that the medical students "were of very low caliber...ignorant, undisciplined, [with] shocking illiteracy" (M. F. Nigro 1966).

Before initiation of Eliot's rigorous reforms, students were taking advantage of the system's laxities, which included two plus one years in school without definite requirements and oral examinations, often less than five minutes long, given by professors to whom the student paid for the course. Only about one-third of the students enrolled in the summer recitation exercises. Oliver Wendell Holmes wrote in a letter that "our new President Eliot has turned the whole University over like a flap-jack" (T. F. Harrington 1905b). During the Eliot years (1869–1909), the approach to instruction and examination changed substantially, and the course of studies for a medical degree was set first at three years and then eventually increased to four years in 1880.

According to the "Catalog of Officers and Students of Harvard College" HMS began to provide lectures in otology and laryngoscopy in 1871. The field of orthopaedics, however, was not mentioned until the 1872 edition of the catalog; it was listed under "examination papers" that were required for all students. At that point in time, first-year students in anatomy now had to "describe the structure of bone [and] describe the scapula and its connections to the trunk" (*Nineteenth Annual Catalog of the Medical School (Boston) of Harvard University* 1872–1873). The questions for the third-year students were obviously influenced and most likely written by Henry J. Bigelow. He asked the students to "describe the different dislocations of the hip-joint; what constitutes the difficulties in their reduction; what are the symptoms of hip disease; what are the symptoms of caries of the vertebrae; what are the symptoms of an impacted fracture of the neck of the thigh-bone; describe a club-foot briefly; and how would you amputate a thigh?" (*Nineteenth Annual Catalog of the Medical School (Boston) of Harvard University* 1872–1873). Each subsequent year, additional musculoskeletal questions were added to the students' examinations.

Between 1871 and 1877, the new curriculum in surgery—required of all students—included anatomy, physiology, and chemistry in the first year; surgery and clinical surgery in the second year; and surgery and clinical surgery in the third year. The number of exercises in surgery increased by 35% and the number of exercises in clinical surgery increased by 54%. The school now required three-hour written examinations; the students had to pass most subjects each year. By 1901, an academic degree would be required for admission to Harvard Medical School.

In 1878, the examination in clinical surgery included an orthopaedic case: a five-year-old boy with a compound fracture of the tibia and fibula treated with reduction and a cast. In this case, the patient became ill with a fever and diarrhea and died 10 days after injury. The leg remained unchanged. The students were asked to discuss the cause of the boy's death. Surgery courses continued to increase. In addition to anatomy in the first year, a practical topographical anatomy course was added to the second year as well as a course on surgery and clinical surgery at the Massachusetts General Hospital and Children's Hospital. In the third year, another course on surgery and clinical surgery was given. In the fourth year, a new course was added entitled clinical and operative surgery (at the Massachusetts General Hospital and Children's Hospital) as well as specialty courses in ophthalmology, otology, laryngology, obstetric and operative obstetrics. Despite increasing time spent addressing orthopaedic content, a dedicated course in orthopaedic surgery was not yet listed in the catalog.

INTRODUCING ORTHOPAEDICS AS A SPECIALTY COURSE

At the centennial celebration in 1881 of the Massachusetts Medical Society, President Eliot spoke at the dinner stating: "This century completed will be looked back upon as the birth of medicine as a learned and liberal profession" (J. J. Byrne 1981). Nevertheless, orthopaedics had remained a part of the anatomy lectures and surgical lectures and demonstrations for almost 100 years at Harvard. General anesthesia and aseptic technique had spurred rapid growth in surgical advancements more generally during this time. Orthopaedics

was not separated from surgery until 1881 when Dr. Bradford (an assistant in clinical surgery; see chapter 15) was granted purview over teaching the specialty. Dedicated coursework in orthopaedics began small and was overshadowed by other classes until, according to Bradford, orthopaedic surgery became "regarded as one of the most important specialties in the Surgical Department" (quoted in H. K. Beecher and M. D. Altschule 1977). By that time, the medical school had relocated five times; it was now on North Grove Street, adjoining the Massachusetts General Hospital.

After March in the academic year of 1881–1882, Bradford taught a course on orthopaedic surgery to the fourth-year class, giving two lectures per week. The course was approximately two to three months in length; sometimes held in the fall instead of late winter/spring. In 1882 and 1883, he also taught the course "Applications of Bandages and Apparatus" with Dr. Coll Warren (12 practical sessions). Textbooks in various subjects, including surgery, had been recommended reading for the students; an orthopaedic text was first recommended in 1885, "Humphrey's Human Skeleton" (Catalog of the Officers and Students 1885).

From 1881 through 1893 Bradford gave this same orthopaedic course to the fourth-year students. In 1893, he was named the first faculty member to have a teaching appointment in orthopaedic surgery, as assistant professor of orthopaedics. In addition to this fourth-year course (two lectures/week for two months), he taught another required course (one hour) in orthopaedics and a fourth-year elective in orthopaedic surgery (two hours). Both written and oral exams were required in these latter two courses. At this time, Dr. Lovett was listed on the faculty teaching clinical surgery for second-year students at Boston City Hospital, and in 1893 he taught the course "operative surgery" for third-year students. In this course, the students were required to do 15 practical exercises; although orthopaedics was not listed, it most likely was included among these practical exercises.

During this time period, an editorial was published in the *Boston Medical and Surgical Journal* in response to an 1893 article in *Lancet* that was critical of medical education in the United States (Harvard and Yale are the best examples) in comparison to England. The editorial stated that medical education in the American schools was

far ahead of that in the English schools...there can be no doubt that the decadence of medical science in England during the last forty years has been most marked...at the very time when medical science began to bloom in Germany... The stimulus which was given medical education in Germany...was due to the greater use of the experimental method...leading to a closer investigation of the problems of disease. The

falling off in England has been largely due to the small place given in medical education to the laboratory and to research...in Germany there is the further advantage of a close union between general and medical education...the faculty of medicine of a great university profits by the stimulus which it receives from other branches of learning...[However] our medical schools have been hampered...by the absence of a close and integral union with those other branches of learning which compose the faculties of a university, by being more or less technical schools where the art of medicine is taught; secondly, by the absence of endowment, making the remuneration of the teachers dependent on the fees of the students, and the work of research almost impossible. (*Boston Medical and Surgical Journal* 1893)

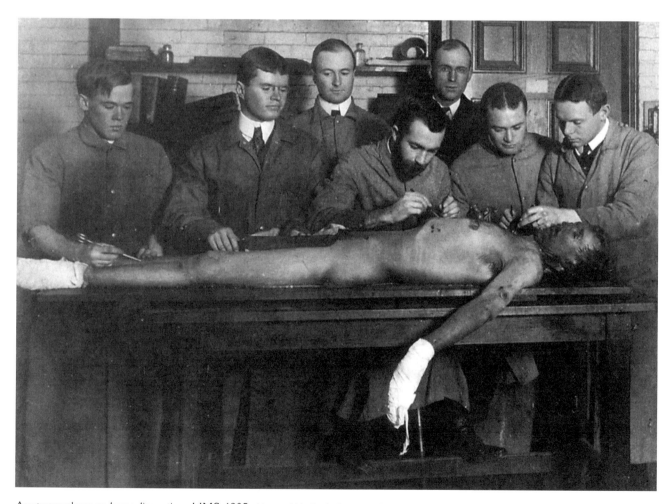

Anatomy class: cadaver dissection, HMS, 1905. Harvard Medical Library in the Francis A. Countway Library of Medicine.

In the 1895 Catalog, orthopaedic surgery (previously listed under surgery) was now listed under "instruction" for the first time, distinctly separate from surgery. Bradford continued to teach his course to the fourth-year class. It was required; one lecture per week for four months at either HMS or Children's Hospital. The students (in sections of four students) attended clinics at Children's Hospital (three times per week) during the academic year (September 26–June 19). A two-hour examination was held in June. An elective in orthopaedic clinical exercises was also offered. Dr. Lovett was listed as teaching clinical surgery and minor surgery at the Boston City Hospital, as well as children's surgery at Boston Children's Hospital. Two orthopaedic summer courses were offered at Children's Hospital: Dr. Bradford on Monday and Wednesday, July 1–August 29 (four hours); followed by Dr. Lovett on Tuesday and Saturday, August 17–October 1 (four hours). Bradford's required course continued, although the length and times changed, and additional faculty were added until he became dean in 1912. Other courses in orthopaedics were also added during this period.

During the next decade, rapid changes occurred within the orthopaedic curriculum. These changes included the following additions:

- *1899*: an elective in clinical exercises in the fourth year in which the students measured apparatus and assisted a few times at surgery
- *1900*: a required course of lectures (1x per week in Room A or at Children's Hospital) and clinical exercises (3x per week) at Children's Hospital followed by an examination in February
- *1901*: a one-hour clinical elective in the fourth year increased to two hours while elective summer courses at Children's continued; a course on fractures offered for the first time by Dr. Scudder at MGH with his book as recommended reading for the students

- *1902*: Drs. Lovett, Brackett, Goldthwait, and Dane as assistants in orthopaedics who taught the clinical exercises at Children's Hospital
- *1904*: orthopaedic courses again listed under the category "Surgery" with the following books as recommended reading: Whitman's *Orthopedic Surgery*, Bradford and Lovett's *Orthopedic Surgery*, and Hoffa's *Orthopädische Chirugie*; graduate courses were also offered in orthopaedic surgery, deformities, curvatures, bone pathology, skiagraphy, and tuberculosis of joints; a new course on fractures for graduates was offered by Dr. Cotton at Boston City Hospital; and a required course in orthopaedics was given in the first half of the academic year (Stevenson's book on *Fractures and Dislocations* was recommended)

See **Box 9.3** for an example of the development of examination questions during this period.

The number of orthopaedic courses continued to increase. The course catalog in 1905 included a description of the required orthopaedic courses in the third and fourth years:

Half courses, afternoons throughout the year. The instruction will consist of ward and out-patient work, the taking of histories, the witnessing and assisting at operations, the reporting of the progress of cases, and seeing the end results. Conferences with the student will be held from time to time.

In 1906 even more courses were offered. There was one other significant change in 1906: fourth year students were no longer required to take a course in orthopaedic surgery; the required course was moved to the third-year class. **Table 9.2** outlines the curriculum at the beginning of the twentieth century. No additional changes occurred over the next five years.

Box 9.3. Examples of HMS Examination Questions

The following is an example of Bradford's examination for the fourth-year students, excerpted from the 1901 *Catalog of the Officers and Students*:

1. How is hip disease to be recognized?
2. How is caries of the spine to be recognized?
3. How is tubercular disease of the knee joint to be recognized?
4. How is tubercular disease of the ankle to be recognized?
5. Describe the condition known as club-foot, — the important anatomical relations, and give the principles of treatment.
6. What are the causes of the curves in rickets?
7. What are the most important curves in rickets?
8. What is meant by weak foot, and what is meant by flat foot?
9. What are the principles of treatment of hip disease?
10. What are the principles of treatment of caries of the spine? (Catalog of the Officers and Students 1900)

Bradford also wrote the questions for the examination at the end of the elective course in 1901. Example:

1. Upon what physical signs can a diagnosis of tubercular disease of the hip joint be made?
2. How is a diagnosis of congenital dislocation of the hip to be made?
3. Give the characteristic symptoms of cervical and lumbar Pott's disease.
4. Mention the different surgical measures which can be employed in the treatment of deformities and disabilities following anterior poliomyelitis.
5. What are the anatomical changes found in pronounced knock-knee?
6. Describe McEwen's operation for knock-knee.
7. Describe the most convenient apparatus to be used in the convalescent stage of hip disease.
8. Describe the most convenient apparatus for the convalescent stage of tubercular disease of the knee.
9. Describe the best retentive apparatus for club foot.
10. What pathological changes are found in scoliosis?

Table 9.2. Medical School Curricula for Third- and Fourth-Year Students in 1906

	Topic/title	Faculty	Location
Required course (third year)	General orthopaedic surgery*	Bradford, Lovett, Brackett, Thorndike, Soutter, or Adams	Children's Hospital
Electives (third and fourth years)	Orthopaedic surgery	Brackett, Soutter, or Lovett	Children's Hospital
		Goldthwait	MGH
	Pott's disease	Thorndike	Children's Hospital
	Flat foot and lateral curvature	Soutter	Children's Hospital
	Deformities	Brackett and Adams	Children's Hospital
	Deformities	Osgood	MGH
	Lateral curvature	Lovett	Children's Hospital
	Research and special work in orthopaedic surgery	Bradford	Children's Hospital
	Surgery of the joints	Codman	MGH
	Diseases of bones and joints	Goldthwait and Osgood	MGH
	Fractures and dislocations	Crandon	Boston City Hospital
	Summer courses in orthopaedics	Brackett, Soutter, Adams, Bradford, Lovett, Dane, Low, and Brown	Children's Hospital, Boston Dispensary, and Warren Museum

*Upon completing this required third-year course, students had to participate in a 15-minute examination.

Third-year Orthopaedic Surgery
Required Course (1906)
Section 25 and 26
Exercises daily from 9 until 11:30 A.M.
Students will meet their instructors promptly at nine o'clock in the Basement of Ward I at the Massachusetts General Hospital and in the Amphitheatre of the Children's Hospital

Date / Place	Topic	Instructor
Tues, Nov. 6 Mass. Gen. Hosp.	Bodily Mechanics. -Methods of Joint Exam.	Dr. Brown
Wed, Nov. 7 Peabody Home	Tuberculosis, Pyogenic Bone and Joint Infections in Children	Dr. Allison Dr. Ghormley
Thurs, Nov. 8 Mass. Gen. Hosp.	Tuberculosis of Joints in Adults Pyogenic Bone, Joint Infections in Adults	Dr. Smith-Petersen Dr. Wilson
Fri, Nov. 9 Children's Hosp.	Spastic and Obstetrical Paralysis	Dr. Sever
Sat, Nov. 10 Children's Hosp.	Scoliosis: Anatomy, Etiology, Diagnosis Clinical Treatment	Dr. Brewster
Mon, Nov. 12	holiday	
Tues, Nov. 13 Children's Hosp.	Congenital Deformities	Dr. Soutter Dr. Ober
Wed, Nov. 14 Mass. Gen. Hosp.	Foot Strain, Anatomy, Dx, Clinical Treat. Methods of Exam. - Spine, Back Strain	Dr. Ghormley Dr. Smith Petersen
Thurs, Nov. 15 Robt. B. Brigham Hosp.	Chronic Non-Tubercular Arthritis	Dr. Brown Dr. Swaim
Fri, Nov. 17 Children's Hosp.	Poliomyelitis: Anatomy, Dx, Clin. Manifest. Non-Operative and Operative Treatment	Dr. Ober Dr. Legg
Sat, Nov. 17 Mass. Gen. Hosp.	Func., Mechan Treatment of Fractures Traumatic Lesions of Joints	Dr. Wilson Dr. Allison
Mon, Nov. 19 Children's Hosp.	Congen. Bone Diseases-Achondroplasia Rickets, Torticollis, Epiphy. Lesions-Coxa Plana	Dr. FitzSimmons Dr. Legg
Tues, Nov. 20	Visit to Warren Museum and Conference	Dr. Osgood

Third-year Orthopaedic Surgery
Required Course (1906)
Sections 1 and 2
Exercise daily from 9 until 11.30 A.M.
Students will meet their instructors promptly at nine o-clock in the Class Room of the Out-Patient Department of the Massachusetts General Hospital and in the Amphitheatre of the Children's Hospital.

Date / Place	Topic	Instructor
Wed, Nov. 21 Mass. Gen. Hosp.	Bodily Mechan. -Methods of Joint Exam	Dr. Brown
Thurs, Nov. 22 Peabody Home	Tuberculosis, Pyogenic Bone and Joint Infections in Children	Dr. Allison Dr. Ghormley
Thurs, Nov. 23 Mass. Gen. Hosp.	Tuberculosis of Joints in Adults Pyogenic Bone, Joint Infections in Adults	Dr. Smith-Petersen Dr. Wilson
Sat, Nov. 24 Children's Hosp.	Scoliosis: Anatomy, Etiology, Diagnosis Clinical Treatment	Dr. Brewster
Mon, Nov. 26 Children's Hosp.	Spastic and Obstetrical Paralysis	Dr. Sever
Tues, Nov. 27 Children's Hosp.	Congenital Deformities	Dr. Soutter Dr. Ober
Wed, Nov. 28 Mass.Gen.Hosp.	Foot Strain, Anatomy, Dx, Clinical Treat. Methods of Exam. -Spine, Back Strain	Dr. Ghormley Dr. Smith Petersen

Thurs, Nov. 29 Thanksgiving	holiday	
Fri, Nov. 30 Children's Hosp.	Poliomyelitis: Anatomy, Dx, Clin. Manifest. Non-Operative and Operative Treatment	Dr. Ober Dr. Legg
Sat, Dec. 1 Robert B. Brigham Hosp.	Chronic Non-Tubercular Arthritis	Dr. Brown Dr. Swaim
Mon, Dec. 3 Children's Hosp.	Congen. Bone Diseases-Achondroplasia Rickets, Torticollis, Epiphyseal Lesion-Coxa Plana	Dr. FitzSimmons Dr. Legg
Tues, Dec. 4 Mass. Gen. Hosp.	Func., Mechanical Treatment of Fractures Traumatic Lesions of Joints	Dr. Wilson Dr. Allison
Wed, Dec 5	Visit to Warren Museum and Conference	Dr. Osgood

Deans Files, Harvard Medical School

Contrast **Table 9.2** with **Box 9.4** later in this chapter to assess curriculum changes over the course of the twentieth century.

MEDICAL EDUCATION REFORM AND THE FLEXNER REPORT

The same year that HMS listed the required orthopaedic course separately under orthopaedic surgery, the American medical education system as a whole underwent a renaissance in response to the now famous Flexner Report. Two years before Bradford became dean and 41 years after Eliot had begun his educational reform efforts at HMS, Abraham Flexner published his report, "Medical Education in the United States and Canada" in 1910. Sponsored by the Carnegie Foundation at the request of the American Medical Association Council on Medical Education, Flexner surveyed the 155 existing medical schools in North America. Flexner recommended that most medical schools, especially the proprietary schools, be eliminated. He suggested decreasing the number of existing schools from 155 to 31 and preserving the university schools that were committed to academic excellence and research. When he completed his research, he had discovered that most medical schools lacked educational admission requirements; in fact, only five of the schools surveyed required two or more years of college education for admission. As a direct result of President Eliot's reforms, the standards at HMS were far superior; when Flexner inspected HMS in 1909, 60 of the 62 members of the entering class had college degrees. Nevertheless, Flexner chose only Johns Hopkins as a model medical school and not Harvard.

Although Harvard and Johns Hopkins were both among the elite medical schools of the early twentieth century, each school valued distinctly different pedagogies; Flexner was biased in his promotion of Johns Hopkins and his neglect of Harvard because his own views coincided more closely with the Johns Hopkins approach. Kenneth Ludmerer raised two relatively unknown issues about Flexner; he stated, "Flexner had already developed a[n]...educational philosophy that emphasized the importance of...'learning by doing' at every level of study...and that professional schools had the duty to promote original investigation, not merely to teach...from his experiences as a college student at the Johns Hopkins University" (K. M. Ludmerer 2010). In contrast, the Eliot reforms focused on academic training and scientific inquiry. While developing his report, Flexner's biases were no more clearly on display than in his response to Frederick T. Gates (the business advisor for John D. Rockefeller) when Gates asked, "What would you do if you had a million dollars...to...start...reorganizing medical education in the United States?" (quoted in H. K. Beecher and M. D. Altschule 1977). Flexner recommended donating any funds available to the Johns Hopkins Medical School, and, as a result the Rockefeller Foundation created an annual $65,000 provision for Johns Hopkins for full-time clinical medical faculty.

Flexner preferred Johns Hopkins' emphasis on the German model of medical education rather than Harvard's emphasis on the French one. Flexner did have one specific criticism of Harvard; he believed it bad practice to appoint heads of services based on hospital seniority rather than academic accomplishments. Flexner believed this practice caused a "noticeable lack of sympathy" between hospital laboratory staff and the university (quoted in H. K. Beecher and M. D. Altschule 1977). The president of the Carnegie Foundation, Henry S. Pritchett, mirrored Flexner in snubbing President Eliot's successful reforms. In 1913, Pritchett wrote that "Credit for the progress achieved in the field of medical education in the United States belongs in the first instance to the American Medical Association and its Council on Medical Education" (H. K. Beecher and M. D. Altschule 1977).

Despite his biases and criticisms, however, Flexner did briefly acknowledge President Eliot (and therefore Harvard) in his writings when he mentioned President Eliot among the four great leaders of medical education. These leaders included Eliot, Gilman, Welch, and Pritchett. Furthermore, Edsall—Dean of both Harvard Medical School and the School of Public Health—most likely was pleased with the part of Flexner's Report that emphasized the physician's role in advancing science that discouraged disease and social promotion of healthy environments. The report stated, "the physician's function is fast becoming social and preventive, rather than individual and curative" (quoted in K. M. Ludmerer 2010). In direct response to the report, proprietary for-profit medical schools were closed across the United States, and schools began to emphasize scholarly and academic work. Dean Edsall and his successors continued reform at Harvard Medical School.

EVOLUTION OF ORTHOPAEDIC SURGERY CURRICULUM

In the same year the Flexner Report was published, the required orthopaedic course was listed separately under orthopaedic surgery and no longer under the courses listed in surgery. At this time, two books were recommended to the students: *Fractures and Dislocations* by Stimson and *Treatment of Fractures* by Scudder.

Earlier in this chapter, Table 9.2 outlines the medical school's curricula in the early 1900s. Except for changes in faculty and new additions to the faculty, the course catalogs show Harvard made minimal changes to its teaching of orthopaedic surgery over the next decade. Box 9.4 highlights some main changes to that curriculum through the year 2000.

Dr. Lovett became the professor of orthopaedics in 1915, and few changes were made to the fourth-year electives O.S.1 and O.S.2. At this time, clinical exercises were limited to small numbers—eight men in the O.S.1 course at Children's and Massachusetts General Hospital and two men in the O.S.2 course at Children's Hospital. The students served as dressers and assistants, following the course of assigned cases. In addition to serving as a dresser, students assisted in the operating room and were given instruction in the use of plaster and apparatus. Lovett (1917) noted, "The amount of teaching is more than doubled" (Children's Hospital Archives). When course O.S.3 was added in 1918, the students (limited to two men) served as assistants in the outpatient department.

During WWI, two orthopaedic surgeons remained on staff at Children's Hospital, resulting in "a great depletion of the department," according to an August 1, 1919, letter from Dr. Lovett to Dr. Bradford; five were on leave of absence to serve in the military (Deans Files, Harvard Medical School). And yet Lovett noted in the same letter that teaching had not decreased, that he gave most of the lectures, and that teaching in the fourth year

Box 9.4. Developments in Third- and Fourth-Year Medical School Curricula throughout the Twentieth Century

The curriculum at Harvard Medical School (HMS) evolved throughout the twentieth century as broad developments advanced the medical field. Courses were added and removed, instructors came and went, and the process of student assessment varied.

1910

- Third-year students were required to take an orthopaedics course during the first half of the academic year. Lectures and demonstrations were given at HMS and Children's Hospital. The students completed clinical exercises at both Children's Hospital and MGH. A 15-minute examination was administered to students upon completion of this orthopaedic course.
- Two courses were added for fourth-year students at MGH and Children's Hospital:
    - O.S.1, which provided daily teaching each afternoon throughout the year
    - O.S.2, a quarter course held afternoons in October, December, February, and April (only at Children's Hospital)

1911

- The 15-minute examination administered upon completion of the required orthopaedic course was discontinued.

1916

- "O.S.2" was a "quarter course" (two–eight-weeks long, earning two credits) and was held in the afternoons, rather than the mornings, from October to April on the wards at Children's Hospital.
- A bone and joint rotation was added as a special service at Boston City Hospital.

1917

- Four orthopaedics courses, four–eight-weeks long, were taught at the MGH and Children's Hospital. Military surgeons attended these before being deployed overseas in World War I.

1918

- An "O.S.3" course was added. This was a quarter course held in the afternoons during January, July, September, October, and December at Children's Hospital. (The O.S.1 course was a prerequisite.)

1924

- Fourth-year electives were expanded to include:
    - O.S.3, held in the outpatient department at Children's Hospital
    - O.S.4, held in the outpatient department at MGH
    - O.S.5, held in the outpatient department at Children's Hospital and in the wards and outpatient department at MGH

1929

- Boston City Hospital was added as a site for the third-year required clinical exercises.
    - O.S.6, a one-half course held in the afternoons all year, was added as an elective to the fourth-year curriculum

1931

- Peter Bent Brigham Hospital was added as a site for the third-year required clinical exercises.
- Electives were added for fourth-year students:
    - A special one-half course ("Spinal Course: Orthopaedics") for a minimum of 10 students at MGH in December; this course earned four credits
    - An all-day or half-day Orthopaedic Clinical Course at Children's Hospital and MGH (entire year)
    - A half-day Orthopaedic Clinical Course in the mornings in the outpatient department at Children's Hospital (entire year)
    - A half-day Orthopaedic Clinical Course in the mornings in the outpatient department at MGH (entire year)
    - A clinical clerkship (part of the Orthopaedic Clinical Course) with Dr. Ober and his staff in the afternoons at Children's Hospital (entire year)
- Third-year students spent five weeks on each of the wards of the medical, surgical, and orthopaedic services at Children's Hospital.

1935

- Charles Mixter taught the first surgical course for third-year students at Beth Israel Hospital; this course in orthopaedic surgery comprised eight hours of lectures and 30 hours of section work (25 hours at Children's Hospital, two-and-a-half hours at the Peabody Home, and two-and-a-half hours at the Robert Breck Brigham Hospital).

- Additional teaching in orthopaedics was included as a part of surgery: 25 hours at the Peter Bent Brigham Hospital and specific times at both Children's Hospital and the Massachusetts General Hospital.

1936
- Required courses added in orthopaedics:
  - Daily lectures at Children's Hospital (from 10:00 a.m. to 12:30 p.m.) for half of the third year
  - Clinical exercises throughout the third year at Children's Hospital, MGH, PBBH, and Boston City Hospital
- Elective courses added in orthopaedics:
  - Three year-long orthopaedic clinical courses (Children's Hospital, MGH, and MGH/Children's Hospital)
  - Special orthopaedic courses (limited to 10 students) at MGH in December

1938
- Orthopaedic clinical exercises now included industrial surgery at MGH, PBBH, and Boston City Hospital; students were assigned to one hospital for three months.

1946–1947
- The required course in orthopaedics for the third-year students remained without any changes (except faculty: Green taught it in 1946 and Barr in 1947).
- Orthopaedic electives in the fourth year included three all-day courses:
  - An orthopaedic clinical course under Dr. Green at Children's Hospital (two students; one-month long)
  - An orthopaedic clinical course at both Children's Hospital and MGH (two students each month; one month long) a spine course under Dr. Barr at MGH (two students each month; one-month long)

1953
- Clinical exercises for third-year students were added at Beth Israel Hospital.
- Fourth-year students were required to do clinical exercises in orthopaedics during their surgical rotation at the Peter Bent Brigham Hospital.
- Peter Bent Brigham Hospital added an elective in orthopaedic clinical exercise.

1954
- A fourth-year elective in anatomy was added.

1958
- Third-year students were required to attend eight hours of lectures and complete a total of 65 hours of clinical exercises (35 of which were spent at Children's Hospital).

1960
- The required lectures for third-year students remained at eight hours, but the clinical exercises were increased to 80 hours (now 45 hours were spent at Children's Hospital and 35 hours at MGH, the PBBH, or BIH).
- MGH, PBBH, and BIH began requiring a clinical rotation in orthopaedics for fourth-year students on a surgical clerkship.

1964
- Required lectures in orthopaedics for the third-year class increased to 12 hours.
- The program began ward clerkships for third-year students, who spent two weeks at MGH or PBBH and one week at Children's Hospital (three weeks total).

1966
- A new elective course was added for fourth-year students: "Skiing Injuries," taught by Ellison and Wolf.
- A longitudinal course was added for fourth-year students: "Fractures and Related Trauma," taught by Green, Banks, Trott, Quigley and others.

1967
- The section on pathophysiology of the musculoskeletal system included 42 hours (up from 18 hours the previous year).
- The course on patient examination now lasted nine hours (the original duration is not known).
- One additional elective was added: "Orthopaedic Aspects of Rehabilitation," taught by Turner, Nalebuff, and Chandler at MGH.

1975
- Third-year students were required to take a three-month rotation in medicine and a two-month rotation in surgery.
- Students had to attend three core clerkships of their choice: dermatology, ophthalmology, otolaryngology, neurology, obstetrics and gynecology, orthopaedic surgery, pediatrics, psychiatry, radiology.
- Orthopaedic surgery was no longer required for all third-year students.

1977

• "General Orthopaedic Surgery," taught by Gillies and Scott, was now available at the West Roxbury Veterans Administration Hospital.

1979

• A one-month-long course in sports medicine was added as an elective: "Adult Orthopaedics and Sports Medicine," taught by Lowell, Sledge, Boland, and others. Two students attended each month, spending mornings at the PBBH and RBBH; during football season, afternoons were spent at the Dillon Field House with Dr. Boland.

1980

• A month-long "Introductory Orthopaedic Clerkship" was offered under Dr. White at BIH. Three students per month were accepted in November, February, and May.

1982

• Third-year students selected five areas—dermatology, neurology, obstetrics and gynecology, ophthalmology and otology, orthopaedic surgery, pediatrics, psychiatry, or radiology—and attended a one-month-long rotation in each at BWH and Children's Hospital.

1983

• The orthopaedic clerkship offered at BWH and Children's Hospital was reduced to two weeks after two months of surgery.

1987

• No core clerkships were offered (the two-week clerkship was discontinued).

• The "Hand Surgery" course taught by Nalebuff and Millender at both the RBBH and BIH was revised to "Hand Surgery and Rehabilitation" under Simmons at BWH and Children's Hospital.

1988

• The Hand Surgery clerkship at MGH, formerly led by Dr. Richard Smith, was now under the direction of Gelberman.

1990

• A two-month core clerkship in surgery began at MGH under Dr. W. G. Austin; at BWH under Dr. Mannick; at BIH under Dr. L. Goldman; and at Mt. Auburn, Faulkner, and New England Deaconess Hospitals. Orthopaedics

was not listed as an elective in any of these core surgical clerkships.

• The surgical clerkship at MGH now included a two-week elective in burns, urology, thoracic surgery, cardiac surgery, plastic surgery, or pediatric surgery.

• A one-week elective in either urology, plastic surgery, neurosurgery, or cardiac surgery was offered to third-year students in the surgical clerkship at BWH. (The other two surgical clerkships offered no electives.)

1991

• The clerkship at the BIH was now led by Dr. Meeks, who took over from Dr. Harris Yett.

1992

• No clerkship was offered at the WRVAMC.

• A new one-month clinical clerkship at the BWH was led by Yodlowski.

• A new course, "Problems in Osseous Reconstruction," was offered by Dr. Glowacki at the BWH. Four to eight students per month were assigned research topics and presented their research at weekly meetings. Each student was required to submit a proposal for an in-depth research project, and some went on to perform the research they proposed.

1993

• The course "Musculoskeletal Pathophysiology" was new in the Health Sciences and Technology program, under the direction of D.R. Robinson, a rheumatologist at MGH. Members of the orthopaedic departments participated (Drs. Glimcher, Sledge, and Hayes). The course was offered to 30 students for one month.

1994

• The rotation at the West Roxbury VA Medical Center was restarted under the direction of Dr. Minas.

• Pediatric orthopaedic rotations at Children's Hospital were now under the direction of Dr. Hresko. (Previously, the department chairman had supervised these rotations.)

• Glowacki's course titled "Problems in Osseous Reconstruction" was categorized under Basic Science rather than Orthopaedics.

1995

- Gelberman's elective clerkship in hand surgery at the MGH was discontinued.

1996

- Orthopaedic surgery was now offered to third-year students as an elective within the three-month core clerkship in surgery at the MGH, BWH, and NEDH.

- At the NEDH (course director: Dr. Stone), a one-month rotation through office practices was available for six to twelve students in orthopaedics, urology, or ENT.

- At the BWH (course directors: Drs. Soybel and Zinner), the final four weeks now included an outpatient experience in orthopaedics (two weeks), urology (one week), and head/neck surgery (one week).

- At the MGH (course director: Dr. W. G. Austin), students rotated for two weeks on orthopaedics, one week on urology, and one week on ENT.

- The director of the orthopaedic clerkship electives at MGH changed from Dr. Curtiss to Dr. Kornack.

- The third-year core clerkship in surgery included one month at BIDMC (six–twelve students), a required two-week outpatient rotation at the BWH, and a required two-week rotation at the MGH.

1999

- Among the orthopaedic clerkship electives, Dr. Ready became director of the VA rotation; Dr. Wright became director of the orthopaedic clinical clerkship at BWH; and Dr. Gill now directed the orthopaedic clerkships at MGH.

1999/2000

- Third-year students attended a Saturday morning session (three hours) that reviewed standardized cases presented by the faculty.

2000

- Students were expected to follow the clinical course of three inpatients each week. They obtained histories and performed physical examinations, participated in rounds, and functioned as interns on the service, writing notes and observing cases in the operating room. Each student was evaluated by a written examination and oral exit evaluation.

---

had "improved." The biggest change he described was the large number of surgeons from the army studying orthopaedics in the Harvard Graduate School (see chapter 16). In the 1917 annual report, he explained, "The hospital [Children's Hospital] has been one of the centers selected for the intensive training of military surgeons in orthopaedic surgery" (Children's Hospital Archives). Lovett stated in the report that courses for third- and fourth-year students were "satisfactory" but teaching to graduates "has fallen off very much" (Children's Hospital Archives). By July 30, 1919, 100 men had completed the course.

Following WWI, Lovett continued to give the third-year lectures (weekly from September 25 through December 22), and, with his assistants, was responsible for the clinical exercises (12 required for each student) at Children's and the MGH. In the annual report of 1922, Osgood noted that "His cosmopolitan viewpoint and his services to medical education in general, beyond the confines of his specialty, have been of inestimable value to the hospital. The heritage which he leaves must be wisely conserved" (Children's Hospital Archives). Orthopaedic teaching increased on the wards and in the outpatient departments. Osgood reported that the orthopaedic staff gave an average of 15 hours per week "of actual clinical and didactic instruction to undergraduates of the third and fourth years of the Harvard Medical School" (Children's Hospital Archives). Dr. Osgood replaced Dr. Lovett as professor of orthopaedics in 1924. Osgood's lectures were always at 2:00 p.m. and section work from 9:00 a.m. to 11:30 a.m. He also expanded the fourth-year electives (see Box 9.4).

The curriculum committee had considered additional changes since 1928. In a letter June 7, 1928, Dr. Allison, the chief of orthopaedics at MGH, commented upon the committee's report when he wrote the following to Dean Edsall:

There seems little to add [to the committee's report] beyond praise for the thoroughness with which the subject is handled. It boils down all the conversations, kinks, fault findings, destructive remarks, etc. that one has heard in the last ten years into tangible form, so that one may say yes or no to many of the propositions...contained in the report...they are much to be congratulated, as the report is free from the exaggeration or foolishness which is often encountered in articles recently written on the subject. I...feel that all of the tentative recommendations...should be tried out, as I am very much in favor of making the student educate himself, not only in the medical school, but throughout his professional life. 'Self-starting' and 'self-propelling' education is what we need...I find that their [students] powers of observation have been sadly neglected. They are not asked often enough what they see, hear, or feel...when they do see or feel something, they try to remember what it means rather than to think what it means. Of course, I find my activity in a special field, and the part of the report which is concerned with the specialist is not half forceful enough to suit my taste. A subject such as orthopaedic surgery should not be taught to medical students except as part of general surgery and general medicine. The undergraduate student is not concerned in any way with the special methods of treatment and technique used in orthopaedic surgery. If we might get the student to bear in mind the importance of tuberculosis of the bones and joints as a general affair so that he would not forget it when he sees a child complaining of pain in the abdomen or extremities, we will have accomplished more that has

yet been accomplished in medical teaching...I am all for having one year or preferably eighteen months, or best of all, two years of hospital experience required by state boards before a man may enter medical practice...I do not believe that the specialist can contribute anything to undergraduate medical education by demonstrating instruments for examination, or showing how patients are treated. His value is solely confined to the importance of finding out what is the matter with...the patient...the importance of early and accurate diagnosis... get them [medical students] to frown upon any attempt made by us at 'spoon fed correlation' we will have accomplished something...I am all for carrying out as speedily...without resolutions, all of recommendations...contained in...this report. I believe we are doing better... towards accomplishing some such results than are other schools... (Deans Files, Harvard Medical School)

On June 2, Osgood also responded to the Curriculum Committee's report:

I have been over the tentative report...and discussed it with Dr. Blackfan and Dr. Allison at some length...The proposed change in the curriculum appeals to me very strongly as a change in the right direction. The Orthopaedic Department for the last five years has had no didactic lectures. In the time allotted to the Department in the third year class, once a week during the first half year for twelve lectures, the men have given a directional lecture in mimeographed form a week before the lecture was due, and the hour has been used for demonstrated clinical cases, a quiz of the students on the subject and a conference with the students in which they asked questions of us. I should personally be very sorry to see this type of exercise in Orthopaedic Surgery cut down very materially, for the students have seemed to find it very profitable. They have certainly cooperated in the exercise very heartedly and it has greatly simplified the teaching in clinics. In these lectures to the whole class and in the clinics we make no attempt to teach the specialty of Orthopaedic Surgery, but only the contacts which every practitioner ought to be ready to meet between Orthopaedic Surgery, General Surgery and General Medicine...I am sure each specialist feels that his own specialty is of extreme importance to the general practitioner and I feel strongly that this is the fact with Orthopaedic Surgery. It is not an anatomic specialty, but it deals with the function of the whole locomotive apparatus...with many types of chronic lesions of the bone and joints. The problems of chronic diseases are those which the general practitioner is constantly called on to solve and which must make up a considerable portion of his practice. In any survey of chronic disease, bone and joint conditions loom large. The Orthopaedic Department will be glad to cooperate most heartily in this proposed change in the curriculum. (Deans Files, Harvard Medical School)

In 1931, Ober became the professor of orthopaedics and gave the required third year orthopaedic surgery lectures. He too made changes in the electives (see **Box 9.4**). In 1935, Dr. Elliott Cutler published a paper, "Undergraduate Teaching of Surgery" in the *Annals of Surgery* (E. C. Cutler 1935). He wrote:

Unfortunately, the impetus toward improvement [in medical education] has been entirely upon undergraduate education and we have now reached the peculiar position...where we turn out...well trained men from our medical schools, but have a totally inadequate mechanism for giving them the necessary practical and special training and experience during the first few years after graduation, so that they may practice the dangerous specialties of their profession with safety...perhaps more glaring in

relation to surgery and its specialties...Legally there are no restrictions once a graduate has passed his state licensing board examinations... Thus the American public may be legally cared for, indeed, subjected to a dangerous surgical procedure, by a student who has just been graduated from medical school. This creates an entirely anomalous situation, for...every teacher of repute in...surgery agrees that it is not his duty to teach the undergraduate medical student practical surgery. He feels it is his task to train the young student in the principles of surgery...our good teachers are about unanimous in their opinion that...teaching...the technical steps of major surgery is a postgraduate problem. This means that we teach much less technical surgery than 20 years ago...Surgery is definitely a postgraduate problem...The curriculum in practically all medical schools follows the block system. The basic sciences occupy the greater part of the first two years... The curriculum for the last two years is given over to clinical study...The curriculum for the last two years is well standardized. Didactic lectures and clinics give to the student a skeleton of regional surgery on which to hang his varied ward and outpatient experiences. The exact order of these last two years is somewhat divided...in the majority of schools...the third-year students in small groups with an instructor are acquainted with disease in the out-patient departments, spending their fourth year on the hospital wards as clinical clerks...The standardization of undergraduate education is almost startling. It is true that the teaching of fractures, anesthesia and the amount of time given to the surgical specialties all vary widely, but that is largely because of the type and supply of material, not because the teachers themselves have a divergent opinion of what it is wisest to teach. [A]...questionnaire [was] sent out to the Class A medical schools [surgery chiefs in 51 schools]...the answers are summarized [as follows]:

What Are the Important Matters to Teach the Undergraduate Medical Student?

Surgical Diagnosis	32
The Principles of Surgery	30
Keep Specialties in the Background	28
The Basic Courses	16
Trauma and Sepsis	13
Clinical Surgery	8
The Indications for Surgery	5
Ambulatory Surgery (minor surgery)	5
Prospective and Postoperative Care	4

Orthopaedics was not taught in the first two years of any of the 51 schools in Cutler's survey of Class A medical schools (these were standard four-year medical schools as defined by the AMA in about 1920), and most of the surgical chiefs saw danger in students specializing too early in their career. Orthopaedics was taught in the third year in only five schools and in the fourth year in two schools, Cutler stated:

Some specialties creep in as special courses...only a negligible percentage of teachers feel that they should teach practical operative surgery...It is obvious that there is great unanimity in keeping the education general, avoiding emphasis on the specialties, and that the curriculum...is set up to ground the students in the essentials and to acquaint them specifically with methods of caring for trauma and sepsis... [and] teaching of anesthesia is inadequate and should be remedied...the real education of the surgeon is a postgraduate affair. (E. C. Cutler 1935)

On November 16, 1934, Dr. George A. Leland Jr. proposed the following schedule for teaching the topic of fractures for the second-, third-, and fourth-year students (Deans Files, Harvard Medical School):

PROPOSED SCHEDULE FOR TEACHING OF FRACTURES IN THE HARVARD MEDICAL SCHOOL

	Lectures MGH	Lab. HMS	Clinic MGH BCH
SECOND YEAR			
1. General Principles—Nomenclature and Repair	●		
2. General Principles—Dx, Treat., Prog.	●		
3. Clavicle, Scapula, Ribs, Emerg. Splinting U.E.		●	
4. Shoulder, Humeral Shaft. Non-Union	●		
5. Elbow, Condyles, Epicondyles, Rad. Head, Neck		●	
6. Both Bones Forearm, Malar, Jaw			●
7. Colles'		●	
8. Carpus, Metacarpus, Phalanges		●	
9. Hip and Trochanters	●		
10. Femoral Shaft and Condyles	●	●	
11. Patella and Olecranon			●
12. Both Bones Leg and Compound Fractures	●		
13. Ankle, Emergency Splinting L.E.		●	
14. Foot and Pelvis			●
15. Dislocations, Sprain and Strains		●	

THIRD YEAR

a) Eight Fracture Clinics for each section. M.G.H. and B.C.H. (one clinic each month)

b) One Group Clinic per week for each Surgical Sub-Section.

FOURTH YEAR

One Group Clinic per week for each Surgical Sub-Section.

Little change occurred in the curriculum for undergraduates in orthopaedic surgery in the medical school for the rest of the duration of Dr. Ober's tenure as professor and chief at Children's Hospital. In the annual report of 1935, Ober noted that the bulk of the orthopaedic teaching to medical students was "carried out at Children's Hospital" (Children's Hospital Archives). Ober wrote that each third-year student spent "five weeks on the wards of the medical, surgical and orthopaedic services...monthly conferences are held throughout the year [house officers also participate], attended by medical students and many outside practitioners" (Children's Hospital Archives). However, as assistant dean, he felt strongly about the importance of continuing medical education after medical school (see chapter 8). In an address to Tufts Medical School Alumni, he stated:

Your capital is your brain...One of the great weaknesses in medicine today is that failure of the doctor to go to school after he has

graduated. There are probably many reasons for this; but most of them boil down to inertia, disinclination to spend the necessary money, or self-satisfaction. Inertia may be overcome. The money can be saved for postgraduate courses out of income...you owe it to yourself and your patients to do so. Self-satisfaction is an unrealized sin and no amount of praying will cure such a disease; it must be plucked out! Increasing your capital can be done only by education...Remember this,—there is no short cut to knowledge...To be successful...there are three good rules for success: To be on time, do your job better today than yesterday and above all, be human. Finally, no one should go into the study of medicine unless he wants to do that more than anything else in the world. (F. R. Ober 1939)

Dr. Ober sent the following schedule of teaching clinics for the third-year class at the Peter Bent Brigham Hospital to the dean in 1939 (Deans Files, Harvard Medical School):

SCHEDULE OF ORTHOPAEDIC CLINICS THIRD YEAR STUDENTS P.B.B.H.
9:45–12:00
September 26, 1939 to December 9, 1939

Monday			Thursday	
Sep. 28	Dr. Elliston, Dr. Green			
Oct. 2	Dr. Karp, Dr. Hugenberger		Oct. 5	Dr. Elliston, Dr. Brewster
Oct. 9	Dr. Karp, Dr. Hugenberger		Oct. 12	HOLIDAY
Oct. 16	Dr. Karp, Dr. Hugenberger		Oct. 19	Dr. Elliston, Dr. Brewster
Oct. 23	Dr. Karp, Dr. Hugenberger		Oct. 26	Dr. Elliston, Dr. Green
Oct. 30	Dr. Karp, Dr. Hugenberger		Nov. 2	Dr. Elliston, Dr. Brewster
Nov. 6	Dr. Karp, Dr. Hugenberger		Nov. 9	Dr. Elliston, Dr. Green
Nov. 13	Dr. Karp, Dr. Hugenberger		Nov. 16	Dr. Elliston, Dr. Brewster
Nov. 20	Dr. Karp, Dr. Hugenberger		Nov. 23	Dr. Elliston, Dr. Green
Nov. 27	Dr. Karp, Dr. Hugenberger		Nov. 30	HOLIDAY
Dec. 4	Dr. Karp, Dr. Hugenberger		Dec. 7	Dr. Elliston, Dr. Green

TOPIC ASSIGNMENTS
Monday Afternoon Exercises
Third-Year Students P.B.B.H.
1:15–1:50

Oct. 2	Introduction	Dr. Green
Oct. 9	Posture: Its Evaluation and Clinical Importance	Dr. Hugenberger
Oct. 16	Low Back Pain: Dx and Treatment Sciatica	Dr. Karp
Oct 23	Feet: Pronation, Foot Strain, Bunions	Dr. Elliston
Oct 30	Internal Derangements of the Knee. Joint Mice Osteo-chondritis Dissecans	Dr. Green
Nov. 6	Pain in Region of the Shoulder: Subacromial Bursitis, Ruptured Supraspinatus, Calcification of Supraspinatus Tendon, Tennis Elbow, etc.	Dr. Hugenberger
Nov. 13	Arthritis: Atrophic and Hypertrophic: Pathology, General Considerations, Therapy, Coxae Morbus Senilis	Dr. Karp
Nov. 20	Dislocations and Sprains	Dr. Elliston
Nov. 27	Tumors of Bone	Dr. Green
Dec. 4	Osteomyelitis: Diagnosis and Treatment	Dr. Hugenberger

The orthopaedic section of third-year students in 1939 had the following schedule at Children's Hospital (also supplied by Dr. Ober):

ORTHOPAEDIC SECTION—THIRD YEAR STUDENTS
September 26, 1939, to October 31, 1939

Tues. Sept. 26	9:45–12:00	ABCD	Introduction—Amphitheatre Drs. Diamond, MacCollum, Green
Thur. Sept. 28	9:45–10:45	AB	Poliomyelitis—Amphitheatre—Dr. Brewster
	10:45–1:00	AB	Rounds—Ward—Dr. Sever
	10:45–1:00	CD	Apparatus-Amphitheatre Annex and Ward V—Dr. Karp
Fri. Sept. 29	9:45–12:00	CD	Rounds—Ward V—Dr. Elliston
Mon. Oct. 2	4:00–5:30	ABCD	Combined Clinical Conference Amphitheatre—Dr. Ober
Tues. Oct. 3	9:45–12:00	AB	Out-Patient Depart.—Dr. McDermott
Thur. Oct. 5	9:45–12:00	AB	Apparatus—Amphitheatre Annex and Ward V— Dr. Hugenberger
	9:45–12:00	CD	Out-Patient Depart.—Dr. McDermott
	12:00–1:00	ABCD	Developmental and Congenital Diseases Dr. Green, Amphitheatre
	2:00–3:00	AB	Scoliosis—Dr. Kuhns—Bader Building
Fri. Oct. 6	9:45–1:00	CD	T.B. Bones and Joints—Peabody Home—Dr. Cave
Tues. Oct. 10	9:45–1:00	AB	Arthritis—Robert Brigham Hospital—Dr. Swaim
Wed. Oct. 11	2:00–3:00	ABCD	Obstetrical Paralysis—Bader Building—Dr. Kuhns

ORTHOPAEDIC SECTION—THIRD YEAR STUDENTS

Thur. Oct. 12			HOLIDAY
Fri. Oct. 13	9:45–12:00	CD	Infantile Clinic—Bader Building
Tues. Oct. 17	9:45–12:00	AB	Infantile Clinic—Bader Building
Wed. Oct. 18	2:00–3:00	ABCD	Spastic Paralysis—Bader Building—Dr. Karp
Thur. Oct. 19	9:45–10:45	ABCD	Septic Joints—Dr. Green—Amphitheatre
	10:45–12:00	ABCD	Presentation of Cases—Amphitheatre— Dr. Green
Fri. Oct. 20	9:45–1:00	CD	Arthritis—Robert Brigham Hospital—Dr. Swaim
Mon. Oct. 23	3:30–5:30	ABCD	Orthopaedic Clinical Conference Amphitheatre—Dr. Morris
Tues. Oct 24	9:45–1:00	AB	T.B. Bones and Joints—Peabody Home—Dr. Brewster
Thur. Oct. 26	9:45–1:00	ABCD	Final Conference—Warren Museum—Drs. Ober, Hugenberger and Brewster
Fri. Oct. 27	9:45–10:45	CD	Body Mechanics and Statics Amphitheatre—Dr. Brown
	10:45–12:00	CD	Gymnasium—Dr. Brown
Tues. Oct. 31	9:45–10:45	AB	Body Mechanics and Statics Amphitheatre—Dr. Brown
	10:45–12:00	AB	Gymnasium—Dr. Brown

About this same time, Dr. Ober proposed his plan for Harvard Medical School's teaching departments using orthopaedics as an example:

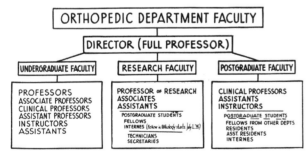

PROPOSED TYPICAL HARVARD MEDICAL SCHOOL TEACHING DEPARTMENT.

ORTHOPEDIC DEPARTMENT FACULTY

DIRECTOR (FULL PROFESSOR)

UNDERGRADUATE FACULTY — RESEARCH FACULTY — POSTGRADUATE FACULTY

PROFESSORS
ASSOCIATE PROFESSORS
CLINICAL PROFESSORS
ASSISTANT PROFESSORS
INSTRUCTORS
ASSISTANTS

PROFESSOR or RESEARCH
ASSOCIATES
ASSISTANTS
POSTGRADUATE STUDENTS
FELLOWS
INTERNES (below a Bkology starts July 1, '35)
TECHNICIANS
SECRETARIES

CLINICAL PROFESSORS
ASSISTANTS
INSTRUCTORS
POSTGRADUATE STUDENTS
FELLOWS FROM OTHER DEPTS.
RESIDENTS
ASST. RESIDENTS
INTERNES

UNDERGRADUATE COURSES LEADING TO M. D. DEGREE
POSTGRADUATE COURSES LEADING TO CERTIFICATES, MASTERS and D.Sc.(ORTHOPEDIC)
RESEARCH: AWARDS OF MASTERS DEGREE. PH.D. and D. Sc.

Office of the Dean subject files, 1899-1953 (inclusive), Box 12, Folder 9:446.

Harvard Medical Library in the Francis A. Countway Library of Medicine.

In his annual department report at Children's Hospital in 1940, Dr. Ober wrote:

The intimate connection of the Children's Hospital with the Harvard Medical School means that the bulk of instruction in orthopedic surgery is carried on in the Out-Patient Department, wards and special allied clinics. The whole third-year class came to the hospital in sections of twenty-four for a period of five weeks. There are always a few fourth-year men who take elective orthopedics and come in small groups remaining for a month. In addition to undergraduates, there are courses in postgraduate work arranged for a large group or for single men who wish to have the contact with the hospital work and members of our staff.
(Children's Hospital Archives)

In 1939, Harvard conducted a student survey to evaluate the curriculum. At the time, orthopaedics was taught at Children's Hospital, the Peter Bent Brigham Hospital, the Robert Breck Brigham Hospital, and Massachusetts General Hospital; nevertheless, orthopaedics was not included in the survey. Dr. Ober complained about this fact in a letter to Dean Burwell, but I could not find any response from the dean. Only 30% of the students filled out the survey, and in their responses requested a need for more teaching in minor surgery and emergency work.

Small stipends that had been paid from Harvard to a special orthopaedic account at the Massachusetts General Hospital for teaching were now paid directly to Dr. Smith-Petersen and Dr. W. A. Rogers after discussions with Dr. Ober and Dean Burwell. This change meant that the two physicians would pay individual taxes on these payments. MGH also had a special teaching fund from special gifts from friends and patients. These funds were not registered at MGH or Harvard University. Dr. Ober was very concerned about the tax issues because the portion paid to him listed as salary was used for course expenses. He cited the following example: with 13 students registered, he made frequent ward rounds and about 30 to 35 instructors (paid $5.00 per hour) were involved with a one-month course; generating $700 or $800 of listed incomes that he used for expenses. He obviously objected to potentially having to pay taxes on this payment, which he did not consider income. Dean Edsall desired to financially support clinicians who "relinquish active practice to teach [required a stipend from both Harvard Medical School and the hospital for department heads and junior members of the department]" and "who are devoting the major part of their time to teaching, investigation and administration" (Deans Files, Harvard Medical School). However, Drs. Ober, Osgood, Barr, and Smith-Petersen and other early orthopaedic leaders were not full-time (without limit of time), but instead clinical professors. They received little, if any, financial support from Harvard. Financial support for orthopaedic surgery has always been a problem in the Harvard system and continues to be in the present.

It was in 1932 that Beth Israel Hospital began courses for Harvard medical students, a particularly bad time for department budgets because of cuts by Harvard Medical School. In 1937, the hospital's board of trustees authorized the hospital director, Dr. Charles F. Wilensky, to move ahead with preparing a budget for a Harvard Surgical Teaching and Research service at Beth Israel Hospital. Dr. Mixter was chief of surgery. The proposal was supported by Dean Burwell and a budget for salaries in surgery at Beth Israel Hospital from Harvard Medical School began in 1939; they had started for medicine in 1934. The dean supported medicine and surgery but not other new specialties like orthopaedics; orthopaedic surgery was not included. Beth Israel Hospital originally "related itself both to Tufts and to Harvard," Dean Burwell wrote December 7, 1939, in a memorandum in his support of Beth Israel Hospital's affiliation with Harvard Medical School: "One of the problems which we face in accepting Jewish students of the first rank, as we are anxious to do, is that there now exists a certain amount of prejudice in hospitals and that they have some difficulty in getting hospital appointments. The Beth Israel Hospital offers first-rate opportunities in Medicine and Surgery for the training of Jewish physicians and surgeons" (Deans Files, Harvard Medical School). At the time, Jewish physicians were not permitted to practice in many US hospitals.

In 1934 the total number of hours in orthopaedic surgery for third-year students was 38; in surgery the total was 175 hours. However, in 1937, Dr. William T. Green wrote that the students at Children's do "not [work] as many hours as [those at the] Peter Bent Brigham Hospital [and those students at Massachusetts General have] adequate teaching but [I do] not know the number of hours" (Deans Files, Harvard Medical School). As chief resident, he noted he would "be glad to submit a written report on Orthopaedic Surgery Teaching" (Deans Files, Harvard Medical School). In 1946, Dr. Green was appointed professor of orthopaedic surgery at Children's Hospital; in 1947, Dr. Barr was appointed professor of orthopaedic surgery at the Massachusetts General Hospital.

In 1947, Dr. Barr was a member of the American Orthopaedic Association's Committee on

Undergraduate Training. The AOA held a Conference of Teachers of Orthopaedic Surgery in conjunction with its combined meeting (American, British and Canadian Orthopaedic Associations) in Quebec, Canada, on June 5, 1948. In addition to AOA members, invitations were sent to deans of medical schools in the United States and Canada, the Association of American Medical Colleges, and the AMA's Council on Medical Education and Hospitals. One hundred fifty-five leaders in education attended. Dr. Green presented a paper, "The Well-Balanced Curriculum in Orthopaedic Surgery" (W. T. Green 1949a), in which he stated:

> It is quite obvious to all of us that in many schools…orthopaedic surgery does not receive its due. In most schools, a representative of the departments…does not serve on the curriculum committee…Often to those serving in such a position, orthopaedic surgery represents a specialty of very limited nature, and it is awarded the same amount of time as is given a specialty limited in scope and confined to one small anatomical area. My remarks are made with the understanding that orthopaedic surgery is a major branch of surgery and… the problems in this field are some of the most common in medical practice…the purpose of undergraduate teaching in orthopaedic surgery is…to teach…basic principles…essential to a balanced education. It seems to me that somewhere between 20 and 25 per cent of the teaching time in surgery should be assigned to the department of orthopaedic surgery…One of the main difficulties, other than too little time… is that it is frequently worked into the curriculum in haphazard fashion…Frequently lectures in the clinical years are scheduled without regard to the time of sectional instruction… In our experience students arrive…to…orthopaedic surgery in the third year with little background leading to its understanding. The time to start the teaching of orthopaedic surgery is in the first year…the Department…should take part in first-year and second-year teaching… correlated with the instruction given in the departments of basic science. I should like to present a sample curriculum…

The First Year

In the first year, instruction by the department of orthopaedic surgery should be correlated with the work in anatomy and physiology. Six or seven lectures may be given, as follows:

1. General: musculoskeletal system, body mechanics
2. The trunk and neck; the back.
3. and 4. Upper extremities
5. and 6. Lower extremities; gait.
7. Abnormalities in embryological development; bone growth

All of these lectures should stress normal musculoskeletal mechanisms…Visits of the orthopaedic surgeon with the students in the dissection room at appropriate times is also most helpful.

The Second Year

If pathology has been taught in the first semester of the second year, it is desirable to have a schedule of orthopaedic exercises in the second half year. These should be designed to acquaint the student with a basic concept of abnormalities of the musculoskeletal system and to show him patients with these problems. Ten lectures, appropriately illustrated, might be given during this second year and might be listed as follows:

1. The problems arising in the musculoskeletal system; examination of a patient.
2. The trauma of bones.

3. Infections of bones.

4. Joint phenomena, infection, trauma; tendons, bursae, and tendon sheaths.

5. Abnormalities of growth, tumors.

6. Paralysis.

7. Developmental and congenital diseases and abnormalities.

8. Mechanical abnormalities.

9. Metabolic disease (probably by division of medicine).

10. Therapeutic measures, general, in relation to pathological processes; traction, casts, exercises, etcetera.

In addition to these lectures, there should be sectional work in physical diagnosis of the musculoskeletal system, taught by an orthopaedic surgeon. These sections should not contain more than six students for certain of the activities, but the sectional work may well be combined with demonstrations in larger groups... There should be approximately four exercises, — that is, four mornings of sectional instruction in relatively close continuity, occupying a total of twelve hours. In addition to these exercises, it is highly desirable to arrange for a single visit of each section for two to three hours to the orthopaedic out-patient department to illustrate the problems that arise. This visit should be supervised by an instructor, as should another morning exercise at which the section should make ward rounds to see the problems that are represented and the techniques of treatment. Another exercise may well be instruction in basic first-aid, bandaging, and other details, if they are not otherwise covered in the curriculum. In all, then, we have had nine or ten lectures of one hour each, and six morning sectional periods of three hours each, totaling eighteen hours of sectional work and ten hours of lecture.

The Third Year

This is the time when the students become more intimately acquainted with the patient, with orthopaedic surgery, and the problems of the musculoskeletal system. The purpose is not to teach orthopaedic surgery as a specialty, but to give an understanding of the musculoskeletal system in its relation to the patient as a whole, which is applicable to medicine in general.

The third year should emphasize sectional work with patients, but some teaching can well be performed in large groups, particularly with visual aids. There is much to be said for and against the lecture including whole classes at this time...The ideal would be to present the subjects, well illustrated and in lecture form, to the whole group and to correlate the sectional work with it;...Translated into detail, there could well be about twenty lectures or exercises corresponding to lectures...These lectures might be tentatively listed as follows:

1. The patient and the musculoskeletal system.

2. and 3. Congenital anomalies (specific problems, congenital hip disorders, club-foot, other anomalies).

4. Development diseases (miscellaneous, coxa plana, slipped epiphysis, et cetera).

5. 6. and 7. Neuromuscular abnormalities, including poliomyelitis, obstetrical paralysis, cerebral palsy, et cetera.

8. and 9. The joints: arthritis, trauma, other conditions.

10. Specific infection of bone,—osteomyelitis, tuberculosis.

11. and 12. The back: the spine, including cervical spine, mechanical difficulties, back pain, sciatica, scoliosis.

13. Tumors and related abnormalities.

14. Upper extremity, general.

15. Lower extremity, hips to knees inclusive.

16. Leg and foot.

17. Fractures: general management, simple, compound.

18. Fractures, upper extremity.

19. Fractures, spine.

20. and 21. Fractures, lower extremity...

This sectional assignment should approximate four weeks and should certainly not be less than three weeks.

The Fourth Year

In our experience this has been planned in correlation with general surgery, when the students have their long sectional assignment in this field. If four months are assigned to surgery, the student's total time in orthopaedic surgery, including fractures, should be not less than two weeks...Likewise all the students in the large surgical section should make regular teaching rounds with the orthopaedic service, perhaps once a week...The students should be responsible for the work-up of patients, they should "scrub up" for the operations on their assigned cases, and participate in all the activities affecting these patients. In addition, it is our belief that one month of elective orthopaedic surgery should be offered in the fourth year...performing many of the duties of a junior house officer.

It has not been our purpose to outline these details with the idea that they should be followed, but merely to represent a pattern of instruction and to emphasize that the teaching of orthopaedic surgery should start in the first year and should be gradually woven into the fabric of the curriculum.

At the same conference, Dr. Barr presented a paper on "The Use of Audio-Visual Aids in Teaching" (J. S. Barr 1949). Briefly, he stated:

The "chalk talk" is the simplest example of audio visual education. Roentgenograms, dissected specimens, the articulated skeleton, et cetera, may be used as visual material can be seen by only a handful of students at one time. To overcome this...the visual image is enlarged by projection from lantern slides...motion-picture films of operative procedures...in my opinion, have little or no place in undergraduate teaching. There does seem to be a place for a few well-made basic films on orthopaedic subjects...such films...would improve the general quality of our teaching and give the student a far better concept of orthopaedic disabilities...such as "The Locomotor System"...include[ing] film[s] on "physical examination"..."trauma and repair,"...on "the aging process"...on "normal and abnormal gaits," and...one on "poliomyelitis"...This appears to be a field in which carefully planned, concerted action [including fundraising] is necessary. I suggest that the time for action has arrived.

In the decade following WWII, a medical school survey evaluated who treats and who teaches about fractures. The survey, organized by the AAOS Fracture Committee (H. R. Johnson and S. L. Stovall 1949), reported the following results:

Answers	Number of Schools	Percentage
Total Schools	70	100
Schools heard from	67	95.7
Fractures treated on orthopaedic service	40	57.1
Fractures treated on general surgery service	27	38.6
Teaching by orthopaedic surgeons	37	52.9
Teaching by general surgeons	9	12.8
Teaching by both orthopaedic and general surgeons	22	31.4

During this decade little, if any, changes occurred in the medical school curriculum in orthopaedics.

Orthopaedic surgery was listed separately and not under surgery in the 1962 catalog of courses. In 1960, the third-year course at Children's Hospital increased both the total number of hours spent teaching and added the use of small groups with the approval of both students and faculty. In the annual report that year, Dr. Green wrote: "Trauma and orthopedic diseases of the skeletal and neuromuscular system are forming a larger and larger portion of medicine; expansion in instruction in the area is greatly needed" (Children's Hospital Archives). Beginning in 1940, there were teaching sections of 25 students, each that lasted for five weeks, with a small number of subsections. The fourth-year course in orthopaedics was an elective.

In 1961, Dr. Green was chairman of the AAOS subcommittee on undergraduate teaching in the Committee on Education. The committee members were: Thomas D. Brower, Guy A. Caldwell, Eldon G. Chuinard, J. William Hillman, Carroll B. Larson, H. Relton McCarroll, Robert D. Ray and Fred C. Reynolds. Appointed in 1958, the committee was charged to make recommendations about teaching orthopaedic surgery to medical students. They surveyed the status of orthopaedic courses in medical schools and the opinions of orthopaedic department chairmen. They found the following current practices:

FIRST TWO YEARS...The teaching by orthopaedic surgeons during these first two years was most irregular [34 schools had orthopaedists participating in the curriculum in the first year; 30 did not; in the second year 50 participated; 14 did not]...In the second year, the most constant activity...was participation in the teaching of physical diagnosis...The average total time of teaching was two- and three-tenths hours in the first year and ten- and three-tenths hours in the second year...

THIRD YEAR: Fifty-four of the sixty-one schools gave instruction in orthopaedics and fractures in the third year...In eight schools the teaching was restricted to the whole class; in twelve...to small groups; and thirty-four schools utilized both small-group and whole-class teaching...The average number of hours...in all schools for the third year was fifty-four...

FOURTH YEAR: Fifty-seven [of 61 orthopaedic departments] participated in the teaching of fourth-year students...In four schools the teaching was confined to the entire class,...thirty-one...to small groups only and in twenty-two the instruction was given to both small groups and the whole class...On the average, each senior student received approximately seventy-five hours of exposure to orthopaedics...Two of the schools had no teaching of fourth-year students except in elective courses...No school rated both its third-year and fourth-year programs as excellent... It was particularly difficult to access accurately the teaching of fractures and trauma... [regarding] 'team approach' in the teaching of trauma...nineteen used...such an approach, and twenty-nine did not...

CONCLUSIONS AND RECOMMENDATIONS...The objective in the teaching of orthopaedic surgery...is to give the student basic concepts, understanding, and knowledge in this area of surgery in proportion to its importance in the total field of medicine and in the balanced education of the student. The first recommendation was that more emphasis should be placed on the neuromusculoskeletal system in the first two years...in the teaching of basic sciences and by providing more teaching by orthopaedic surgeons...In the first year, at least eight hours...most of this time should be related to anatomy...In addition, teaching programs correlated with physiology and biochemistry would be highly desirable...In the second year, twenty hours seems to be the minimum...ten to twelve hours of physical diagnosis taught by orthopaedic surgeons...Also in the second year, lectures and lecture demonstrations to the whole class on the basic phenomena and responses of the musculoskeletal system...on such subjects as the reactions of bone, skeletal growth and development, the neuromuscular system...factors producing deformity, and basic concepts of therapy. Eight such lectures and lecture-demonstrations represent a minimum number...In the third and fourth years, the patient and his diseases are emphasized... distribution of time and assignments between the third and fourth year depends on the general curriculum...we favor...seventy-eight hours of instruction during the third year and two weeks of clinical clerkship (eighty hours) during the fourth year...for the third year...a certain number of lecture-demonstrations and symposia for the whole class, totaling...eighteen to twenty hours...cover[ing] all needs of orthopaedic surgery, including fractures and...rehabilitation... The remainder of the time in the third year would be devoted to small-group teaching... dealing with patients in the out-patient clinic and on the ward...including both children and adults...In the fourth year...the student should be assigned for two weeks...as a clinical clerk. He should live with the Service and participate in its activities in a complete way....an ideal plan would...[include two weeks also in] the emergency room...At the end of...medical school... the student should have enough understanding of fractures and trauma to meet medical emergencies that any physician may be called on to face. A clinical clerkship in orthopaedic surgery for every medical student is considered highly desirable...for eighty hours...It does seem that 186 hours is the minimum amount which will permit adequate instruction...[but] 200 to 220 hours would be an ideal assignment [for orthopaedics in the curriculum]...Teaching should be

the primary interest of a department of orthopaedics, and, indeed, of a medical school. (W. T. Green et al. 1961)

After reviewing the orthopaedic curriculum at Harvard Medical School from 1872 through 1990, I do not believe that Dr. Green's and his committee's recommendations were ever fully accepted at Harvard Medical School.

However, some significant changes in the orthopaedic curriculum for medical students occurred in the mid-1960s. Dr. Green in his annual report of 1963 stated: "orthopaedics is a required part of the curriculum for the first time" (Children's Hospital Archives). Since orthopaedics had been a requirement in the third year, it is not clear what Dr. Green meant. He did state that this change was a great advance and required new and added responsibilities. He may have been referring to the fact that orthopaedic surgery was now responsible for its own course and not just a part of the surgical clerkship.

The new curriculum for the third- and fourth-year students began in September 1964. As Green noted in the 1963 annual report, the clerkship in orthopaedic surgery increased "the responsibilities of our Department and the time which our faculty must devote to students. This change... in our judgment is a great advance, and we are pleased to meet this new and added responsibility" (Children's Hospital Archives). The clinical exercises continued at MGH, CH, PBBH, BIH, and BCH. Clinical exercises in orthopaedics also continued in the general surgery course at BIH, MGH, and PBBH. There were no changes in the electives. In the annual report in 1966, Green noted additionally that "a section of pathophysiology of the musculoskeletal system was added to the second-year curriculum in which our department participated...long overdue and was a recognition of the school of the great void that existed in pathophysiology...[and] the exercises were well received by the student" (Children's Hospital Archives).

Other changes occurred in 1965 when Dr. Glimcher, along with Dr. Green oversaw the orthopaedic courses. The only change in the required third-year course was that orthopaedics was no longer listed in the general surgery course. But electives were expanded as follows:

Block courses:

501M	Children's Ortho	Green, Trott & Assoc. CH
502M	Children's Ortho	Green, Banks & Assoc. PBBH
503M	Adult Ortho	Green, Banks & Assoc. PBBH, CH
504M	Functional Anatomy, Biomechanics, Reconstructive	Kermond and Pierce MGH
505M	Clin Ortho Surg, Fractions, Trauma	Glimcher, Barr & Assoc. MGH

Block Courses—Research:

801	Musculoskeletal System	Banks
802	Musculoskeletal System	Cohen
803	Musculoskeletal System	Green
804	Musculoskeletal System	Pappas
805	Research Problems in Struc. and Function of Bone, Cartilage	Glimcher & Assoc., MGH
806	Electrophysiology of Skeletal Muscle	Pierce, MGH

Longitudinal Course:

701	Trauma	Moore, Green, Banks, Quigley, Matsen, Harrison, Van Dorn, Morgan, PBBH

(Official Register of Harvard University 1965)

Further changes occurred in 1966 in the orthopaedic curriculum. In the second year, a required course was added: a musculoskeletal section in pathophysiology and examination of the patient (total 18 hours). Introduction to the clinics (eight hours) was held in sections at CH, MGH, PBBH, BIH, and BCH for second year students. Course catalogs are not available between 1969 and 1974. In 1969, in his annual department report at Children's Hospital, Dr. Pappas wrote:

Members of our staff instruct Harvard Medical School students during all four years of their curriculum [required courses]: first year, anatomy; second year, pathophysiology of the musculoskeletal system; third and fourth years, Introduction to the Clinic and Principal Clinical Year instruction. Our teaching has been well received by the students; with the ultimate test being the increasing number of students from the Harvard Medical School entering the field of Orthopaedics as the specialty of their choice.

(Children's Hospital Archives)

In 1975 the third-year students were required to take a rotation in medicine and in surgery, but orthopaedic surgery was no longer required for all students in the third-year class. This was a significant change after almost 70 years during which it was required for all students.

Block courses available included:

OS 500M.3:
  • Core Clinical Clerkship
  • One Month at MGH for 6 students: Mankin & associates
  • Included ward work, outpatient,
  • ER (H & Ps and patient care),
  • OR Experience,
  • Students take ER call.

OS 500M.J:
  • Core Clinical Clerkship
  • One month for 4 students at CH, PBBH, RBBH: Glimcher & assoc.
  • Includes ward service at PBBH; primary
  • Experience: outpatient clinics (do H & Ps),
  • OR and ER call
  • Specialty clinics at CH and RBBH

[Elective opportunities after completing one of the core clerkships:]

OS. 506M.3
- Preceptorship in Ortho: Mankin MGH
- 1 student/faculty/month: private office

OS 506M.7
- Preceptorship in Ortho: Hall and Watts CH
- 1 student/month
- Outpatient, inpatient and OR

OS 506M.13
- Preceptorship in Ortho: Sledge & associates, PBBH and RBBH
- 4 students/month
- Work in private practice in a university setting

OS 508M.40a
- Skiing Injuries: Glimcher, Ellison, Wolf
- 1 student /month @ Haystack Mountain
- Work with ski patrol

OS 508M.40b
- Skiing Injuries: MacAusland, Otis and Assoc.
- 2 student/month Stratton Mountain

Longitudinal
701M.4 Fractures and Related Trauma: Sledge & Assoc., PBBH
Course: Demonstrations and Conferences
    2 days/week (2–3-hour sessions)

(Official Register of Harvard University 1975)

The Introduction to Clinical Medicine course was held in the spring of the second year in 1977, three days per week, followed by the three-month medicine clerkship and the two-month surgical clerkship. That same year, the required core

courses in orthopaedics remained unchanged. Some new electives were added to those electives already in existence:

OS 501M.1   Clinical Ortho Surgery: Yett & Assoc, BIH
- 2 students/month
- Workup elective admissions and ER patients
- 3 clinics/week and frequent conferences

OS 502M.14   General Orthopaedic Surgery: Gillies & Scott, WRVAH
- 2 students/month
- Students are part of the care team (2 staff & 2 residents)

OS 502M.13   Medical and Surgical Care of Patients with Rheumatoid Arthritis: Sledge, Austin & associates, RBBH
- 2 students/month

OS 504M.7   Children's Ortho: Glimcher & associates, CH
- 2 students/month

OS 505M.3   Hand Surgery: Smith, Leffert, Cannon & associates (plastics) MGH
- 1 student/month

OS 505M.J.   Hand Surgery: Nalebuff & Millender, RBBH and BIH
- 2 students/month

OS 510M.14   Rehabilitation of the Spinal Cord Injury Patient: AB Rossier & Associates, WRVAH
- 1 student/month

(Official Register of Harvard University 1977)

The next change in the orthopaedic curriculum occurred in 1979 with the addition of a new course in sports medicine as an elective. Students attended Saturday pregame clinics and the game; on Sundays they attended the morning clinic. After the football season, they met with Dr. Boland on Monday, Wednesday, and Friday. They also assisted Dr. Boland in the emergency department and in the operating room.

The following electives were included for orthopaedics in 1990, which required that the student complete the Patient-Doctor Year II course (709.M. JB):

OR 501M.1   Introductory Ortho Clerkship: Knirk & assoc., BIH
- 2 students/month: Nov., March, May only

OR 501M.3   Clinical Clerkship: Curtiss, Jr. & assoc., MGH
- 6 students/month

OR 501M.14   General Orthopaedic Surgery: Wilson WRVAMC
- 2 students/2 or 4 weeks (not offered in Sept.)

OR 501M.23   Clinical Clerkship in Ortho: Sledge & assoc., BWH
- 2 students/month (prerequisite: ortho course)

OR 502M.3   Adult Ortho: Curtiss, Jr. & assoc., MGH
- 1 student/month

OR 502M.23   Adult Ortho: Sledge & assoc., BWH
- 2 students/month (not offered in August)

OR 503M.23   Med. and Surg. Care of Pts w/ Arthritis: Anderson & assoc., BWH
- 1 student/month

OR 504M.7   Children's Ortho: Hall & assoc.
- 1 student/month (not offered in August)

OR 505M.3   Hand Surgery: Gelberman & assoc., MGH
- 1 student/month

OR 505M.J.   Hand Surgery and Rehabilitation: Simmons & assoc., BWH, CH
- 2 students/month

OR 506M.3   Preceptorship in Ortho: Curtiss, Jr. & assoc., MGH
- 1 student/month (not in June, July, August)

OR 506M.7   Preceptorship in Children's Ortho: Hall & assoc., CH
- 3 students/month (not offered in July)

OR 508M.40b   Skiing Injur. and Fam. Prac.: MacAusland, Jr., & assoc, Stratton Mt.
- 2 students/month (Dec. through March)

OR 511M.J.   Sports Medicine: Boland & assoc., MGH/UHS
- 1 student/month (not in June, July, August)

(Harvard Medical School Course Catalog 1990–1991)

Significant changes developed for orthopaedics in the curriculum in 1996. Orthopaedic surgery was now offered as an elective within the three-month core clerkships in surgery at the MGH, BWH, and BIDMC.

The last printed Harvard Medical School course catalog was in 1999–2000. Consequently, the subsequent course catalogs were published online and are not available. In 1998, Dr. Tim Hresko at Children's Hospital was appointed as chair of the Medical Student Undergraduate Education Committee. Dr. Wright had overseen the students at BWH, Dr. Lipson at BIDMC and Dr. Perlmutter at MGH. In addition to shadowing the surgeons in clinics and on the wards, each hospital's staff and residents gave lectures to the students.

During 1999–2000, the orthopaedic faculty prepared a new addition to the teaching program for third-year students: a Saturday morning session that consisted of a review of standardized cases presented by the faculty. The purpose was to ensure that all third-year students received the same basic core instruction in orthopaedics because their experiences varied widely at each of these teaching hospitals. "A team of faculty members will generate case studies in the following areas: Hand and Upper Extremity—David Ring; Spine—Steve Lipson; Sports Medicine—Tom Gill; Reconstructive Adult—Dick Scott; Pediatrics—Tim Hresko; Infection, tumors—John Ready; Metabolic Bone Disease—Sam Doppelt; Trauma—Mark Vrahas" (MGH HCORP Archives). The case-based discussions (one or two cases per specialty) were led by three faculty (rotating) per Saturday session. Imaging studies and lab data were presented to the students, along with the history and physical findings. A brief discussion of management followed each case. Each hospital was provided with two copies of Salter's book, *Textbook of Disorders and Injuries of the Musculoskeletal System* and Ron McRae's book, *Clinical Orthopaedic Examination* for student use. The students were also given a copy of the *Journal of Bone and Joint Surgery* article "The Adequacy of Medical School Education in Musculoskeletal Medicine" by Freedman and Bernstein (1998). As the Harvard Orthopaedic Residency Program Director, I participated in the study in which 81% of the 154 orthopaedic program directors responded to the survey.

During the same period, the third-year student evaluations at MGH had improved. Dr. Charles McCabe, who was the surgical core clerkship director at MGH, emailed Dr. Gary Perlmutter, November 18, 1998, stating: "the students were incredibly enthusiastic about their experience on Orthopaedics" (MGH HCORP Archives). At a meeting of the Surgical Clerkship Committee (headed by Dr. William Silen at BIDMC) on February 24, 1999:

The committee expressed general dissatisfaction with the orthopedic rotation during the third core-based year:

a) at BWH…85% of students stated the rotation is not well organized and does not meet their educational goals.

b) at MGH…Silen thought that things were going well at MGH (Six months ago this committee claimed the MGH rotation was doing poorly).

c) at BIDMC…the student rotation is variable depending on the staff attending…

They requested that a greater emphasis be placed on medical student education by the orthopedic department…[and] asked what [curriculum] would be appropriate for the two weeks? (MGH HCORP Archives)

The next year it was noted that the orthopaedic faculty were not consistently attending their Saturday morning conferences for students at BWH and BIDMC. In March 2000, Silen wrote to Hresko: "There have been significant problems because cancellations of teaching responsibilities continue to plague us, and some faculty have not been as assiduous as they should be in meeting their current obligations. These issues need urgent attention now, but as we think of instigation of your five-year plan, it is vital that teaching assignments be taken seriously" (MGH HCORP Archives).

The orthopaedic clerkship remained a required outpatient experience in the third-year core surgical clerkship. An example of the fourth-year elective orthopaedic surgery rotation at the MGH included four weekly rotations on the trauma, hand, joints, and sports services. Beginning in 2001, the students attended the 6:30 a.m. daily morning trauma reports. They also attended the teaching conferences of their subspecialty rotation and were given one or two lectures each week on common orthopaedic problems and injuries. Around the same time (1999), orthopaedic faculty also began to voluntarily participate in the Objective Structure Clinical Examination (OSCE), a series of practice stations that tested the students' knowledge and skills necessary for Harvard Medical School IV's expected competence. The orthopaedic stations were knee and back, both with simulated patients.

A perfect storm developed that allowed for major changes in musculoskeletal education for medical students at the turn of the last century. In 1998, Freedman and Bernstein published their classic article on graduating medical students' knowledge of orthopaedics:

> In summary, seventy (82 per cent) of eighty-five medical school graduates [PGY1 residents at the University of Pennsylvania] failed a valid musculoskeletal competency examination. We, therefore, believe that medical school preparation in musculoskeletal medicine is inadequate...Our findings suggest the need for two educational reforms: an increase in instructional time and a revision of the content of the curriculum. One week of required orthopaedic training is probably insufficient...an ideal required rotation in musculoskeletal medicine would be at least two weeks...and would emphasize common outpatient orthopaedic problems, orthopaedic emergencies, and physical examination for musculoskeletal problems... all students must be instructed in musculoskeletal medicine...Medical schools must reform their curricula by adding more contact hours with broader content...steps...necessary for optimum patient care. (K. B. Freedman and J. Bernstein 1998)

In January 2000, the World Health Organization launched the Bone and Joint Decade "to raise awareness of the increasing societal impact of musculoskeletal injuries and disorders, to empower patients to participate in decisions about their care, to increase funding for prevention activities and research, and to promote cost-effective prevention and treatment" (S. L. Weinstein 2000).

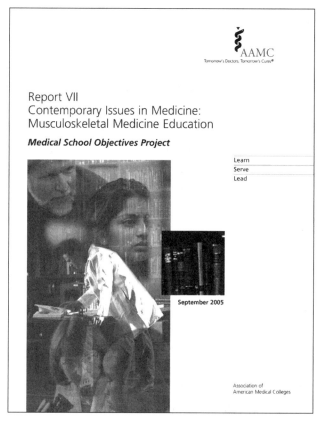

Cover: "Report VII: Contemporary Issues in Medicine: Musculoskeletal Medicine Education." The AAMC recommended that musculoskeletal medicine be added to medical schools' curriculum in the US, 2005.
Association of American Medical Colleges.

The final and most significant component of the perfect storm that led to real musculoskeletal curricular changes in medical schools in the United States was the American Association of Medical Colleges Medical School Objectives Project in September 2005, which published, "Report VII. Contemporary Issues in Medicine: Musculoskeletal Medicine Education." This report recommended that an expert panel add learning objectives on musculoskeletal conditions to the curriculum for undergraduate medical students; their findings noted the time spent on the curriculum in medical schools did not correlate with the prevalence of musculoskeletal conditions among the general populace, which had led to practicing physicians who were poorly equipped to evaluate these conditions. The report summarized the learning objectives in three categories: attitudes, knowledge and skills. The report stated:

> Accordingly, medical schools should strive to integrate learning experiences relevant to musculoskeletal medicine throughout the curriculum...as part of a coherent...component...It is essential that Medical Schools strive to create a more organized approach to how musculoskeletal medicine is practiced within an academic environment...[and] address fragmentation of musculoskeletal content in the curriculum...[to help students begin to recognize and associate the musculoskeletal thread between the disciplines...[using] teaching cases...illustrating the integration of core principles and fundamental skill sets. (Association of American Medical Colleges 2005)

Finally, the report recommended use of appropriate assessment tools to evaluate students in the three categories as well as to "integrate musculoskeletal conditions into existing OSCEs and/or create OSCEs with musculoskeletal conditions (Association of American Medical Colleges 2005).

This perfect storm culminating in the AAMC's endorsement of adding musculoskeletal medicine to the curriculum in all medical schools; it also provided a great opportunity for change at HMS. This opportunity was seized by Dr. Charles Day, a young faculty member of orthopaedic surgery at the BIDMC. During the year following the publication of the AAMC on Musculoskeletal Medicine (2005), Dr. Day identified the total musculoskeletal content taught during the four years of medical school at Harvard, then assessed each medical school class's knowledge by having all students take the Freedman and Bernstein's basic competency examination in musculoskeletal medicine

(online). With an overall participation rate of 73%, "compared with a national validated passing threshold of 70%, only 2%, 6%, and 26% of the second-, third-, and fourth-year students, respectively, passed the musculoskeletal competency examination...86% of the fourth-year students suggested additional curricular time be spent on this topic" (C. S. Day et al. 2009). Following the AAMC medical School Obstetrics Project Report on musculoskeletal medicine and with the support of the leadership at Harvard and its teaching hospitals—especially the Vice Chair of the Curriculum Committee with his appointed Musculoskeletal Task Force, Dr. Day developed a longitudinal curriculum for the four years of medical school. Some course directors allowed musculoskeletal education in their curriculum:

> The Human Body Course...required for all first-year medical students, added ten hours to the traditional curriculum...an additional six hours of limb dissection time and four hours of small group sessions on limb surface anatomy...[a] 10:1 student-faculty ratio was requested...[in] the second-year curriculum...directors of three [courses] (Human Systems, a year-long pathophysiology course; Patient-Doctor II, a year-long physical diagnosis course; and Human Development)...responded with increased structured time devoted to the musculoskeletal education objectives...[totaling] twenty-seven hours... seven hours were added to Patient-Doctor II... four hours were added to Human Development...[and] sixteen hours were devoted to a new musculoskeletal-orthopaedic pathophysiology block in Human Systems. (C. S. Day et al. 2009)

Dr. Day had the cooperation and commitments of the orthopaedic faculty, department chairs, as well as other specialists to provide the new demands for teaching medical students. However, the two-week required third year orthopaedic clerkship remained only at the MGH.

During this time, about 29% of the fourth-year classes took a clinical orthopaedic elective. Continuous improvement in musculoskeletal education is needed by additional increases in instruction time as well as "improving the integration of musculoskeletal medicine into the four-year medical curriculum" (Yeh, Franko, and Day 2008).

Research and reform throughout the twentieth century led to significant changes in medical school admission requirements, pedagogy, and curriculum and also gave rise to the specialty of orthopaedics. Although orthopaedic surgeons have long argued the importance of their specialty, power at HMS resided in the basic sciences; orthopaedics was viewed as a specialty, and even today it is not given its due academic credit. Arguments for musculoskeletal education in medical school has been critical not just for the field of orthopaedics but also for diverse practicing physicians—general practitioners, emergency room physicians, and hospitalists alike. For many minor conditions, a remedy could have been applied earlier with a simple splint, bandage or a cortisone injection, but care for simple conditions continues to be delayed until the patient sees a specialist. These reforms and advancements led by HMS, Flexner and other education researchers, the AMA, and the AAMC transformed the field as we know it today.

CHAPTER 10

The Evolution of the Organization and Department of Orthopaedic Surgery

Each of Harvard's teaching hospitals eventually approved independent orthopaedic surgery departments as permanent fixtures—in 1903 at Children's Hospital, in 1907 at Massachusetts General Hospital, in 1970 at Peter Bent Brigham and Robert Breck Brigham Hospitals, in 1978 at Beth Israel Deaconess Medical Center, and in 1980 at Brigham and Women's Hospital. However, department status for orthopaedic surgery has changed and fluctuated at Harvard over the past two centuries. Tracing its evolution can be confusing, but it's clear that specialized departments emerged from the general department of surgery at Harvard Medical School (HMS) and as a result of the early seeds planted by Buckminster Brown.

Initially, orthopaedic surgery comprised a branch of the Division of Surgery. Although it is not entirely clear what a "branch" designated, Beecher and Altschule (1977) explained that its organization included a full professor and four assistants. The branch was led in 1906 by E. H. Bradford, who was assisted by R. W. Lovett, E.G. Brackett, A. Thorndike, and R. Soutter. Harold Ernst (1906) stated:

> The "Department" in the Medical School has always had a somewhat different significance from that attributed to it in other parts of the University, and has been, loosely, held to indicate a branch of instruction of sufficient importance to have its Head rank higher than an annual appointment. Some years ago, the Faculty expressed its approval of a grouping of allied Departments into Divisions, but the only one yet in existence is the Division of Surgery.

In a report of the committee of education in medicine in 1904, Ernst, Mallory, and Bradford recommended changing the four existing departments (medicine, surgery, pathology and anatomy, and physiology) into divisions for simplicity and thereby placing the departments of orthopaedic surgery, clinical surgery, surgery, otology, ophthalmology and laryngology under the division of surgery. They stated the following reasons for organizing the clinical departments into four divisions:

1. The simplicity of the method…It is hoped that the Divisions would become units of effort and active stimulation.

2. The representatives of the Divisions together with the Dean may be substi-tuted for the present Administrative Board producing a small and compact Executive Committee for the School.

3. If this system of four Divisions be adopted, the interests of the different Departments and smaller branches will be entirely safe-guarded…each of those Divisions shall have an executive head or chairman, to be appointed by the President and Dean at intervals of two or three years; questions of policy affecting any Department of the Divi-sion shall be discussed in the Division; any teacher above the rank of assistant may take part in the discussions and have the right to vote; recommendations from the Division…come to the Faculty of Medicine through the Chairman, but the head of the Depart-ment shall have the right of appeal to the Faculty from the decisions of his Division.

4. If an attempt at further sub-division be made, the difficulty of knowing where to stop arises…the only alternative—if every one is to be satisfied—[is to make] each full professor or head of a Department repre-sent a Division.

(Deans Files, Harvard Medical School)

A department of orthopaedic surgery at Har-vard Medical School was first mentioned in the article, "Methods of Treatment in Infantile Paral-ysis. Summarized by the Department of Ortho-pedic Surgery of the Harvard Medical School" by Bradford et. al. in 1910. In 1915, the depart-ment's annual report at Children's Hospital stated:

Article in the *Boston Medical and Surgical Journal*: "Sum-marized by the Department of Orthopedic Surgery of the Harvard Medical School," (Bradford et al. 1910).
Bradford, et al. *Boston Medical and Surgical Journal*, 1910; 162: 881.

"These two departments of the work [teaching students at MGH and Children's Hospital] consti-tute the relation of the Orthopedic Department to the Harvard Medical School" (Children's Hospital Archives). However, in 1923 in the HMS Course Catalog, Dr. Osgood was listed as professor of orthopedic surgery and chairman of the depart-ment. After reviewing documents and publications during the early twentieth century, I believe that the department of orthopaedic surgery at HMS and Boston Children's Hospital were either con-fused or were one and the same department.

When Bradford became dean of HMS in 1912, he functioned as dean only half time. Because of increased growth, troubled finances, and increased demands on the dean, two alternatives were con-sidered: hire a full-time dean or add an executive officer or business director to assist the dean. The latter was chosen. The medical school was orga-nized with an administrative board, a faculty coun-cil, and the committee of professors. There were eight members of the administrative board (six fac-ulty appointed annually by the Corporation plus the president and dean, both ex officio), and this board functioned as an executive committee of the medical school. The faculty council (one elected member of each of six divisions plus the president and dean ex officio) reported to the administrative board. It dealt with the curriculum and arrange-ment of courses. The committee of professors consisted of all professors, associate professors, and clinical professors whose appointments were without limit of time plus the president and dean ex officio. The committee was responsible for appointments and promotions at the associate professor or professor level.

At a meeting of the
President and Fellows of Harvard College
in Boston, May 3, 1916

Voted to approve the following by-laws, as amended, for the conduct of the affairs of the Harvard Medical School:

Departments   1. The Faculty shall be divided into the following departments:

Anatomy,   Medicine,
Warren Museum,   Surgery,
Physiology,   Orthopaedic Surgery,
Comparative Physiology,   Obstetrics and Gynaecology,
Biological Chemistry,   Pediatrics,
Bacteriology,   Dermatology and Syphilis,
Pathology,   System,
Comparative Pathology,   Diseases of the Nervous
Preventive Medicine   Ophthalmology,
   and Hygiene,   Otology,
Pharmacology,   Laryngology

2. No new departments shall be created or existing departments combined except by a two-thirds affirmative vote of the Faculty.

3. Each department shall consist of all teachers included in the department (Faculty members, Instructors, and Assistants).

Orthopaedic Surgery is listed as one of the 20 departments in the medical school, 1916. Meeting of the President and Fellows of Harvard College. May 5, 1916. Office of the Dean subject files, 1899–1953 (inclusive). Box 18, Folder 13: 779. Harvard Medical Library in the Francis A. Countway Library of Medicine.

Notes from the bylaws meeting of the president and fellows in 1916 indicate that there were monthly faculty meetings and 20 departments (no divisions named); orthopaedic surgery was listed as one of the 20 departments. Other departments of surgery included ophthalmology, otology, obstetrics and gynecology, and laryngology. The bylaws stated: "no new departments should be created, or existing departments combined except by a 2/3 affirmative vote of the faculty" (Deans Files, Harvard Medical School). To add to the confusion, at the same meeting, departments were grouped into six divisions; the surgical field (Division E) included surgery, orthopaedic surgery, obstetrics, and gynecology. Each division was to select a chairman and a secretary to serve for three years. Department heads were appointed

by the president and fellows, usually upon the recommendation of the dean. A chairman led at the department level. At the division level, departments were grouped together to effectively decrease the number of professors sitting on the faculty council. Each division selected a chief and secretary, one member of each (n=6) to serve on the faculty council along with the president and dean, both ex officio. The dean of HMS "is the financial officer" (Deans Files, Harvard Medical School). The department head "makes recommendations in his group and is responsible for the conduct of teaching and research" (Deans Files, Harvard Medical School).

In 1908, Dr. Henry Christian, dean of HMS, proposed a new medical faculty organization consisting of 22 departments, including the Warren Museum as a department. In the surgical field, Christian recommended the following departments: surgery, orthopaedic surgery, laryngology and rhinology, obstetrics and gynecology, ophthalmology, and otology. Organized like the college of arts and sciences, each department selected a chairman and determined length of service; the department consisted of all teachers and only faculty who had served for more than three years could vote. Each department had divisions, and chairs and secretaries were selected by the division to serve for three years. New departments or divisions were created at any time by a 2/3 vote of the faculty. However, President Eliot had trouble with Christian's proposals. He made several modifications including that the chair of departments or divisions be appointed by a committee consisting of the president, the dean, and three professors named by the president.

Department status remained confusing throughout the first quarter of the twentieth century. In 1909, the Corporation voted to establish a Harvard clinic. Christian was dean, and, as a member of the staff at Peter Bent Brigham Hospital, he was concerned about the effects of this clinic on the outpatient services at the Peter Bent Brigham Hospital. On October 1, 1909, Bradford requested space for the orthopaedic department. The purpose of the clinic was to act as a charity, not only providing care for patients but also using patients for teaching medical students. The clinic included three physicians, three surgeons, and three assistants, but no orthopaedic surgeon. Lovett, chief at Children's Hospital, was happy to send patients who were "too old for Children's Hospital" to this university clinic (Deans Files, Harvard Medical School). The orthopaedic clinic at MGH was already in existence.

While dean, Bradford wanted to maintain and improve relations with the major teaching hospitals. He began the so-called Harvard Medical Meetings; the first one was held in Amphitheater A on Friday evening, 8:00 p.m., December 15, 1916. His vision was to have different departments "explain the work of their respective departments" (Deans Files, Harvard Medical School). The first department to report was pathology. The meeting was followed by light refreshments. It was strongly supported by Dr. Christian. I was unable to find any documentation of other meetings, or, if held, when they were stopped.

In an early attempt to organize the department of surgery, Dean Bradford described his plan in a letter to President Lowell, which included a full-time professor of surgery at each of the following teaching hospitals: the Peter Bent Brigham Hospital (H. W. Cushing), the MGH (G. A. Porter), and Boston City Hospital (E. H. Nichols). Previously, there had been no full-time professors, and Bradford's goal was to have these men work together for the interest of the school. In fact, staff (faculty) at MGH were appointed without the input from HMS. A few years later, Dean Edsall in a letter to President Lowell wrote that the "tendency of the MGH staff [is] to be cautious about too intimate a cooperation with HMS" (Deans Files, Harvard Medical School).

After Dr. Bradford retired in 1918, David L. Edsall became dean. During Bradford's tenure as dean, the Harvard Medical School budget had only increased from $251,389 to $270,000 over a span of 10 years, which failed to account for the cost of living increase during the period or for department growth. The budget became Edsall's immediate priority (Beecher and Altschule 1977).

In June 1918, about to be forty-nine years old... [Dr. Edsall] had become part-time dean, along with his position as chief of a medical service at the Massachusetts General Hospital. In November the European war ended, and during the early postwar years, the medical school had such serious financial problems that "it was quite uncertain whether [the school] would not go downhill rather than forward." Both senior and junior staffs were in a "state of dangerous dissatisfaction and depression because of the limited opportunities for carrying on their activities with the funds available..." Furthermore, a number of other medical schools tried to attract "distinguished personnel" from Harvard offering "much better conditions"...by 1928 [Dr. Edsall] could identify major accomplishments. Most importantly, the financial situation of the medical school had improved. Although the budget was three times larger than before, it was now balanced, whereas previously there had been a deficit...the Harvard Medical School had "obviously become a School of national influence"...The Dean had also done research to improve relations between the medical school and its affiliated hospitals. (A. J. Linenthal 1990)

In 1923, HMS listed 26 departments, including six in surgical fields: surgery, orthopaedic surgery, obstetrics, gynecology, laryngology and otology. Most of the departments had a head and a secretary. "Each department does its own business and is independent of the other departments" (Deans Files, Harvard Medical School). Osgood was listed as head of the orthopaedic surgery department. His private office was listed as his address at 372 Marlborough Street, whereas the

Office Memo
Date : 1923

OUTLINE OF ORGANIZATION OF HARVARD MEDICAL SCHOOL

PRESIDENT OF HARVARD UNIVERSITY - - President A. L. Lowell

Personal Secretary to President Lowell - - Miss Dwyer

President Lowell has a Board of Overseers who meet once a month and a Corporation who are sort of an Executive Committee and who are responsible for the policies of the University.

School Departments   The School has the following 26 Departments:

Administration: Dr. David L. Edsall - Room 103

Anatomy: Dr. J. Lewis Bremer - Room 301 - B II

Bacteriology: Dr. Hans Zinsser - Room 364 - D I

Physical Chemistry: Dr. Lawrence J. Menderson - Room 366- C I   *acting Dr. E. J. Cohn*
Biological Chemistry: Dr. Otto Folin, Rooms 334 - 335 - 336 - C - I

Dermatology: Dr. Charles J. White, 269 Marlborough St., Boston

Gynaecology: Dr. William P. Graves, 198 Commonwealth Ave., Boston

Laryngology: Dr. Algernon Coolidge, 613 Beacon St., Boston
Dr. Harris P. Mosher, 828 Beacon St., Boston

Medicine: Dr. Henry A. Christian, Brigham Hospital

Neurology - (Nervous System): Dr. Edward W. Taylor, 457 Marlborough St. Boston

Neuropathology - (Nervous System): Dr. Stanley Cobb, Room 104 - D II

Obstetrics: Dr. Franklin S. Newell, 443 Beacon St., Boston

Opthalmology: Dr. George S. Derby, 23 Bay State Road, Boston

Orthopedic Surgery: Dr. Robert B. Osgood, 372 Marlborough St., Boston

Otology: Dr. D. Harold Walker, 390 Commonwealth Ave., Boston

Pathology: Dr. S. Burt Wolbach, Room 393 - D I

Comparative Pathology: Dr. Ernest E. Tyzzer, Room 229 - E II

Pediatrics: Dr. Kenneth D. Blackfan, Children's Hospital, Longwood Ave. Boston

Pharmacology: Dr. Reid Hunt, Room 202 - E I

Physiology: Dr. Walter B. Cannon - Room 301 - C I
Dr. Alfred Redfield, Bldg. e. secretary

Comparative Physiology: Dr. William T. Porter, Room 351 - C I

Preventative Medicine & Hygiene: Dr. Milton J. Rosenau, Room 238 - E II

Psychiatry - (Nervous System): Dr. C. Macfie Campbell
Boston Psychopathic Hospital
74 Fenwood Road, Boston

Surgery: Dr. Harvey Cushing, Brigham Hospital, Boston

Syphilology: Dr. C. Morton Smith, 437 Marlboro St., Boston

Tropical Medicine: Dr. Richard P. Strong, Room 246 - D I

Orthopaedic Surgery is listed as one of the 26 departments in the medical school, 1923. Dr. Robert B. Osgood is chairperson. "Outline of Organization of Harvard Medical School." Office of the Dean subject files, 1899–1953 (inclusive). Box 18, Folder 13; 781.
Harvard Medical Library in the Francis A. Countway Library of Medicine.

DEPARTMENT OF ORTHOPAEDIC SURGERY
HARVARD MEDICAL SCHOOL
240 LONGWOOD AVE.,
BOSTON, MASSACHUSETTS

June 7th, 1928

Dr. David L. Edsall, Dean,
Harvard Medical School,
Boston, Mass.

Dear Dr. Edsall:

I have been over the tentative report of the Curriculum Committee and discussed it with Dr. Blackfan at some length. I was reserving my comments until a little more detailed scheme had been worked out for the teaching at the Children's Hospital to be divided between the Pediatic, Orthopaedic and Surgical Services. The proposed change in the curriculum appeals to me very strongly as a change in the right direction....

In a tentative scheme which Dr. Blackfan showed me for teaching at the Children's Hospital it appears that there will be about the same amount of time, possibly a little more, given to the clinical teaching of such contacts in Orthopaedic Surgery. I am sure each specialist feels that his own specialty is of extreme importance to the general practitioner and I feel strongly that this is the fact with Orthopaedic Surgery. It is not an anatomic specialty but it deals with the function of the whole locomotive apparatus and peculiarly with many types of chronic lesions of the bones and joints. The problems of chronic disease are those which the general practitioner is constantly called on to solve and which must make up a considerable portion of his practice. In any survey of chronic disease, bone and joint conditions loom large.

The Orthopaedic Department will be glad to cooperate most heartily in this proposed change in the curriculum.

Very sincerely yours,

[signature]

Letterhead of Dr. Osgood states: "Department of Orthopaedic Surgery, Harvard Medical School." Letter to Dr. David L. Edsall, Dean HMS, from Robert B. Osgood, June 7, 1928. Office of the Dean subject files, 1899–1953 (inclusive). Box 12, Folder 9: 454.
Harvard Medical Library in the Francis A. Countway Library of Medicine.

heads of medicine and surgery had their hospitals listed as their address. Each department chief or head had his own budget under the Dean.

Previously, Dean Edsall had noted the large growth of specialty departments, the importance of hospital connections and the fact that governance was difficult. He wanted an increased participation in governance by the professors. His plan for the clinical departments contrasted with the departmental organization at Johns Hopkins where the faculty were strictly full-time; it included the following:

1. **Department heads**—with their offices in the hospitals—were in charge of the department organization, and they received salaries from HMS or both HMS and the hospital. They spent the majority of their time teaching and in research and had small consulting practices.

2. **Junior faculty** instructed part-time, had a consulting practice, and were on a career track to become department chairs. Edsall disliked the full-time system, which he felt wouldn't allow for these junior positions.

3. A limited number of practitioner-teachers admitted patients who would become cases for students to examine and treat under supervision as well as be used for teaching purposes by the practitioner.

Edsall believed that HMS could not support a full-time system like Johns Hopkins, stating it was "unwise and unnecessary" (Deans Files, Harvard Medical School). He said, "To do it all well with our conditions here, in medicine and surgery alone would cost at least a million and a half dollars" (Deans Files, Harvard Medical School). Lovett in a letter to Dr. Cabot objected to the phrase: "the professors…who are giving the larger portion of their time to the affairs of the school" because he felt that this would limit people on the new administrative board to laboratory or full-time positions (Deans Files, Harvard Medical School). Cabot agreed with Lovett.

Dean Edsall thought of two different methods to raise the money needed for hiring faculty at HMS. He rejected raising significant money from foundations like the Rockefeller or Carnegie foundations and chose a less difficult, incremental approach by raising money periodically for specific individual department purposes. He realized the importance of combining and amalgamating the interests of the school and the hospitals. For example, when he arrived he had one full-time member on his staff, but he had no additional salaries available to him. Whereas, at MGH the hospital added a full-time assistant and three residents to his and Dr. Cabot's service. These men spent half of their time teaching and doing research. Edsall began hiring new faculty by combining a small salary from HMS with an additional salary provided by the hospital, a model that continued to grow over time. In medicine, he planned to have seven or eight new faculty by the following year with half in full-time work at the hospital and school also being given room, board, and laundry (like the residents). Christian developed similar plans at the Peter Bent Brigham Hospital. I could not find any such program for the development of orthopaedic

surgery. In fact, Drs. Bradford, Lovett, Osgood, and Ober were all in private practice to a large extent. The first full-time faculty member in orthopaedics was Dr. William T. Green. Ten years after Edsall had become dean, he remained concerned about the development of the medical science departments because the "organization [HMS] was not very satisfactory" (Deans Files, Harvard Medical School) and that the committee of professors didn't meet frequently enough. Lowell responded to Edsall's concerns, saying that they were not training the best and they needed to give faculty more independence and weed out the weaker individuals.

The historical record supports the fact that there was an orthopaedic department at HMS in the 1920s. For example, Osgood discussed the

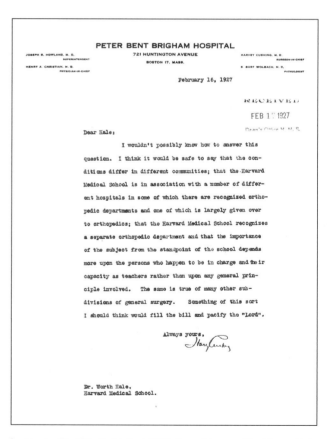

Letter to Dr. Worth Hale, HMS, from Harvey Cushing which states "Harvard Medical School recognizes a separate orthopedic department." February 16, 1927. Office of the Dean subject files, 1899–1953 (inclusive). Box 14, Folder 11: 568. Harvard Medical Library in the Francis A. Countway Library of Medicine.

spelling of orthopaedics in a letter to Worth Hale in the dean's office; he strongly supported spelling it with an "ae," not just an "e" (Deans Files, Harvard Medical School). Osgood's letterhead also clearly stated: "Department of Orthopaedic Surgery. Harvard Medical School, 240 Longwood Avenue." Dr. Cushing's response to a Dr. Lord—who had complained to the dean that orthopaedics was encroaching on surgery by treating fractures, arthritis, and osteomyelitis—further supports the existence of a distinct department of orthopaedics. Cushing wrote that "HMS recognizes a separate orthopaedic department," the same as in the hospitals (Deans Files, Harvard Medical School). In another letter from Osgood to Dean Edsall, with the same letterhead, he stated: "The Orthopaedic Department for the last five years has had no

February 24, 1927.

Dr. J. P. Lord,
482 Aquila Court,
Omaha, Nebraska.

Dear Lord:

In answer to your circular inquiry as to Orthopaedic Surgery, the Medical School here is an association of a number of different hospitals, in some of which there are recognized orthopaedic departments – and in one of which the clinic is largely given over to orthopaedics.

This school recognizes a separate orthopaedic department, probably because of the individuals connected with it and the high development of orthopaedic surgery in this city. Our Professor of Orthopaedic Surgery is one of our most capable instructors.

Yours very truly,

Worth Hale, M. D.
Assistant Dean.

WH:MH

Letter to Dr. J. F. Lord from Worth Hale, MD, Assistant Dean (HMS), which states "This school recognizes a separate orthopaedic department." February 24, 1927. Office of the Dean subject files, 1899–1953 (inclusive). Box 14, Folder 11: 568. Harvard Medical Library in the Francis A. Countway Library of Medicine.

didactic lectures" because the faculty distributed copies of the lectures to the third-year students before the scheduled lecture, then presented cases and held quizzes during the allocated lecture time (Deans Files, Harvard Medical School). Curriculum changes were under development, which Osgood supported, but because the students liked the new method of instruction in orthopaedics, he didn't want orthopaedic lecture time decreased. As Dean Edsall continued to be concerned about governance issues at HMS, a committee chaired by Bradford reported in 1920 that, in contrast to HMS, other medical schools were led by department chairs and one compact body controlled activities of the school. These schools included Johns Hopkins, Washington University, Columbia, Western (Canada), Rush, Northwestern, Wisconsin, Michigan, California, Cornell, and the University of Pennsylvania. Christian stated concern in a letter that both Bradford and Edsall were "afraid to engage the faculty" (Deans Files, Harvard Medical School).

To add further to the confusion, Dean Edsall described the HMS system to Dr. Beene at the University of Michigan in a letter, stating "the system we use: modified full-time" (Deans Files, Harvard Medical School). He explained they had two chairs in medicine and two in surgery as well as three chairs in surgery in hospital units, but he did not mention orthopaedic surgery. He planned to allow clinicians to head departments until researchers became available, which was "a compromise between ideal and practical necessity" (Deans Files, Harvard Medical School). Clinicians who were department heads received a salary of $10,000 to $12,000. The professors were allowed to perform consultations for limited number of patients in order to charge fees to increase their income (not to exceed their salary) as well as to be in touch with the problems of private practice. In 1922, Osgood received a salary of $4,200 as the John Ball and Buckminster Brown Clinical Professor and apparently had no limits on the number of patients he could see.

Dean Edsall was not supportive of department status for orthopaedic surgery. When he wrote about surgery, he said, "Obstetrics is looked upon as being a major subject and orthopaedic surgery and genitourinary surgery are in some degree part of the general subject of surgery itself" (Deans Files, Harvard Medical School). He established a faculty council in 1934, which included two representatives from medicine and two from surgery, representatives from each of the basic science departments at HMS, heads of pediatrics, obstetrics, neurology, and psychiatry. According to the faculty council's final report in 1934, "clinical subjects should not be represented at all times, but should have representatives in the group (two representatives chosen from orthopaedic surgery, gynecology, dermatology, ophthalmology, otology, tropical medicine and physical chemistry) to serve for three years. Representatives of major hospitals would rotate every three years, giving all full professors a chance to serve" (Deans Files, Harvard Medical School). Dr. Ober was chief at Children's Hospital at the time and the John B. and Buckminster Brown Clinical Professor. He was not full-time, but he was a clinical professor as were his predecessors, which suggests that, since orthopaedics was only clinical (not research oriented) and its professors only clinical, orthopaedic surgery was not seen as a significant department or a scholarly field by the leadership at HMS and the university. Dr. Kenneth D. Blackman, pediatrician at HMS, recommended to Edsall that a representative be included from each of the following specialties: orthopaedic surgery, ophthalmology, otolaryngology, gynecology, and dermatology; he felt that otherwise "too large a distinction is made between the so-called major departments and minor departments" (Deans Files, Harvard Medical School). Edsall responded, "some of these men are not full professors...time may come...if the school...has full-time professors in these fields" (Deans Files, Harvard Medical School). The author could find no comments or objections by Dr. Ober about this new faculty council membership.

Edsall also expressed his opinion about different faculty ranks in a letter to Dr. Frothingham at the Peter Bent Brigham Hospital in 1927. He wrote that clinical professors were those who spend "only a moderate portion of their time in the Medical School services"; associate and full professors had roles such that "the major portion of their time is devoted to the school and its correlated activities"; adjunct professors and associate professors were titles only for a short time, "probably three years," and were not on the committee of professors (Deans Files, Harvard Medical School). In another letter, Edsall commented on the committee of professors and said, "it was established long before I came here" (Deans Files, Harvard Medical School). Professors and associate professors were life appointments (without limit of time), but in 1934 associate professors were no longer life appointments and instead were three-year appointments. Interestingly, 20 other representatives were chosen (including instructors). Together with the dean and assistant dean serving as ex officio, the total number of members of the faculty council was 40 (no orthopaedic surgeon)—far too many to be effective in governance. In 1931, there were no orthopaedic representatives on the administrative board; only two representatives were selected from nine clinical departments that included orthopaedics. President Lowell told Edsall that he felt the recommendations to the administrative board were reasonable. However, all administrative boards at Harvard were appointed by the Corporation, who would take the recommendations to the administrative board as a "guide." Edsall changed the title "Clinical Professor of Surgery" to "Professor of Clinical Surgery" because he wanted researchers to head clinical departments.

Between 1930 and 1933, salaries for faculty in 13 departments ranged from $100 to $12,000. Clinical faculty received less because the administration felt they were not giving more than a fraction of their time to the school. Orthopaedic surgeons were included, as seen by the few known

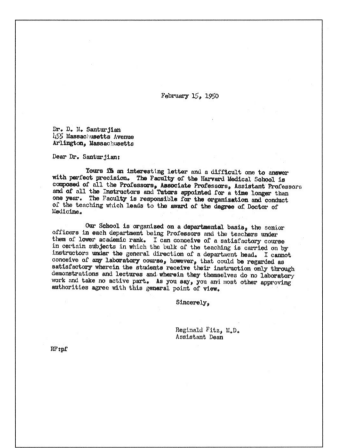

February 15, 1950

Dr. D. N. Santurjian
455 Massachusetts Avenue
Arlington, Massachusetts

Dear Dr. Santurjian:

Yours is an interesting letter and a difficult one to answer with perfect precision. The Faculty of the Harvard Medical School is composed of all the Professors, Associate Professors, Assistant Professors and of all the Instructors and Tutors appointed for a time longer than one year. The Faculty is responsible for the organization and conduct of the teaching which leads to the award of the degree of Doctor of Medicine.

Our School is organized on a departmental basis, the senior officers in each department being Professors and the teachers under them of lower academic rank. I can conceive of a satisfactory course in certain subjects in which the bulk of the teaching is carried on by instructors under the general direction of a department head. I cannot conceive of any laboratory course, however, that could be regarded as satisfactory wherein the students receive their instruction only through demonstrations and lectures and wherein they themselves do no laboratory work and take no active part. As you say, you and most other approving authorities agree with this general point of view.

Sincerely,

Reginald Fitz, M.D.
Assistant Dean

RF:pf

Letter to Dr. D. N. Santurjian from Reginald Fitz, Assistant Dean (HMS) which states "our school is organized on a departmental basis." Office of the Dean subject files, 1899–1953 (inclusive). Box 18, Folder 13: 779.

Harvard Medical Library in the Francis A. Countway Library of Medicine.

examples: Assistant Cave $100 and Assistant Green $250. In 1916, Instructor Osgood was paid $500 by HMS; in 1922, as the John B. and Buckminster Brown Professor, he received $4,200.

Assistant Dean Reginald Fitz explained in a letter that "our school is organized on a departmental basis, the senior officer in each department being Professors and the teachers under them of lower academic rank" (Deans Files, Harvard Medical School). Nevertheless, when referring to the 1939 HMS catalog, Dr. George B. Wislocki observed to Dean Burwell that the administrative head of a department should be listed after the person's name; he noted that orthopaedic surgery was not listed. Dr. Cutler was listed after surgery as the administrative head

of the department of surgery at the Peter Bent Brigham Hospital, and the department of surgery's chairman was designated as "secretary" of the department. This all adds further confusion to the departmental organization and leadership of departments at HMS.

In 1949, Dean Burwell wrote the following memorandum:

Orthopaedics has existed as a separate department in the HMS for a long time, but it has almost no financial support from University funds…(total: $2,700 per year)…For a long time it was taught chiefly at Children's Hospital and until recently the endowed professorship, the John B. and Buckminster Brown professorship, was held by the incumbent at the Children's…As adult orthopaedics became more important and particularly as Dr. Smith-Petersen developed orthopaedics at the MGH, the teaching of adult orthopaedics became increasingly important. Some years ago, a small budget was divided so that there were two budgetary units: one for Children's and one at the General, on the ground that the administration of budgets in Hospital B by a man whose appointment in Hospital A doesn't work…When Dr. Ober and Dr. Smith-Petersen retired recently, two relatively young men were made heads of these two departments. Dr. William T. Green at the Children's Hospital is a man with a considerable private practice who also receives a salary of some $10,000 from the Children's Hospital and who could on that account perhaps be classified as Hospital Full-time, although up to now his classification has been part-time. Dr. Joseph Barr is the head of the department at the Massachusetts General and now holds the title John Ball and Buckminster Brown Clinical Professor of Orthopaedic Surgery (Dr. Green is also a Clinical Professor). These two men and their departments work well together, and I believe have rotated training of house overseerships [residency program director]. They act as a division in recommending appointments and in organizing teaching. (Deans Files, Harvard Medical School)

I was unable to determine why Dr. Green did not receive the John B. and Buckminster Brown Chair as chief at Children's Hospital, following Dr. Ober.

Seven years later, confusion persisted. Mr. Fred A. Rogers, vice president of Year Book Publishers, wanted to donate one of the company's recent orthopaedic publications—*Atlas of Plaster Cast Techniques* by Dr. E. E. Bleck—to the individual at HMS who was in charge of teaching fractures to the students. Dean Berry's secretary replied that "Harvard's Department of Orthopaedic Surgery is headed by two members of the faculty: Dr. J. S. Barr at the MGH and Dr. W. T. Green at the Children's Hospital" (Deans Files, Harvard Medical School)"; the secretary requested that a copy of the book be sent to each. In a letter to Dean Berry, Dr. Barr wrote that:

The Chief of the Orthopaedic Service at the MGH has always held a part time appointment. The increasing demands of this position, particularly in view of the anticipated expansion of both our teaching and research programs, have convinced me that eventually this post must be a Hospital full-time appointment. (Deans Files, Harvard Medical School)

When asked by Alfred Shands (President, OREF) about teaching students and residents orthopaedics because the OREF was planning to help fund education, Dean Berry asked both Dr. Green and Dr. Barr about the most pressing needs of the orthopaedic department before responding.

During the late 1950s, Dr. Barr made a significant effort to develop research laboratories and programs at MGH. He invited Dean Berry to support a fundraising campaign and requested additional funds from HMS. The department's budget support from HMS was $12,000 in 1957–1958. Dr. Barr had requested additional money from HMS's unrestricted funds in 1956, but I could find no reply. The total department budget at MGH was $48,500. Dr. Barr planned for a research budget of $300,000 per year. Barr believed that "The amount contributed by Harvard is disgracefully small" (Deans Files, Harvard Medical School).

In 1959, Barr wrote to Dean Berry about plans at MGH for the orthopaedic department, including teaching 3rd year residents. He said:

I am exploring with Dr. Green the possibility of having all third-year students assigned to the Orthopaedic Department at the MGH for their training in adult orthopaedics and in trauma. We have ample clinical material in the Emergency Ward, in the Ambulatory Clinics and on our hospital wards and we have a sufficiently large staff. (Deans Files, Harvard Medical School)

I could not determine whether Barr was partnering with Green as two hospital department chiefs or whether Barr was seeking Green's approval because Green was the head of the orthopaedic department at HMS. Both were full professors. In 1962, Dean Berry stated, "This appointment [Dr. Green as the Harriet M. Peabody Professor] will bring into being for the first time a full-time Department of Orthopaedics at Harvard Medical School and the Children's Hospital"—further adding to the confusion about the status of orthopaedics as a department at Harvard Medical School (Children's Hospital Archives).

Orthopaedics at HMS functioned without departmental status or a chairperson after Dr. Green retired and Dr. Glimcher moved to Children's Hospital. At the time, Dr. Sledge was appointed chair of orthopaedics at BWH and Dr. Mankin was recruited as chair of orthopaedics at the MGH. Leadership consisted of an executive committee, which initially included Dr. Sledge as secretary, Dr. Mankin as residency program director, and Dr. Hall and later Dr. White (see chapter 11). In 1998, when I was recruited to the new position of chairman of the Partners Department of Orthopaedic Surgery (MGH and BWH), I had an agreement from Dean Joseph Martin that I would be chairman of the HMS orthopaedic executive committee, program director of HCORP, and after my arrival Dean Martin would restore department status to orthopaedic surgery at HMS with myself as chairman. This latter position was important, just as it was when Dr. Bradford was Dean and Dr. Lovett, the John Ball and Buckminster Brown Professor, became the department head, because the chairman: "makes recommendations in his group and is responsible for the conduct of teaching and research" (Deans Files, Harvard Medical School), including the responsibilities of recruiting and promoting academic faculty, the orthopaedic curriculum for the medical students, organizational structure and operations, oversight of the residency and fellowship training programs, developing research and clinical budgets, leading a practice plan of the faculty and developing endowment funds and endowed professorships.

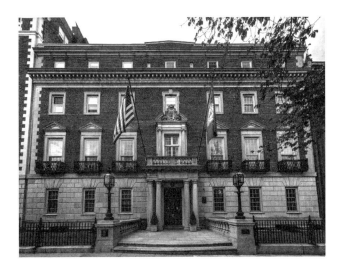

Harvard Club on Commonwealth Avenue, Boston.
Kael E. Randall/Kael Randall Images.

The dean fulfilled his commitment by naming me chairman of the HMS orthopaedic executive committee while holding the partners chairmanship; it was not to be rotated every three years as it had in the past. He also named me as HCORP's director. However, he never fulfilled his commitment to re-establish a department of orthopaedic surgery at HMS, with me as chairman. After over two years in my new position, I requested a luncheon meeting at the Harvard Club with the dean to address this remaining important unfulfilled commitment. The dean was noncommittal, stating: "Jim, you knew what you were getting into" (J. Martin, pers. comm.). Harvard Medical School's 2019 preclinical and clinical departments are listed in Box 10.1.

Of the 18 clinical departments, four have a single department head: ophthalmology, otology-laryngology, physical medicine and rehabilitation and population medicine. Of the other 14 clinical departments, the leadership consists of an executive committee. Twelve of these—including surgery and neurosurgery (an academic department established in 2013)—have an executive committee chairperson. Only two of the 14 clinical departments—anesthesia and orthopaedic surgery—have a secretary of the executive committee as the head of the committee. The executive committees of each clinical department include the heads of the services of their specialty in each of the major teaching hospitals. The executive committee's secretary position rotates every three years. The chairperson of clinical departments maintains that position for only three years.

The former administrative board of the medical school no longer exists. The committee of professors and the faculty council remain; the faculty council meets monthly. As of 2019, it consists of elected members of the voting faculty (three-year terms), representing all institutions and specialties. The council is chaired by the dean. It receives reports from committees of the dean and submits policy recommendations to the dean. There are

Box 10.1. Harvard Medical School's Preclinical and Clinical Departments

PRECLINICAL
    Biological Chemistry and Molecular Pharmacology
    Biomedical Informatics
    Cell Biology
    Genetics
    Health Care Policy
    Microbiology and Immunobiology
    Neurobiology
    Global Health and Social Medicine
    Systems Biology
    Stem Cell and Regenerative Biology

CLINICAL
Anesthesia—Executive Committee Secretary
    BIDMC Chair, BWH Chair, BCH Chair, MGH Chair
Dermatology—Executive Committee Chairperson
    BIDMC Chair, BWH Chair, MGH Chair
Emergency Medicine—Executive Committee
    Chairperson
Ob, Gyn and Repro. Biology—Executive Committee
    Chairperson
    BIDMC Chair, BWH Chair, MGH Chair

Ophthalmology—Chairperson
Orthopedic Surgery—Executive Committee Secretary
    BIDMC Chair, BWH Chair, BCH Chair, MGH Chair
Otology–Laryngology—Chairperson
Pathology—Executive Committee Chairperson
    BIDMC Chair, BWH Chair, BCH Chair, MGH Chair
Pediatrics—Executive Committee Chairperson
    BCH Chair, MGH Chair
Physical Medical & Rehabilitation—Chairperson
Population Medicine—Chairperson
Psychiatry—Executive Committee Chairperson
    BIDMC/MMHC Chair, BWH Chair, VA Boston
    Health Care System Chair, Cambridge Health Alli-
    ance Chair, BCH, McLean, MGH
Radiology—Executive Committee Chairperson
    BIDMC Chair, BWH Chair, BCH Chair, MGH Chair
Radiation Oncology—Executive Committee Chairperson
    BIDMC Chair, BWH/CH/DFCI Chair, MGH Chair
Surgery—Executive Committee Chairperson
    BIDMC Chair, BWH Chair, BCH Chair, MGH Chair

numerous standing committees (including the committee of professors). There is no council or committee of clinical department chairs. There are four advisory councils that provide strategic advice to the dean and faculty: Discover, Education, Global Health and Service, and Health Care Policy. The medical school also has a board of fellows, which includes leaders in different professions who serve as external advisors and council to the dean. In addition, there is a visiting committee that is appointed by the Harvard University Board of Overseers to report on each school, department, or administrative unit.

Leadership at the department level is important for a medical school. The chairperson is responsible for the department's academic mission and is necessary for establishing a culture of significant research productivity and quality education—especially in teaching medical students. The curriculum in musculoskeletal medicine is important and should not waver or be diminished as it has been in the past when the department lacked necessary leadership. Teaching, research, and faculty recruitment priorities—essential for the academic mission of any department—are dependent on leadership that is not influenced by a hospital's competing priorities.

CHAPTER 11

The Harvard Combined Orthopaedic Residency Program

(HCORP)

The current Harvard Combined Orthopaedic Residency Program (HCORP) has evolved over more than a century to provide residents with unparalleled education and training. This evolution was shaped by early eighteenth-century instruction in medicine and surgery, by changing surgical practices and standards, and by the specialization of medicine in general and of orthopaedics in particular. Numerous influential physicians and orthopaedic surgeons had a hand in creating the orthopaedic residency program and the curricula for the education and training it provides; their beliefs and goals for providing residents with the necessary foundational knowledge, experience in patient care, and surgical expertise profoundly influenced the process of specialization in orthopaedics at Harvard Medical School.

EARLY SURGICAL TRAINING

Internship, the transition between graduating from medical school and becoming a practicing physician, has its origins in hospital apprenticeships, a concept that began in the eighteenth century and transferred to the United States from Europe. Some medical historians, such as Dr. Douglas Guthrie of Edinburgh University,

believed that such physician and surgeon apprentices were called "residents" because they lived in the hospital (Wentz and Ford 1984). Overall, historical documentation of the global and domestic development of hospital positions and apprenticeships is sparse. In the United States, however, hospital apprentices were first appointed at the Pennsylvania Hospital in Philadelphia in 1773. By 1846, Massachusetts General Hospital (MGH)

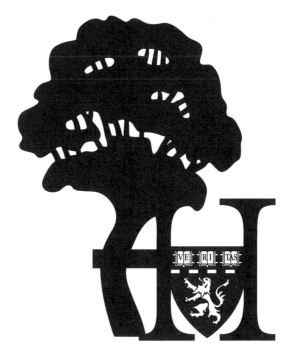

HCORP logo. MGH HCORP Archives.

was appointing graduate "house physicians" and "house surgeons" (Wentz and Ford 1984).

In the early 1800s, the Massachusetts Medical Association licensed physicians practicing in Massachusetts. The terminology used to refer to licensed physicians who were receiving postgraduate training has evolved but is poorly documented. For example, shortly after opening in 1821, MGH appointed its first house officer, who was referred to as an "apothecary." This individual had completed one year of medical school and worked under the supervision of a physician or surgeon. The apothecary was responsible for preparing and dispensing drugs and surgical instruments. By 1828, "house physicians" took over the apothecary's duties. Around 1830, both a house physician and a house surgeon were on duty at MGH. They lived in the hospital and were paid a small salary ($50 per year).

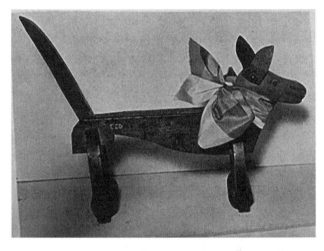

Wood carving of a "pup." A gift from the MGH nurses.
Massachusetts General Hospital, Archives and Special Collections.

Grillo (1999) notes this as the point when surgical training within hospitals began evolving. Physicians began surgical training directly after medical school, as house surgeons. These young house surgeons (later called interns or residents) often became overly independent and arrogant, assuming the care of patients while ignoring the advice of staff. Leadership at MGH responded

by replacing these house officers with third-year medical students, or house pupils, nicknamed "pups"—a term reminding them of their lower status in the hospital's hierarchy. Over time, however, the name "pup" evolved into a source of pride for generations of student physicians (Grillo 1999). I remember being called a "pup" when I started the orthopaedic program in 1967; I was a PGY3 but a first-year resident in orthopaedic surgery.

By 1872, pups were living onsite, sleeping and eating in the hospital. By 1901, MGH had eight house pupils, and over the subsequent decade that number increased as the hospital added inpatient departments. According to Grillo (1999), MGH had twelve pups, each in one of four positions—an "etherizer," the role in which students began their tenure; a pup, who acted as an assistant in the clinics and ran errands; a junior, who cared for patients on the ward and was second assistant in the operating room; or a senior, who scheduled and assisted during surgeries, eventually operating alone—across three surgical services (East, West, and South). House pupils moved through the ranks over 16 months. The schedule was unrelenting and rigorous, providing the groundwork for a career in surgery. Most graduates, however, apprenticed to a more experienced surgeon after completing their tenure as a house pupil. The term "resident in surgery" was first documented at MGH in 1911, in a role that was the forerunner of today's "chief resident" (Grillo 1999).

The French term *interne* had been used since before 1859 to refer to hospital interns, but it was not until the 1880s that the term was documented in the US. On the basis of recommendations from its board of trustees, Children's Hospital in Boston first appointed house officers, called "internes" or "externs," in 1882 (F. H. Brown 1882). These house officers were "to assist the Medical Officers in the care of patients" (F. H. Brown 1882), particularly outpatients. "Interne" was first mentioned at MGH in 1913, in a report of the MGH General Executive Committee. The French *interne* and the US "intern" refer to different stages of training:

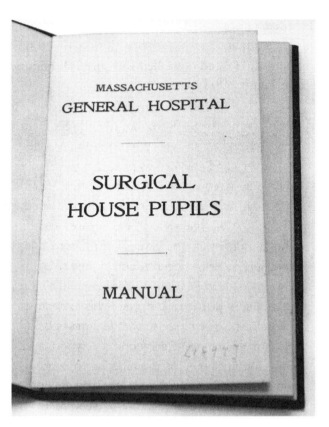

MGH Surgical House Pupils' Manual.
Massachusetts General Hospital, Archives and Special Collections.

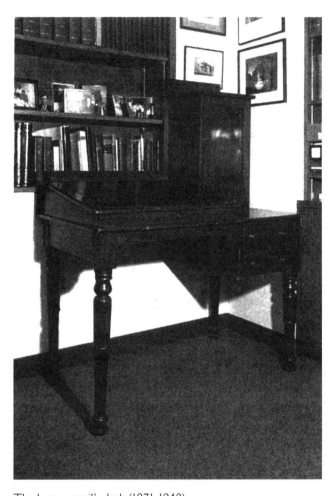

The house pupil's desk (1871-1940).
Massachusetts General Hospital, Archives and Special Collections.

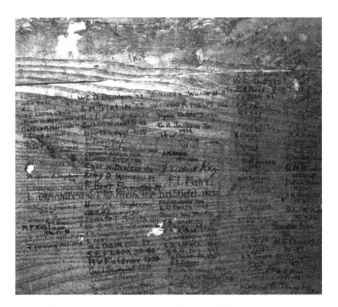

Surgical residents' signatures under the desk top.
Massachusetts General Hospital, Archives and Special Collections.

a French interne has a status similar to that of a resident in the US system. Curran (1959) theorizes that Dr. William Halsted adapted the French term to refer to medical school graduates in their first year of training in the new residency system he created at Johns Hopkins Hospital in 1899—a system that today is ubiquitous throughout the US. Around the time Halsted began his program, surgical training programs lasted 21 months. Over the subsequent 35 years, this training period increased to at least three years.

Halsted's residency program at Hopkins greatly influenced the development of surgical training throughout the twentieth century. In 1889, both Dr. William H. Welsh and Sir William Osler, professor of medicine at Johns Hopkins, chose Halsted, who had graduated from Yale and been trained in Germany, to head the department of surgery. Halsted modeled surgical training at Johns Hopkins on the German system, which included education in basic science and, importantly, graduated responsibility during the training period. Halsted described this surgical training program in a 1904 speech:

> Pain, hemorrhage, infection, the three great evils which had always embittered the practice of surgery and checked its progress, were, in a moment, in a quarter of a century [1846–1873] robbed of their terrors. A new era had dawned; and in the 30 years which have elapsed since the graduation of the class of 1874 from Yale, probably more has been accomplished to place surgery on a truly scientific basis than in all the centuries which had preceded this wondrous period. The *macula levis notae* [stigma of being illegitimate] clung to surgeons the world over until the beginning of the nineteenth century, although distinguished and scholarly men, as well as charlatans and barbers, have practiced the art in almost unbroken succession from the time of Hippocrates [460–375 BC] to the present day. A warning for all time against satisfaction with present achievement and blindness to the possibilities of future development in the imperishable prophecy of the famous French surgeon, Baron Boyer, who over a hundred years ago declared that surgery had then reached almost, if not actually, the highest degree of perfection of which it was capable.
> (W. S. Halsted 1904)

Polavarapu et al. (2013) enumerate three "principles of surgical training" for residents under Halsted's program:

1. Numerous opportunities to provide care to patients, with guidance from an experienced surgeon
2. A foundational knowledge of pathophysiology
3. Experience managing patients and the development of surgical skills until independent

Halsted specified the importance of incremental increases in authority and autonomy as residents gain experience.

> Were it not for the unattainable the world would indeed be a poor place. Those qualities that make the true man in any walk of life are doubly necessary to the making of the real surgeon:
> "Self-reverence, self-knowledge, self-control…
> Yet not for power (power of herself would come uncalled for) but to live by law.
> Acting the law we live by without fear;
> And, because right is right, to follow right
> Were wisdom is the scorn of consequence."
> —Peter P. Johnson, MD, Presidential Address, American Surgical Association, 1918, quoting from Alfred, Lord Tennyson, "Oenone," 1829

EARLY TRAINING IN ORTHOPAEDIC SURGERY

Historically in the US, postgraduate training comprised apprenticeships in which a recent medical school graduate spent one or two years working with and learning from an established practitioner, usually in general medicine with some minor surgery. Some—beginning with Buckminster Brown in 1844 (see chapter 6) and then Edward H. Bradford in the 1870s (see chapter 15)—began to study the specialty of orthopaedics in Europe. Others, like Robert Lovett in the late 1880s (see chapter 16), did an orthopaedic apprenticeship in the United States as a few physicians began to practice the specialty in hospitals, focusing their clinical work on orthopaedic surgery.

Residency, i.e., specialty, training was not available until the first quarter of the twentieth century. At the turn of the century, however, internships became increasingly available in many hospitals. For example, 6–12-month internships were offered not only at Children's Hospital but also at MGH, Boston City Hospital, the House of the Good Samaritan, Carney Hospital, and others. These internships were available to fourth-year medical students and to medical-school graduates.

Physicians would often extend their internship (for example, up to a total of 18 months) in order to receive additional training in different fields of surgery—although many specialties (except medicine and surgery) were not defined until later.

Some physicians began to focus or limit their practice to orthopaedics after internships. For example, after graduating from Harvard Medical School in 1889, Joel E. Goldthwait did two internships: one at Children's Hospital in 1890 and a second at Boston City Hospital in 1891 (see chapter 30). The influence of Dr. Edward H. Bradford and Dr. Robert W. Lovett at both hospitals led Goldthwait to eventually limit his practice to orthopaedic surgery. In the first decade of the twentieth century, Children's Hospital offered two options for additional surgical training: a six-month internship in surgery or a six-month internship with three months in surgery and three months in orthopaedics. Two positions were available in each of the years 1910, 1911, and 1912. Dr. J. W. Sever, who had been a house officer at Children's Hospital in 1901, learned from and worked with both Bradford and Lovett. As noted before, documentation of postgraduate training in the late-nineteenth century and the first two decades of the twentieth century is inadequate, and examples of individuals such as Dr. Sever and Dr. Goldthwait are difficult to discover.

Although orthopaedics had been a separate department from the department of surgery at Children's Hospital since 1903; internships were surgical or medical and usually six-months long, as noted in the orthopaedic department's 1912 annual report:

A great improvement has been made by the appointment of a Resident Surgeon, a policy which is being adopted by many of the more modern hospitals. The service of the house officer in our hospital is six months...their stay at the hospital has been too short and the change in personnel too frequent to secure that continuity and experience which are for the best interest of the patients. The presence of a permanent resident surgeon of large experience... in addition to the surgical house officers has proved of the greatest use in standardizing and elevating the practical and scientific work of the institution. No change of recent years has been of more direct practical value. (Children's Hospital Archives)

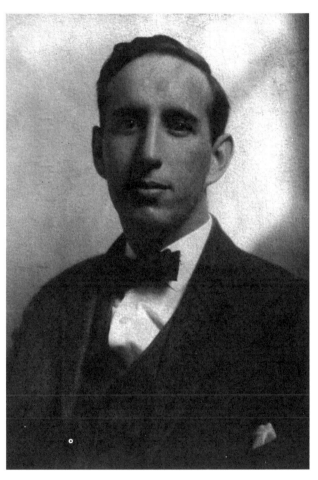

Henry FitzSimmons. He preferred to spell his name with a capital "S" after Fitz, instead of Fitzsimmons (commonly used). Courtesy of Henry J. FitzSimmons Scannell.

In 1910, Henry J. FitzSimmons became a surgical house officer at Children's Hospital (see chapter 23). He chose to spend his entire six-month internship in orthopaedics and not rotate to surgery, as he had completed an 18-month surgical internship at Boston City Hospital and afterward spent time as a resident surgeon at the

East Boston Relief Station. During FitzSimmons' internship, Dr. Bradford was chief of the orthopaedic service. After completing the internship, FitzSimmons spent two years visiting prominent orthopaedic surgeons in Europe and leading orthopaedic centers in the United States. He returned to Children's Hospital in 1913, according to the orthopaedic department's 1935 annual report, as the "first chief resident" and was referred to as the "House Staff Resident"; he "served in that capacity for two years and demonstrated very well the need for the position" (Children's Hospital Archives).

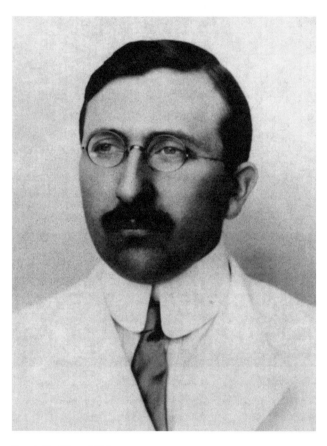

Frank R. Ober, 1914.
Boston Children's Hospital Archives, Boston, Massachusetts.

Also, in 1913, Dr. Frank R. Ober (see chapter 20) was a house surgeon; in 1914 he was recorded as being both a graduate house surgeon and house staff resident. He had been accepted into a one-year training program in orthopaedic

surgery, which he completed in September 1915. At the time, Dr. Lovett was head of the orthopaedic department. Dr. Ober remained on staff at Children's Hospital, and John T. Hodgen of Grand Rapids, Michigan, filled the position of house officer (or resident) in orthopaedic surgery. Other than these details about Ober and Hodgen, the records from Lovett's tenure as professor and chief reveal little about the new required year of training as a house officer (resident) in orthopaedics. I was unable to identify any orthopaedic surgeon between 1916 and 1924 on the 1924 list of former house officers at Children's Hospital.

Dr. Ober's appointment was a significant change in surgical training at Children's Hospital, as noted in the 1914 orthopaedic department annual report:

> A step in the way of advance has been made by the separation of the orthopedic and general surgical services, as far as house officers are concerned. Formerly house officers served on both, and under the new conditions it was found impractical to go on with this. Now separate house officers give their entire time, one set to the orthopedic service and the other set to the general surgery service. In this way greater concentration of work has been accomplished...More instruction is given at the hospital than formerly. (Children's Hospital Archives)

According to F. A. Washburn (1939):

> In 1901, Medical House Pupils [at MGH] were increased to eight...Beginning in 1909 the number grew with the addition of special departments with beds in the Hospital. Two orthopaedic House Pupils were added in that year, and in 1910 one for the Dermatological and one for the Children's Department...in 1911 the South Surgical Service was given up, and House Officers reverted to the two services East and West, there was no lessening of numbers but an increase.

In 1911, the first House Surgeon was appointed.

Between 1910 and 1915, Boston was becoming a center of orthopaedic institutions. A weekly short course in orthopaedics for medical graduates had been started at Children's Hospital in 1911; attendees came from all over the United States. In 1912, this course came under the control of the new Graduate School of Medicine at Harvard University. A nominal fee was charged. In 1913, courses at Children's Hospital were also available to general practitioners, specifically eight lectures on common orthopaedic problems. According to the annals of orthopaedic department for that year, "Grand rounds were established as a training experience" (Children's Hospital Archives).

In 1913, the number of surgical interns who spent three months on surgery and three months on orthopaedics increased from two to three per year, and the length of their internship increased to nine or twelve months; interns could choose how they spent their time among the various services. Because of an increase in the volume of orthopaedic outpatients being seen at Children's Hospital—5,000 more visits in 1915 than in 1914—the orthopaedic leadership believed that more house officers were needed.

At MGH, Dr. Osgood was a surgical intern in 1904 (see chapter 18). In the years 1908 through 1916, two or three surgical house officers were on the orthopaedic service at MGH under the leadership of Dr. Goldthwait and then of Dr. Brackett.

After 1917 the number of orthopaedic house officers (one-year appointments) at MGH varied yearly. Under the leadership of Drs. Osgood and Allison, the hospital appointed from three to seven officers each year. Some notable graduates of this one-year program include Drs. Charles Scudder, Leroy C. Abbott, Marius N. Smith-Petersen, John C. Wilson Sr., Mark Rogers, Zabdiel B. Adams, Philip D. Wilson Sr., George Van Gorder, and John Albert Key.

THE GROWING SPECIALTY OF ORTHOPAEDICS

During the first quarter of the twentieth century, medicine and surgery were moving toward increased specialization. Physicians practicing specialties established "national boards" to delineate requirements to take the certifying examinations and for being considered competent in the specialty. Rappleye (1935) described "three major phases of training" that physicians must undergo to be appropriately prepared to practice their chosen specialty: (1) foundational medical education and an internship in a hospital; (2) high-level scientific training in the clinical area of focus; and (3) real-world training overseen by experienced clinicians in a hospital—the goal of which is to achieve expertise and proficiency in a specialty.

The number of internships quickly increased across the United States. In Massachusetts, internships existed at the Peter Bent Brigham Hospital, Boston City Hospital, Carney Hospital, and 30 other hospitals. Such internships were becoming required after medical school, as a fifth year of training. To help maintain the quality of these teaching programs and to provide accurate information to medical school applicants, the American Medical Association (AMA) surveyed internships available throughout the country. Among the 2,424 hospitals with more than 25 beds the AMA surveyed, only 852 had interns. This list of hospitals became the first guide for graduating medical students. The AMA then developed a list of "approved" internships—those that met 10 criteria regarding the buildings and grounds; general supervision of the interns; commitment of the hospital to the community; a goal of teaching scientific medicine (versus being solely for the profit of the attending staff); workload of the interns; laboratory and x-ray facilities; recordkeeping; emergency services; and the educational functions (teaching and research) influences on the local physicians. The AMA organized committees in each state (called "State Committees on

Hospitals") whose purpose was to collect information on the aforementioned criteria from the listed hospitals in their state and "grade them on a civil service basis" (*American Medical Association Bulletin* 1914–1915). Dr. Ernest A. Codman, a physician at MGH, was one of three members of the committee in Massachusetts. The AMA concluded that reports of these committees will be used for a "larger list of hospitals which can be approved for the furnishing of internships and may show that the requirement of a fifth year as an intern in a good hospital will soon be fully justified" (*American Medical Association Bulletin* 1914–1915). In 1914, the AMA published the first "Provisional List of Hospitals Furnishing Acceptable Internships for Medical Graduates." In that same year, internships became a requirement for licensure as a practicing physician.

Children's Hospital underwent many changes during Dr. Lovett's tenure as professor and chief of orthopaedic surgery. In 1914, the hospital moved to its new facilities on Longwood Avenue. The number of beds on each ward was reduced to 10 in order to minimize the infection rate, and a ward was isolated if any patient developed an infection. Physicians would no longer treat active tuberculosis in the hospital, so the use of convalescent homes increased. At that time, Children's Hospital was treating only patients younger than 12 years of age, and the children could not visit other children on different wards. Also, in that year, the surgical house officers were separated into two groups: surgery and orthopaedic surgery.

Because of Dr. Lovett's interest in research, the orthopaedic department developed a closer relationship to the scientific departments at Harvard Medical School. The 1914 annual report noted, "Every [visiting surgeon] and house officer in the orthopaedic department has on hand some place of research work" (Children's Hospital Archives). Research was begun to study the effectiveness and outcomes of plaster jackets to treat scoliosis and the results of treatments for club feet and polio.

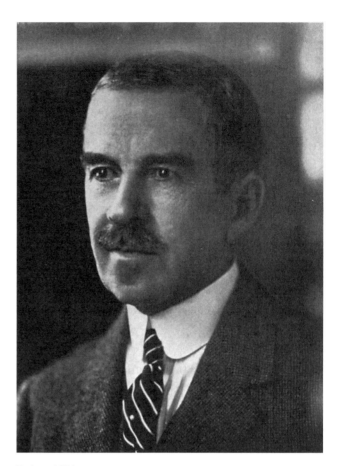

Robert W. Lovett.
Boston Children's Hospital Archives, Boston, Massachusetts.

Lovett, a strong organizer, improved outpatient care. Patients who lived far from Boston were seen and registered in the morning, then given appointments with one of the regular clinics in the afternoon. As the numbers of outpatient and inpatient cases increased, two Harvard medical students were assigned to orthopaedics each month, observed clinical material and followed assigned cases from admission to the end of their treatment. Lovett gave lectures to the two medical students every morning at Children's Hospital and, in alternate months, in the afternoon three or four days each week. Physicians at MGH gave lectures in the afternoon on one or two days each week during the alternate months. By 1915, orthopaedic clinics were held on Monday, Tuesday, Wednesday, and Saturday from 2:00 to 4:00 p.m. The annual report notes that this dual attendance at Children's Hospital and MGH "constitute[d] the relation of the Orthopedic Department to the Harvard Medical School" (Children's Hospital Archives).

During the summer of 1916, hundreds of children were crippled by poliomyelitis; many were treated at Children's Hospital. The annual report for the following year reports that, in 1917, Children's Hospital became a center for "intensive training of military surgeons in orthopedic surgery" (Children's Hospital Archives), an effort led by Dr. Lovett (see chapter 55). By 1918, a total of 201 military surgeons had taken the training course. During World War I, many of the hospital's staff were conscripted into the army and sent to Europe, but at Children's Hospital, both inpatient and outpatient cases as well as the numbers of operations done remained stable. Between teaching the third- and fourth-year students as usual and handling the additional courses for military surgeons, the orthopaedic staff, including house staff, were obviously very busy.

In 1920, the American Medical Association formed a committee to define the education and training of physicians who want to specialize in orthopaedic surgery. This committee unanimously established four *minimal* requirements, which were meant to regulate orthopaedic surgery by defining "those who will call themselves orthopaedic surgeons" (Allison 1921):

1. Standard medical school course, Class A school, four years;

2. Surgical internship at least one year;

3. Graduate course, one year as interne on service devoted entirely to orthopaedic surgery;

4. Six months in allied studies, physio-therapy, shop work and schools for cripples.

We will have then, after a total of six and one-half years of medical school and hospital work, our minimum requirement man, about to take up his life work as an orthopaedic surgeon. The committee also recommended that

languages other than our own should be part of this man's accomplishments, and that he should also be versed in anatomy, physiology and neurology, beyond the requirements for the degree in the Class A medical school... it remains for us, as teachers, simply to decide what we shall teach and how we shall teach it...After that, several years as assistant to some of our ablest and best orthopaedic surgeons...Sir Robert Jones...says: "In my early days, under the guidance of H. O. Thomas, part of my daily routine consisted in manually unraveling advanced club-feet, aided, perhaps, by tenotomy; each case representing several months of hard work, consisting of alternate stretching and fixation. The lesson it taught was invaluable in demonstrating the effects of perseverance and patience"...[At that time Sir Robert Jones defined the scope of orthopaedic surgery]: May I therefore venture to suggest the group of cases which a modern orthopaedic surgeon should be prepared to treat? They should consist of:

- Fractures—recent, malunited and ununited
- Congenital and acquired deformities of the extremities
- Paralyses of the extremities
- Diseases, derangements and disabilities of the joint, including the spine

...The war has taught the orthopaedic surgeon that he has to be more of a general surgeon; it has taught the general surgeon that he should be more of an orthopaedist...Our little wars with the so-called general surgeon come from a misunderstanding of terms, and an insistence upon rigid observance of what are regarded as rights and privileges. There is a certain type of so-called general surgeon who desires to operate only. His interest in surgery is largely from the standpoint of operative technique. Such a one will manifest his interest in the operative side of the diseases that affect the bones and joints, but this interest will fail during the long period of treatment necessary in these conditions. He is glad enough after operating, to turn over the case and responsibility to perhaps, an orthopaedic surgeon. Against this attitude in surgery there should be vigorous protest. The rule in surgery should be that unless a surgeon is willing and skillful enough to care for all the phases of diagnosis and treatment that arise in the individual he assumes the responsibility of treating, then he should assume none of the responsibility, but should advise the patient to seek surgical aid from a surgeon who is able to direct the treatment of the condition from start to finish…This principle should pervade all surgery. Unless a surgeon has this point of view, he becomes simply an "operator." We must teach our students that the operative side of surgery is comparatively small, that it is necessary to be able to operate well in order to deserve the name of surgeon, but the ability to operate well alone does not qualify a man as a surgeon… The important thing is that we should train ourselves and our students so that our minds and theirs shall be alive to the ultimate restoration of function…What is orthopaedic surgery? It is simply this—the surgery of the extremities and spinal column, which has the reestablishment of function as its guiding principle.

THE HARVARD "COMBINED" PROGRAM

In 1921, Dr. Lovett was in his final year as chief at Children's Hospital, and Dr. Osgood in his last year as chief at the MGH. The 1921 annual report notes that before they ended their posts, they created "an eighteen-month graduate course" for physicians who aimed to specialize in orthopaedic surgery after already receiving experience in general surgery (Children's Hospital Archives). It combined services at Children's Hospital and MGH; physicians spent six months at each hospital

after receiving six months of basic science education ("fundamentals") at Harvard. As Pappas recalled in the 1969 annual report, "Initially this program was under the auspices of the Harvard Medical School Courses for Graduates, although later it became an independent program" (Children's Hospital Archives). As Dr. Ober would write for the annual report in 1935:

> The House Staff of the [Children's] Hospital continues at a high level since this department formed a gentleman's agreement with the Orthopaedic Staff of the Massachusetts General Hospital giving the House Officers a combined service. There has been no dearth of applications for house appointments. It is safe to say that this is still the outstanding appointment of the country and there are applicants for places from all over the United States. (Children's Hospital Archives)

Dr. Osgood would follow Lovett as the head of orthopaedic surgery at Harvard Medical School as the John Ball and Buckminster Brown Professor of Orthopaedic Surgery, a post to which he was elected on June 21, 1922. This carried with it the position of orthopaedic surgeon-in-chief at Children's Hospital, and he started in that role on September 1 of that year. During his negotiations with Harvard, Osgood changed this arrangement so that future John Ball and Buckminster Brown Professors of Orthopaedic Surgery could reside in any of Harvard's teaching hospitals and not necessarily be the professor in charge of orthopaedic surgery at Harvard Medical School.

During the first year in his new position at Children's Hospital, Dr. Osgood noted increased demands for teaching both medical students and nursing students and the need for additional patient care in both clinics and wards. With money raised through Children's Hospital (not Harvard Medical School), he hired a resident teaching fellow for one year. The position included a salary (paid in part by the medical school) and room and

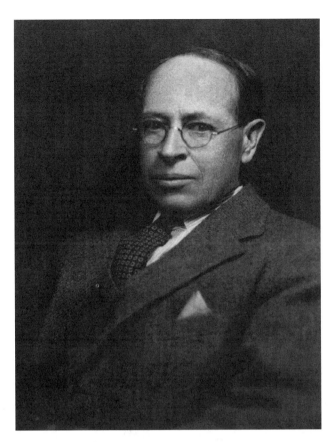

Robert B. Osgood. HCORP Director: 1921–1930.
Boston Children's Hospital Archives, Boston, Massachusetts.

board. The first appointment by both Children's Hospital and Harvard Medical School was Winthrop M. Phelps, one of the first notable orthopaedic surgeons to complete the combined program at Harvard. Phelps was orthopaedic chairman at Yale in 1931 and in 1962 became vice president of the American Orthopaedic Association. The position continued with yearly appointments, and by the second year the fellow was partly responsible for keeping Children's Hospital at the center of orthopaedic education at Harvard Medical School.

In addition to improving education for the students and house officers, Dr. Osgood assigned an orthopaedic surgeon to cover ward cases for three months, followed by six months in the outpatient department to provide follow-up to patients on whom the surgeon had operated. Specialization was increasing within orthopaedics, and Osgood started three specialty clinics: faulty posture, polio, and scoliosis. Osgood changed the

spelling of "orthopedic" to "orthopaedic," adapting the English version in 1924.

He also encouraged and increased the research efforts of the staff. In 1926, he obtained two rooms in the basement for research, where he studied embryology and the etiology of arthritis and nutritional diseases, and Rodney F. Atsalt investigated the early diagnosis of bone and joint tuberculosis. Osgood also provided house officers with protected time for research. For example, Dr. Joseph A. Freiberg, who identified the condition avascular necrosis of one of the lesser metatarsal heads (Freiberg disease), spent eight months on a research project to determine the cause of chronic arthritis, and Dr. John G. Kuhns studied the lymphatic supply to joints.

Following the teaching of Ignaz Semmelweis about the importance of hand washing in preventing infections, Osgood instituted a hand-washing policy outlined in the 1923 annual report: "[W]ash basins have been placed in all the open wards in convenient and conspicuous places and the rules of washing the hands after touching any of the cases is rigidly observed" (Children's Hospital Archives).

In 1925, the resident teaching fellow—now paid by Harvard Medical School rather than Children's Hospital—primarily taught students on the orthopaedic service. Orthopaedics was popular among the students: voluntary evening classes were started for the third-year class, and the number of fourth-year students taking an elective course in orthopaedics (both inpatient and outpatient) increased. Harvard Medical School awarded the first degree in orthopaedic research, a master of arts, to Arthur Van Dessel for his research on osteomyelitis. Van Dessel was a fellow from Belgium supported by the Hoover Foundation. Also in 1925, the number of orthopaedic interns increased by four; they were from the two-year postgraduate course given by Harvard Medical School and the orthopaedic department of MGH. By 1926, Dr. Osgood had started weekly rounds on the orthopaedic ward; these included the entire

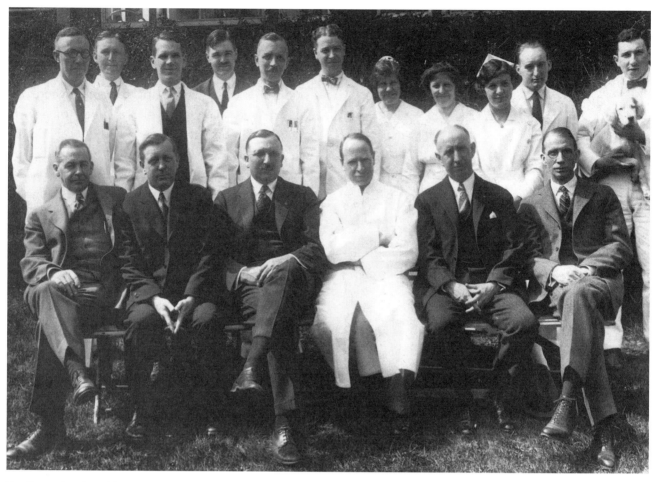

Dr. Osgood with staff and residents at Children's Hospital (ca. 1928). Front row from the left: Drs. Sever, Legg, Ober, Osgood, FitzSimmons, and Phelps. Boston Children's Hospital Archives, Boston, Massachusetts.

staff, a radiologist, a laboratory consultant, Social Services, and a physical therapist, a "Miss Merrill" (Children's Hospital Archives).

Dr. Ernest Codman was Osgood's colleague at MGH, and the 1927 annual report makes clear Osgood was aware of Codman's "end results" idea (Children's Hospital Archives). Osgood put Codman's concept into action, establishing in 1927 a bimonthly end-results clinic for the entire staff at Children's Hospital. All patients who underwent operations in previous years were reviewed and examined by staff who submitted a report of the patient's condition, which was entered into the patient's record. Dr. Robert H. Morris, a junior staff surgeon, and Dr. John G. Kuhns, the resident teaching fellow and a former orthopaedic intern, organized the clinic.

In his orthopaedic department report in 1929, Osgood wrote that he continued the Sunday follow-up clinics (start date unknown) and the weekly ward rounds by all staff (Thursdays at 8:30). The resident teaching fellow was now on duty continuously. Also, the Harvard Medical School curriculum changed: each month, a different group of twenty students began to rotate at Children's Hospital to study pediatric diseases, including orthopaedic-related conditions. He began weekly exchange visits with the surgical service at the Peter Bent Brigham Hospital (Tuesday mornings) to improve communication between hospitals. By 1930, however, the annual report concedes that the teaching needs of the students in orthopaedics continued to be in demand and the department's "most crying need" was more opportunities to do research (Children's Hospital Archives).

Sometime around 1983, Dr. Thornton Brown delivered an Osgood Lecture titled "Orthopaedics at Harvard: The First 200 Years." In this unpublished lecture, Brown credited Osgood with engineering the Combined Residency Program that is currently in place:

> It would also appear that the Combined Residency Program as we know it today emanated from the Children's engineered by the deft diplomacy of Robert Bayley Osgood. In his obituary tribute to Dr. Osgood, Philip Wilson, Sr., wrote: "He was able to arrange the incorporation of the resident training programs of the Massachusetts General Hospital and the Boston Children's Hospital into a single program under the aegis of the Harvard Medical School...It was the most advanced and comprehensive program of orthopaedic training in the U.S. and served as a model for many other medical schools. Dr. Osgood's concern for the residents and their training was legendary and to him goes the credit for the beginnings of the residency as we know it today." (Massachusetts General Hospital Harvard Combined Orthopaedic Residency Program Archives, henceforth: MGH HCORP Archives).

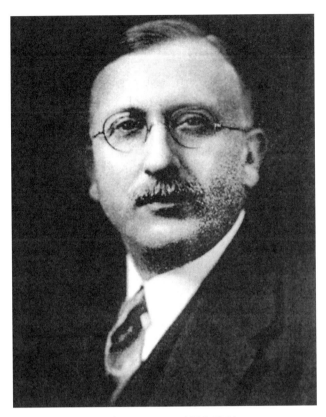

Frank R. Ober, HCORP Director: 1930–1946.
Journal of Bone and Joint Surgery, 1962; 44:787.

In 1930, Dr. Ober followed Osgood as the chief of orthopaedics at Children's Hospital and in 1937 as the John Ball and Buckminster Brown Professor at Harvard Medical School. He began spelling "orthopaedics" without the "a," as "orthopedics." As assistant dean in charge of graduate courses at the medical school, Ober published in 1930 a paper that briefly described orthopaedic training at Harvard:

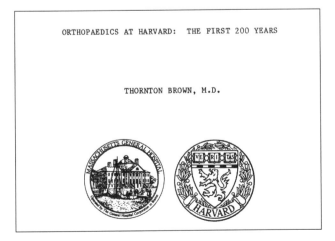

ORTHOPAEDICS AT HARVARD: THE FIRST 200 YEARS

THORNTON BROWN, M.D.

Thornton Brown. Osgood Lecture title: "Orthopaedics at Harvard: The First 200 years," ca. 1983. MGH HCORP Archives.

> The Department of Orthopaedics has organized a two-year course, eight months of which are given at the Mass General Hospital, eight months at the Children's Hospital, and the third eight months are spent in some of the chronic hospitals and in the laboratories at the Medical School. Along with these courses, the men are given clinical instruction by the members of the Visiting Staff, and they are allowed to do operations assisted by the members of the Staff on service in the work of the hospitals. These men

have the care of the patients in the wards under the direction of the visiting surgeons and are held responsible for their care...It has not been thought advisable to give degrees in medicine nor to give certificates for having done work, because there has been a feeling that such degrees and certificates are used for advertising purposes only, and personally, I do not consider it an ethical procedure. (F. R. Ober 1930)

At the time, the Harvard School of Graduate Courses offered four residency programs: neurology, ophthalmology, pediatrics, and orthopaedic surgery; this orthopaedic program lasted two years.

EXPANSION AND REGULATION OF GRADUATE MEDICAL EDUCATION

The Council on Medical Education and Hospitals of the AMA described medical education in a brochure in 1927. In 1934 it published the first list of approved hospitals for residencies in specialties. It included forty-four programs in orthopaedics in the United States, three of which were in Boston; one program on fractures at Cook County Hospital in Chicago was listed independently. The three orthopedic programs in Boston were at Boston City Hospital, Children's and Infant's Hospitals, and MGH. Each had one resident, usually for 12 months, who received a monthly stipend varying from $41.66 to $79.17.

The same council published in 1936 another list of the hospitals approved for training interns in the United States. Specialization had progressed to the point that all internships in Harvard-affiliated hospitals now focused solely on the area of specialization—interns did not rotate among specialties (rotating internships), as commonly offered in other hospitals. Thirty-seven internship programs were available in Massachusetts, 10 of which were in Boston. By that year, MGH had 32 interns, Peter Bent Brigham Hospital had 24 interns, Beth

Israel Hospital had 11 interns, and Boston City Hospital had 93 interns. Children's Hospital of Boston was not listed. **Box 11.1** lists important publications and milestones regarding the regulation of graduate medical education in the United States from 1914 through 1936 and onward.

Box 11.1. Regulations and Milestones of Graduate Medical Education in the United States

1914	"Provisional List of Hospitals Furnishing Acceptable Internships for Medical Graduates" American Medical Association (AMA)
1928	"Essentials in a Hospital Approved for Interns. Prepared by the Council on Medical Education and Hospitals of the AMA"
1934	"Hospitals Approved for Residencies in Specialties" (Council on Medical Education and Hospitals of the AMA)
1936	"Hospitals Approved for Training Interns" (AMA)
1948	"Approved Internships and Residencies in the United States" (the annual report of the Council on Medical Education and Hospitals of the AMA)
1953	First meeting of the Orthopaedic Residency Review Committee (RRC)
1972	Formation of the Liaison Committee for Graduate Medical Education (LCGME)
1981	Formation of the Accreditation Council for Graduate Medical Education (ACGME)

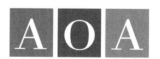

THE AMERICAN ORTHOPAEDIC ASSOCIATION®
Leading the profession since 1887

American Orthopaedic Association. Founded 1887.
The American Orthopaedic Association (aoassn.org.)

In 1933 the American Orthopaedic Association appointed a five-member committee to study graduate education (residency training programs) in the United States. Dr. Ober was chairman;

other members included Drs. LeRoy C. Abbott, William E. Gallie, Edwin W. Ryerson, and DeForest P. Willard. They created a survey of graduate training in orthopaedic surgery. Sixty-two of sixty-four medical schools and 14 hospitals (including Shriners Hospitals) completed the survey. The programs had few similarities: only 15 of the medical schools had orthopaedic departments, and interns spent an average of one to two months on an orthopaedic rotation, although five medical schools with hospital affiliations offered orthopaedic internships ranging from three to six months. The committee presented its findings at the American Orthopaedic Association annual meeting in Philadelphia on June 6, 1935, and published a report in the *Journal of Bone and Joint Surgery* in October of that year:

> The New York Society for the Relief of the Ruptured and Crippled (Hospital for Special Surgery) now has a service of two years for internes, and for resident surgeons a course lasting one year…The interns serving at the New York Orthopaedic Hospital and Dispensary [eight internships of two years], at the New York Society for the Relief of the Ruptured and Crippled, and at Harvard Medical School must be graduates of accredited medical schools and must have served a rotating internship of at least two years or a one-year surgical internship…The course in Orthopaedic Surgery offered at the Harvard Medical School now consists of eight months of pathology, an internship of eight months at the Children's Hospital, and eight months at the Massachusetts General Hospital, making a total of twenty-four months. Both hospitals have a Chief Resident on each service, part of whose time is spent in teaching. These residencies last for one year or more. (Ober et al. 1935)

At this time, graduates of the Harvard program received no diploma. Residencies, as defined by the AMA Council of Medical Education and

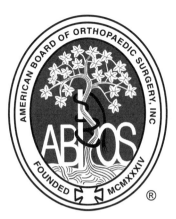

American Board of Orthopaedic Surgery. Founded 1934.
Used with the permission of the ABOS (abos.org.)

Hospitals, were classified as "special internships"; "residency" did not become widely used until around 1940 (Wentz and Ford 1984).

During 1933–1935, when Dr. Ober's American Orthopaedic Association's (AOA) committee was meeting, the American Board of Orthopaedic Surgery (ABOS) was established; the board was incorporated on February 4, 1934.

> In the beginning, the AOA, the newly formed American Academy of Orthopaedic Surgeons (AAOS) and the American Medical Association (AMA) each appointed orthopaedic surgeons to the newly formed ABOS. The ABOS gave its first certification examination in 1935… [which] consisted of four essay questions regarding basic sciences and clinical orthopaedic surgery. (Kettlecamp 2006)

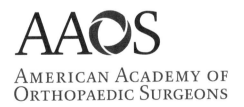

American Academy of Orthopaedic Surgeons. Founded 1933.
The American Academy of Orthopaedic Surgeons (aaos.org.)

The ABOS supplied to the AMA's Council on Medical Education and Hospitals information that identified hospitals suitable for training house officers in orthopaedic surgery; the council included those data when creating its list of hospitals approved for specialty residencies. Around this time, certification and state licensure were inconsistent. As time went on, the ABOS moved away from auditing teaching hospitals and began to conduct certifying examinations.

In 1935, ABOS created new requirements for candidates who wanted to take the certifying exam. To help his residents meet those requirements, in that same year Dr. Ober lengthened clinical service rotations to 24 months (12 months at Children's Hospital, 12 months at MGH) and required residents to spend eight months in pathology before starting clinical duties. In 1936, the house officers' curriculum included two-hour evening lectures every week or biweekly. House staff were accepted from all parts of the United States. By 1944, the ABOS required residents to have (after completing an internship and a year of training in general surgery) a basic scientific knowledge and experience treating fractures (six months for each), and to have spent time managing both pediatric and adult orthopaedic cases (twelve months for each).

Harvard medical students continued to receive the bulk of their orthopaedic education at Children's Hospital. They began to attend the monthly conferences with the house officers. Because of the increased clinical teaching demands, and to improve the research efforts in the department, Dr. Ober hired Dr. William T. Green (see chapter 15) as the first full-time staff member on site; he was paid a small salary to teach.

Dr. Edward Churchill, the John Homans Professor of Surgery, criticized the system in which physicians obtain experience through unsupervised private general practice, advocating instead for supervised training in an institutional graduate program. Thus, as 1940 began, he entirely restructured the surgical internship and surgical residency programs at MGH. The hospital retained its internal medicine and general surgical

training programs, but it began to offer specialized training programs in orthopedics, urology, neurosurgery, and anesthesia, each of which were now considered a separate service. For Churchill (1940), this "technical training under supervision in an institution must replace unsupervised technical experience obtained in private practice at the expense of an unsuspecting public."

Churchill (1940) goes on to describe the results of this restructuring:

> The Orthopedic Service occupies a separate floor of 50 beds. Fractures, certain cases of osteomyelitis and bone tumor, as well as pure orthopedic cases, are cared for on this floor. The Orthopedic Clinic of the Out-Patient Department cares for an average of 51 patients per day. Approximately 350 patients a year receive treatment for orthopedic conditions in the private wards. Third-year assistant residents in general surgery are assigned to this service for two months. Three of the six second assistant residents are assigned to this service for an additional period of four months. The Orthopedic Service in co-operation with the Orthopedic Service of the Children's Hospital offers a formal training for specialists in this field. The curriculum for training as a specialist in orthopedic surgery is as follows:
>
> 1. Preliminary appointment in general surgery of 2 years or its equivalent.
>
> 2. Combined service at the Massachusetts General Hospital and the Children's Hospital of Boston divided as follows:
>
>   8 months—Children's Hospital
>
>   8 months—Massachusetts General Hospital
>
>   8 months—Basic science, pathology and anatomy
>
> (At the present time opportunity for study in basal science cannot be guaranteed to every man by the hospital. Efforts are being

directed toward increasing the opportunities in this field.)

3. Certain men may secure additional training in the position of resident [chief resident]

Maintenance and Stipends. Interns, assistant residents and residents receive room, board and laundry while on clinical service in the hospital. Second assistant residents will receive maintenance during the periods of actual clinical service at the hospital but not during periods of elective study in basal science, laboratory investigation or work in other institutions. Salaries are paid to the Residents, First and Second Assistant Residents. They are determined in each case by vote of the Board of Trustees and vary in amount depending on the length of service in the hospital. No salary is paid during the intern year or to third assistant residents.

Churchill's reorganization of the program was not the only cause of change at this time. The United States declared war on the Axis powers in 1941. Although the US government implemented the draft, Dr. Ober noted, in that year's annual report, only one intern had been lost and thus the orthopaedic service had not been seriously disrupted. He did, however, project some problems for 1942: the visiting staff would be depleted, the number of interns would decrease because the War Department would allow only one intern in each graduating class, and Harvard Medical School would be reduced from four years to three years. Because of this shorter period of study, teaching occurred year-round, and as Ober predicted, the number of staff and resident surgeons in orthopaedics declined quickly. Both of these increased the required amounts of teaching.

Because of this smaller orthopaedic workforce, Dr. Ober discontinued the eight-month requirement in pathology and accepted residents into the orthopaedic program after they had completed a surgical internship. By 1944 the shortage of orthopaedic residents was helped by having surgical

residents spend additional time on the orthopaedic service. To complicate matters, however, the physicians had to deal with a polio epidemic in that same year. All research training for orthopedic residents at MGH and Children's Hospital was suspended until the end of the war.

Further changes in the regulation of resident training programs occurred during and shortly after the war.

From its earliest beginnings in 1936 through the war years to 1945, the ABOS and the AMA collaborated with the inspection of residency programs, as well as with publishing the list of approved programs...charged with maintenance of standards of postgraduate and resident training programs...In 1942 the AMA established the Liaison Committee on Medical Education (LCME) to maintain standards for undergraduate medical programs and to accredit medical schools in the United States and Canada...Subsequently throughout the 1950s, residency review committees were created for all...specialties, and were charged with setting the standards for organized residency programs in each specialty...the residency training program...no longer [was] a function of the Board alone. (DeRosa 2009)

A working group comprising members from the AMA Council on Medical Education and Hospitals, in collaboration with the ABOS Committee on Resident Training, reviewed the institutions to be authorized. The final list of approved residencies, published on May 1, 1948, by the AMA's Council on Medical Education and Hospitals, included the following Harvard teaching hospitals: Children's Hospital (Chief: Dr. W. T. Green; eight residents); MGH (Chief: Dr. G. W. Van Gorder; two residents); Peter Bent Brigham Hospital (Chief: W. T. Green; one resident); Boston City Hospital (Chief: Dr. J. H. Shortell; two residents); and the West Roxbury Veterans Administration (Chief: Dr. J. Barr; one resident). Boston

City Hospital was reported as the only Harvard teaching hospital open to women in orthopaedics. Residents' monthly salaries ranged from $41.67 to $83.33 at all but the West Roxbury Veterans Administration Hospital, where the salary was an extraordinary $275.00. The specialty RRCs in the current Accreditation Council for Graduate Medical Education (ACGME) are responsible for accrediting specialty residency programs, whereas the ABOS is responsible for certifying individual orthopaedic surgeons.

TRAINING UNDER DR. WILLIAM T. GREEN

Dr. Green published his thoughts on "The Ideal Curriculum in Children's Orthopaedic Surgery" in the *Journal of Bone and Joint Surgery* in 1949. Green believed that creating an "ideal" curriculum

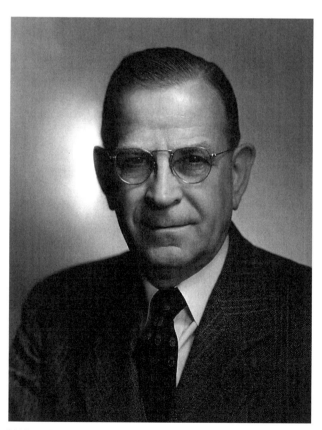

William T. Green. HCORP Director: 1946–1968.
Clinical Orthopaedics and Related Research, 1968; 61: 3.

was difficult because every organization differed. For him, however, any orthopaedic training program must include two essential elements:

> 1. Sufficient diversified representative clinical material; 2. Capable orthopaedic surgeons in the children's field to spend sufficient time in teaching the men who are in training...an ideal curriculum is difficult to discuss. What would be ideal in one situation would not be ideal in another. (W. T. Green 1949b)

Dr. Green did not seem to support a curriculum for graduate training, preferring instead "an ideal plan of training":

> In general, I believe that the best type of training represents an evolution from the apprentice system...apprenticeship is to a hospital service with all its attendant diversification rather than to one individual...problems presented by the patients...serve as the axis about which training revolves. Progressive responsibilities and experience should be given the trainee, as he is ready to receive them. Didactic lectures should be minimal...On the other hand, conferences and exercises in which the trainees participate are valuable, and form an essential part of any program...Ideally, a children's orthopaedic service is best located in a hospital which is concerned with all types of pediatric problems, both medical and surgical...at all times the orthopaedic service must maintain its autonomy...A service employing one resident is at a great disadvantage...It is preferred to have at least two residents on a junior-senior relationship, both in time of service and experience. A service that requires a larger number, however, is much more desirable...provides for a better discussion group. A large part of effective teaching of a trainee is by those residents who are senior to him in the rotation. The timing of the training in children's orthopaedic surgery in relation to the total

program may vary. There is much to be said for a rotation...at the start of the clinical training...it is essential to have...a senior resident or residents...who have completed at least two years of training...[they] have a teaching function and are prepared to receive senior surgical experience. We prefer to have a chief resident who has completed three years of training and is prepared for a position of great responsibility. (W. T. Green 1949b)

Regarding the clinical staff, Dr. Green stated:

It is preferable...to have several visiting men who have periods on house service and off service. This gives diversity to the teaching program, but continuity must be maintained by the orthopedic surgeon-in-chief. Out-patient clinics should be attended by visiting men who consult and advise. The major activities of the clinics, however, should be performed by the resident staff. Clinics integrated toward particular conditions are often desirable. They may be assigned to a particular visiting man, who has this as a special interest. Such an arrangement provides for a continuity of care, concentrates thought, and leads to productive activity. It provides an excellent teaching medium... each [resident] progresses from position to position, each with increasing responsibility. The men in training must do the work; observation has limited value...The teaching of surgery must be well supervised. Training should evolve through assisting, performing operative procedures assisted by a competent teacher, with progression to more independence as a senior resident. A man cannot learn surgery unless he does it...

Formal rounds should be conducted by the chief-of-service at least once a week, at which all members of the visiting staff and house staff are present...Cases should be presented by the house staff and discussed by the house staff and the visiting staff. The residents must be able not only to present cases well, but also to give their ideas and to discuss the problem. "Resident rounds," including the visiting staff and residents, should be made daily with all residents in attendance...They should see the patients, discuss all problems, and consider new admissions...The chief-of-service should have a weekly meeting with the resident staff, both for discussion of administrative problems and to consider any questions brought up by the residents about a patient or not. Regular seminars....should include a presentation of papers prepared by members of the house staff. Ideally, each resident should have a research project for investigation and report. Journal reports may occupy some of the exercises, as well as talks by...members of...the staff or by men in various fields. X-ray conferences may occupy certain of the periods. The chief resident may be made responsible for arranging the exercises...Pathological conferences should not be restricted in their material... [and] include such aspects as pathological physiology and biochemistry. It is our opinion that teaching in basic science...is best integrated with the clinical problems as they arise...A special orthopaedic laboratory, staffed with a director and research fellows, is very desirable [with]...a free interchange between the laboratory and clinical groups...A regular weekly exercise [combined conference], participated in by all the services...is valuable...All trainees should be encouraged to attend the general pathological conference of the hospital...Particularly desirable exercises are follow-up clinics, which are attended by all visiting men and residents...for end-result observations, thus allowing the trainees to observe the results obtained from various types of procedures...it should be emphasized that the program...must be adjusted to its environment. The essentials still remain: adequate clinical material and stimulating teachers who spend time in teaching. (W. T. Green 1949b)

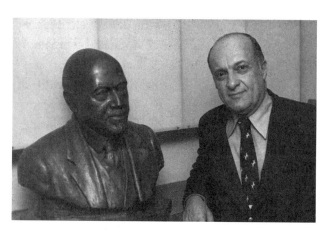

Henry. H. Banks with bust of Frederic J. Cotton.
Digital Collections and Archives, Tufts University.

Dr. Henry Banks, whom I interviewed on July 14, 2009, spoke proudly of his residency training under Dr. Green. He shared many recollections of that time during our conversation and in an unpublished manuscript he wrote and shared with me. For eight months (July 1, 1949–March 30, 1950), he was an assistant resident assigned to the pathology department at Children's Hospital. He spent the first two months in general pathology and the last six in orthopaedic pathology. "The teaching and supervision were excellent" (H. H. Banks, pers. comm., July 14, 2009). During that time, he was not required to work many nights or weekends and had plenty of time to read. He then began his clinical program, initially spending one year as an assistant resident in orthopaedics at Children's Hospital. It was "an intensive and stimulating educational experience...the best I had to that time" (H. H. Banks, unpublished manuscript). He had no salary but was provided a room and given meals and uniforms. He recalled that the hospital had four assistant residents, a few senior residents, and a chief resident.

"For my first three months, I was called a 'pup,' which was the lowest man on the totem pole" (H. H. Banks, unpublished manuscript). His responsibilities included obtaining an initial history from and performing a physical examination on all patients admitted to the ward service, performing all routine laboratory work, and assisting

his senior resident, Richard Kilfoyle. Each morning he and Kilfoyle made rounds among the ward patients. They had to be in the operating room by 7:30 a.m. and thus had to complete orders and test requests for all patients before then. "Those were very early days" (H. H. Banks, unpublished manuscript). Evening rounds started at 5:30 p.m.; in attendance were the chief resident, all residents, and teaching staff. The team saw each patient and reviewed their x-rays (which had been organized by the pup). He was on duty every other night and every other weekend. Even on his evenings off, he never left before 8:00 p.m. He recalled that one day he left the hospital early to help his wife move to their new home. The next day "I was called in to see Dr. Green and properly chastised" (H. H. Banks, unpublished manuscript).

Dr. Banks's spent the second quarter of his clinical program in the plaster room, where he learned how to make casts and bivalve casts—he made casts all day, five days a week. During the next three months, under the supervision of Dr. David Grice, Banks cared for patients on the polio floor, where he oversaw their rehabilitation. This kept him very busy both in the hospital and in the clinics. During the final three months of his first year, he advanced to senior resident and

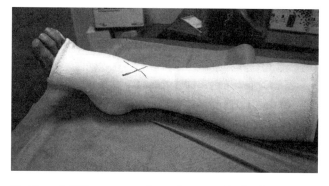

Dr. Green's "X" on a recently made cast with the foot in equinus—unacceptable by Dr. Green—which meant that the resident had to remake the cast before the next morning's rounds. Courtesy of John Burns (orthopaedic technician at MGH for 50 years). He made the cast on the author as an example for the readers. I was unable to locate an original photograph of this constant, forceful, demanding and often necessary oversight by Dr. Green. John L. Burns.

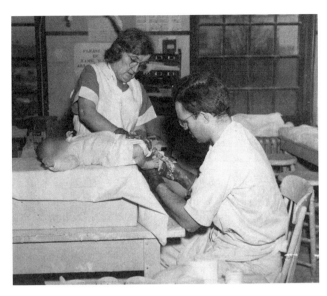

Resident (Thornton Brown) making a cast at Children's Hospital. Boston Children's Hospital Archives, Boston, Massachusetts.

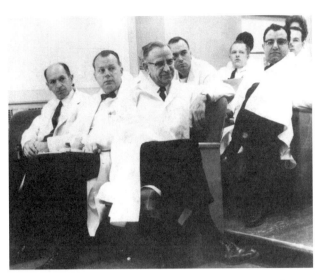

Grand Rounds at Boston Children's Hospital under Dr. Green. Front row, left to right: Drs. Cohen, Trott, and Green. MGH HCORP Archives.

managed the ward service with the assistance of his own "pup." He was then given the opportunity to do more major operations under supervision. He recalled that Ward 5 (the orthopaedic ward) was on the second floor. Older patients were on the first floor, younger patients on the second floor. No orderlies were available to help and the building had no elevator; therefore, the pup had to carry patients up and down the stairs for procedures, cast applications, x-rays, and so on.

He recalled that grand rounds were held every Tuesday morning at 8:00 a.m., followed by bedside rounds until 11:00 a.m. The pups would organize and present the x-rays for each patient. The senior resident on the service presented the cases. In addition, Dr. Green held a weekly "prayer meeting" (one–two-hours long) in which he and the residents discussed any issues of importance. It was called a "prayer meeting" because it was originally held on Sundays after Dr. Green, the staff, and the residents made rounds at the Peter Bent Brigham Hospital and the Children's Hospital. Eventually they were moved to Saturdays and finally, when the author was a resident at Children's Hospital in 1967, they were held on Wednesday afternoons. Dr. Green also held monthly a chief's consultation

clinic that served as a teaching clinic: residents would present complex and unusual cases from the clinics to Dr. Green, and he would give his opinion on further management.

"After this grueling year as an assistant resident at the Children's Hospital, Dr. Green invited Dr. Banks to be chief at the Peter Bent Brigham Hospital for six months, followed by one year as chief resident at Children's Hospital" (H. H. Banks, unpublished manuscript). Banks was in the orthopaedic residency program for a total of four years and two months.

Banks spent his third year at MGH, starting April 1, 1951. He recalled that his "educational experience at the MGH was more relaxed without any of the rigor and tension at Children's [Hospital]" (H. H. Banks, unpublished manuscript). Dr. Barr was the chief at MGH; Banks recalled him as a "superb surgeon and teacher; a giant unassuming man" (H. H. Banks, unpublished manuscript). Dr. Barr was apparently assisted by Drs. Eugene Record and Thornton Brown, who were together in a small group practice on Marlborough Street. Others, also in practice at the MGH, were Drs. Smith-Petersen, Aufranc, and Jones. Drs. Norton, Joplin, Klein, and Rogers

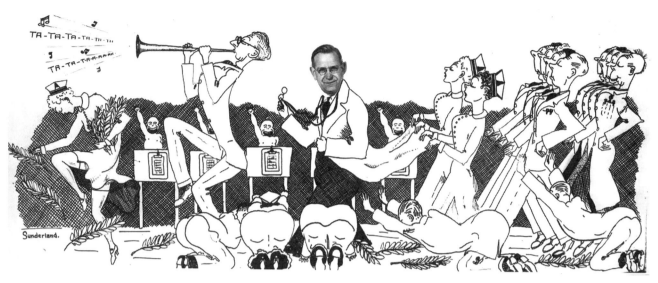

Cartoon of Dr. Green's hospital rounds, artist and date unknown. The artist modified a cartoon of Dr. Blackfan on Grand Rounds, replacing his face with that of Dr. Green. Published in *The Children's Hospital of Boston* by Clement Smith, Little, Brown & Co, 1983. Boston Children's Hospital Archives, Boston, Massachusetts.

practiced alone. Four assistant residents (from Children's Hospital, serving at MGH for three-month intervals) and four junior residents had previous training elsewhere, usually abroad, including Dr. Robert Harris from Toronto. (Harris would become a famous orthopedic surgeon and a leader of orthopaedics in Toronto.)

Banks's assignments at MGH included White 5 (male and female wards), Baker Memorial (patients in semiprivate rooms), and the Philips House ("Gold Coast"). The chief resident was in charge of the White 5 ward service. The visiting orthopaedic surgeons were assigned to supervise but were seen infrequently unless a problem occurred. The chief resident was "highly trained and experienced" (H. H. Banks, unpublished manuscript); he assigned the residents to cases and supervised the assistant residents. On the Baker Memorial or Philips House rotations, the residents provided work-ups of the patients for the attending staff, assisted the staff in the operating rooms, and provided postoperative care to all patients. Banks recalled that when Smith-Petersen operated, Dr. Aufranc assisted and the residents held retractors during the entire surgery. Grand rounds were held Wednesday mornings in the

Bigelow Amphitheater; the staff actively discussed cases that were presented by the residents. Banks remembers them being relaxing and not as stressful as those at Children's Hospital.

Returning to the Longwood-area hospitals for his third year (beginning April 1, 1952), Banks became the chief resident at the Peter Bent Brigham Hospital. At that time, Peter Bent Brigham Hospital had no designated orthopaedic floor. Private patients were scattered across both private and semiprivate areas, and male and female patients were often placed in separate open wards. Banks remembers it as "a small, remarkable teaching hospital. My masters were Dr. Harvey Cushing and Dr. William T. Green" (H. H. Banks, unpublished manuscript). His supervisors for fractures were Dr. Thomas Quigley and Dr. Carl Walter; he had separate visits (orthopaedic staff) with orthopaedic patients. The visiting orthopaedic and fracture staff made infrequent rounds, mainly to review problematic cases. Banks's chief resident at Children's Hospital had been Dr. Albert Ferguson, who had become a full-time attending physician at the Peter Bent Brigham Hospital and was Banks's visiting orthopaedic surgeon.

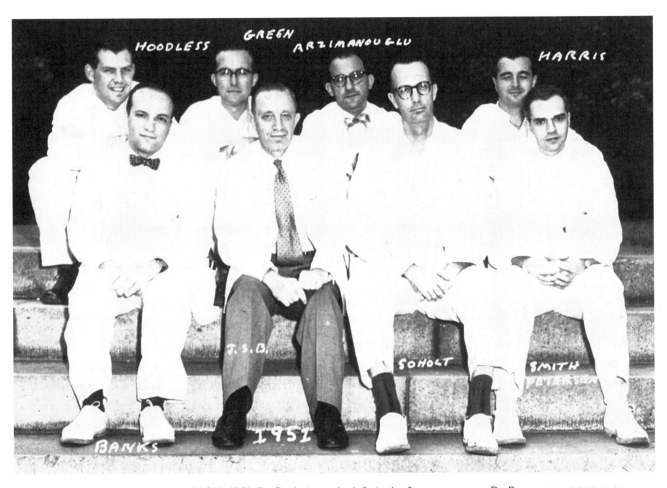

Dr. Joseph S. Barr with residents at MGH, 1951. Dr. Banks is on the left, in the first row, next to Dr. Barr. MGH HCORP Archives.

As chief resident, Banks had a senior assistant resident and intern on his service. They, along with a visiting orthopaedic surgeon, covered three out-patient clinics each week and made rounds twice daily (morning and evening), visiting patients in both private rooms and the wards. It was a busy service. Dr. Green made daily rounds of inpatients at 7:00 p.m. He was also in charge of grand rounds, which were at noon on Thursdays for one hour. (These resembled the grand rounds at Children's Hospital—they were stressful for residents, and Dr. Green could be demanding and intimidating.) After the grand rounds, the residents would present a few ward cases to Dr. Green for his advice. He expected the chief resident to assist him in the operating room. "In the Hopkins' tradition, the chief resident operated independently unless he asked for assistance by the visit...it was

a busy six months" (H. H. Banks, unpublished manuscript).

In his fourth and last year of training, Dr. Banks returned to Children's Hospital as chief resident, beginning October 1, 1952. He was in charge of the orthopaedic ward service and was responsible for supervising and teaching four assistant residents, three or four junior residents, and third-year medical students. His duties included making daily evening rounds, overseeing afternoon outpatient clinics, planning Tuesday's grand rounds, developing the operating room schedule, assigning cases in the operating room and selecting those patients he wanted to operate on, and requesting a visiting surgeon's presence in the operating room when their advice was needed. He was allowed to take calls at home after evening rounds and on weekends after noon on Saturdays. After six months, Dr. Grice

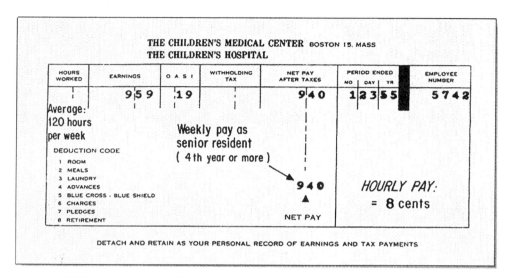

Senior resident pay stub; Children's Hospital, 1955. *Images of America. Children's Hospital Boston.* Charleston, SC: Arcadia Publishing, 2005. Boston Children's Hospital Archives, Boston, Massachusetts.

requested that Banks join him at his monthly disabled children's clinic in Fall River (the first Monday of each month), and Dr. Green asked Banks to join him in his similar clinic in Haverhill (the first Wednesday of each month). Banks recalled that he picked up Dr. Green at his home, and they rode together to Haverhill. Dr. Banks remembered that his salary as chief resident at Children's Hospital in 1952 was $3000 per year—equivalent to $29,091 at the end of 2019.

By 1960—almost a decade after Banks had completed the program—Dr. Green had extended the residency program to three-and-a-half or four years. This was after physicians had completed medical school and at least two years of internship and surgical residency. First-year orthopaedic residents (today referred to as PGY3s) all began their service at Children's Hospital. Second-year residents served at MGH. Third-year residents were scattered among various locations, spending either 12 months at Children's Hospital, six months at Children's Hospital and six months at MGH, or six months at Children's and six months at the Peter Bent Brigham Hospital or the West Roxbury Veterans Administration Hospital. In addition, one or two residents were placed in the orthopaedic laboratories at Children's Hospital or spent time in pathology. Interestingly, although the 1948 list of

approved residencies reported a salary of $41.67 per month at Children's Hospital, the 1960 report from the Orthopaedic Department stated that there was no salary for the first-year orthopaedic resident (PGY3 in current terminology). Second-year residents (PGY4) received a modest salary. Third-year residents (PGY5), however, received a much lower salary than second-years.

The residency program accepted two residents every three months in 1960, for a total of eight residents. All residents had to complete two years of residency training (with one in surgery) before entering the orthopaedic program.

The main financial support for the program came from the clinicians' practice income, and money was limited. Thus, the Children's Hospital staff covered cases and teaching obligations at the Peter Bent Brigham Hospital and the Veterans Administration Hospital. Eventually the leadership had to find potential additional funding sources, and in April 1960 the hospital began charging patients for visits to the large polio clinics.

At a conference on residency training in orthopaedic surgery in 1959, sponsored by the ABOS and the AAOS, Dr. Joseph Barr presented a paper titled "Residency Training in Orthopedic Surgery." He was asked to discuss whether residents in approved programs should have to

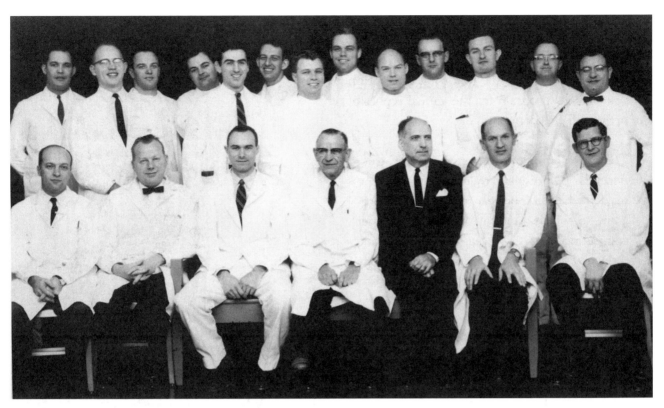

Dr. William T. Green with staff and residents (ca. 1962). Front row, left to right: Drs. Banks, Trott, Eaton, Green, Hugenberger, Cohen, and Griffin. MGH HCORP Archives.

complete a year of general surgical training before receiving specialty orthopaedic training. Barr enumerated the things inexperienced physicians learn during such general training, including important essentials of care of a postoperative patient—how to handle metabolic changes, blood replacement, treatment of shock, and wound care. This is in addition to education received in the operating room, which includes antiseptic techniques, patient positioning, draping, and tissue exposure, handling, and repair. He suggested that residents spend time in various departments and fields, e.g., emergency/trauma, psychiatry, so they could gain insight into their patients' conditions.

Barr (and, he assumed, most other educators) believed that the education students receive in medical school is lacking. Thus, he endorsed general surgical training and a curriculum that would provide it. He suggested a collaborative process between the board, the chiefs of various departments, and leaders in the field of orthopaedics to

develop this curriculum, which students would have to complete before beginning training in their chosen specialty (Barr 1959). For him, this would give potential orthopaedic surgeons more knowledge and allow them to provide better patient care.

By 1962 the residency remained three-and-a-half-years long, but in the last year, half of the residents stayed at MGH and its affiliates and the other half served at the Peter Bent Brigham Hospital, followed by a six-month period as chief resident at Children's Hospital or the Veterans Administration Hospital. In 1963 the program developed a secondary affiliation with the Robert Breck Brigham Hospital. The program occasionally accepted an international applicant, but the leadership mainly appointed only American citizens as residents. At the time Dr. Green felt that the limited time for research was the program's largest weakness. In 1964 residents began taking on a three-month rotation at the Robert Breck

Brigham Hospital; otherwise the residency program did not change.

In 1966—the year I was accepted into the program—Dr. Green wrote the following description of the residency program for the annual report of the orthopedic department:

> The major effort of our postgraduate instruction is in our resident training program. Our residents have a four-year (and 3 ½ year) program to which candidates are eligible after completing at least two years of internship and residency after medical school, including one year of surgical training. In the clinical portion of the orthopedic program, the first year is spent at Children's Hospital, the second year at the MGH and the first six months of the third year back at Children's. During the last year of their program, the residents are divided into two groups: one-half finish their preparation under the auspices of Children's Hospital and the other half under the aegis of MGH. We have enrolled at any one time 14 residents in various stage of training. The Chief Resident is in his sixth year after medical school. In the rotation those individuals under our aegis for the latter part of the program spend three months at the Robert Breck Brigham Hospital and in their final year spend six months at the Peter Bent Brigham Hospital, which includes the position of Orthopaedic Resident at that hospital. In their last six months our residents occupy one of two positions, namely that of Chief Resident at Children's or Resident of the West Roxbury Veterans Hospital. (Children's Hospital Archives)

Pappas further described the program in the annual report a few years later, in 1969:

> In July 1968 the number of incoming residents was increased to twelve per year, three starting every three months…[beginning on January 1, 1969]. They spend the first nine months of

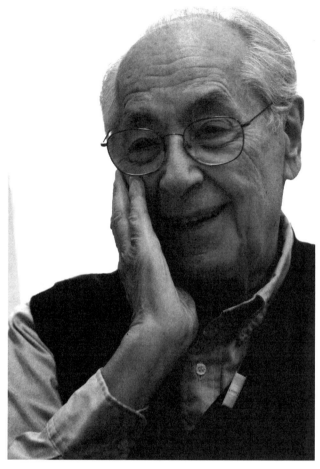

Melvin J. Glimcher. HCORP Director: 1968–1972. Stephanie Mitchell/Harvard University.

their program at the Children's Hospital Medical Center, rotating their experience between the in-patient divisions, the general clinics, and the specialty clinics. After nine months at Children's Hospital, they spend fifteen consecutive months at the Massachusetts General Hospital, and then return to the Children's Hospital for an additional six months of training. The next six-month period is spent at two of six affiliated hospitals: Robert Breck Brigham, Peter Bent Brigham, West Roxbury Veterans Administration, Beth Israel, Lemuel Shattuck, and Lynn Hospitals. Following these rotations, the residents spend six months as Chief Resident at one selected hospital. Therefore, at any one time we will have 42 residents enrolled in our training program, in addition to the

Fellows working in the laboratory or receiving additional training in special clinical areas. We actively encourage the resident orthopedic surgeon to spend time in the laboratory and develop a basic science interest. Many residents choose to spend a period of six months to one year in the laboratory prior to starting their formal orthopedic residency...Our research program has been gradually increasing in scope as new laboratory space has become available to us. We anticipate a greater enhancement of our research efforts when the new Pediatric Service Building opens in 1970. (Children's Hospital Archives)

Several years after Dr. Melvin Glimcher was named chief of orthopaedics at MGH in 1965 (see chapter 25), he was in charge of the residency program for a brief period. Sometime during Dr. Green's tenure as residency program director, Green may have shared the responsibility with Dr. Barr at MGH (Glimcher, pers. comm.). The only clue I discovered supporting this was a statement in a June 29, 1949, memorandum from Dean Burwell to Dr. Berry (the next dean): "These two men and their departments work well together, and I believe have rotated training of house overseerships [residency program director]. They act as a division in recommending

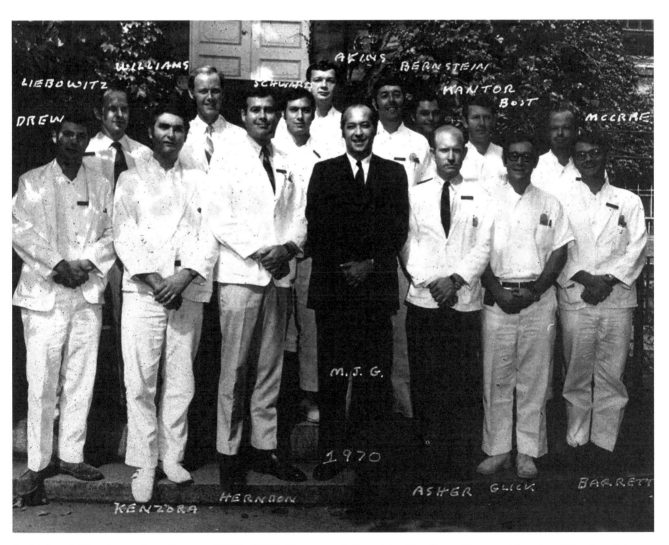

Dr. Melvin J. Glimcher with residents at MGH. (1970). Front row, left to right: Drs. Drew, Kenzora, Herndon, Glimcher, Asher, Glick, and Barrett. MGH HCORP Archives.

appointments and in organizing teaching" (Deans Files, Harvard Medical School).

With the aforementioned recent changes in rotations, residents received more experience with adult patients, while the length of the rotations at Children's Hospital decreased. The ABOS required 12 months of pediatric orthopaedic residency training until 1965; this duration was reduced to nine months from 1966 through 1970, and decreased further to six months in 1971. (I recall doing rotations at both Lynn and Lemuel Shattuck Hospitals before becoming chief resident at MGH in 1970).

Dr. Glimcher organized a series of six oral examinations, 30 minutes each, for third-year orthopaedic residents. The results of the examinations would determine two things: whether the resident would be promoted to the fourth year, and if promoted, at which hospital they would be chief resident. I recall the details of only one examination by Dr. Glimcher, who spent the entire half hour asking questions about the biomechanics of Harrington rod instrumentation in the correction of a scoliotic spine.

Around 1970 or shortly thereafter, the Children's Hospital/MGH program was placed on probation, according to Dr. Sledge (pers. comm., Sept. 18 2009). He informed the author that it was because "Dr. Glimcher, a non-clinician, was running the program" (C. Sledge, pers. comm., Sept. 18, 2009). (I attempted to determine whether the program was ever on probation at any other time. However, the ACGME does not maintain such records from before 1984, and no others were available to me.)

When both Children's Hospital and MGH first shared residents, Dr. Ober had referred to the residency as a "combined" program in 1935 (Children's Hospital Archives). In subsequent annual reports, Dr. Pappas and Dr. Green also called it a combined program, or a "coordinated" or "integrated" program (Children's Hospital Archive). Originally housed in Harvard's Graduate School of Medicine, the program eventually

became an independent hospital program under the MGH—a requirement by the ACGME and, in the 1950s, of its predecessor, the Liaison Committee on Graduate Medical Education (LCGME). I was, however, unable to find the exact date on which this occurred.

PROGRAM CHANGES UNDER DR. HENRY MANKIN

In 1971, Dean Robert H. Ebert and the MGH leadership recruited Dr. Henry Mankin to chair the orthopaedic department at MGH (H.J. Mankin, pers. comm., Dec. 22, 2008). The residency was on probation by the LCGME, and according to Dr. Sledge, Dr. Mankin would take the job only "if he was given charge of the residency program as a combined program in all the major Harvard teaching hospitals...agreed to

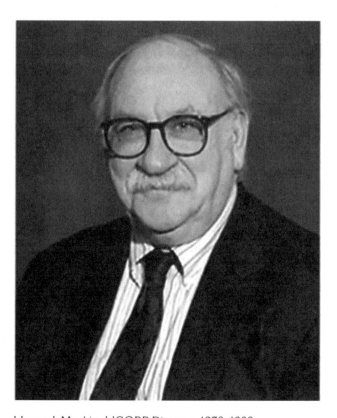

Henry J. Mankin. HCORP Director: 1972–1998.
MGH HCORP Archives.

by the dean" (C. Sledge, pers. comm., Sept. 18, 2009). The main orthopaedic departments at the time were at MGH, Boston Children's Hospital, and the Peter Bent Brigham Hospital. Dr. Sledge told me that the dean consolidated the hospital's orthopaedic departments in order to have just one chair in the medical school. Dr. Mankin was the program director and, together with Dr. Hall and Dr. Sledge, served on the orthopaedic executive committee at Harvard Medical School (C. Sledge, pers. comm., Sept. 18, 2009). Dean Ebert named Dr. Sledge secretary of the executive committee, de facto making him the chairman of the orthopaedic department at the medical school. Dr. Sledge reported directly to the dean.

> We needed a good residency program…it wasn't good enough with Children's and the Massachusetts General Hospital. Both Brigham Hospitals had merged into one…later we added the Beth Israel Hospital…we established a system for the three-hospital residency…Clement and I did the whole work; we put it together. John Hall loved it and subsequently everybody enjoyed working on it. (H. J. Mankin, pers. comm., Dec. 22, 2008)

When I asked him whether Harvard approved of using their name, Mankin replied, "No…no reason to get approval from Harvard…Harvard liked the name, I think" (H. J. Mankin, pers. comm., Dec. 22, 2008).

Dr. Mankin discussed orthopaedic education in an unpublished paper he wrote about orthopaedics in the year 2050:

> Education in Orthopaedics has been a major activity for many orthopaedic surgeons. The teachers teach the students and the students teach the teachers. Everybody wins! In recent years there has been some problems associated with this, chiefly in terms of the impact of health care administrative and funding agencies, which consider education

a less-than-necessary function. Education in the last decade of the 20th century is clearly less directed and less well conducted as it was in the prior decades, despite the fact that there is more to teach, and the students are more capable and avid for knowledge than ever before. If we are to maintain the quality of our orthopaedic care and research, we must make a very strong effort over the next years to maintain and enlarge our educational commitment to medical students, residents, registrars, fellows and, of course, each other. Without research in one generation, the specialty will not grow…without education in one generation there will be no specialty! (MGH HCORP Archives)

In my interview with Dr. Mankin, he said this about the Children's Hospital/MGH residency when he arrived in Boston: "We made a commitment to resident education and their [residents'] ability to become educators and investigators… [it's] not being done well now" (H. J. Mankin, pers. comm., Dec. 22, 2008).

Dr. Mankin accepted the directorship of the orthopaedic residency program in 1972. In the same year, representatives from the AMA, the American Board of Medical Specialties, the American Hospital Association, the Association of American Medical Colleges, and the Council of Medical Specialty Societies joined together to form the Coordinating Council on Medical Education (CCME). Their goal was to regulate graduate medical education through specialty RRCs. The CCME established the LCGME, which initiated the systematization and supervision of the various RRCs, including the orthopaedic RRC. The orthopaedic RRC was accountable to both the ABOS and the AMA through 1981, first under the CCME and then the LCGME. The orthopaedic RRC became a tripartite committee: In addition to the three members of the RRC from the AMA Council on Medical Education and Hospitals and three members from the

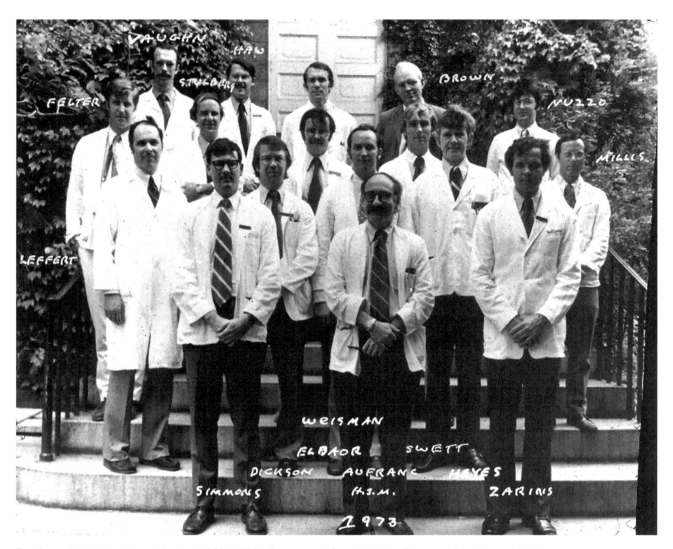

Dr. Henry J. Mankin with residents at MGH (1973). Front row, left to right: Drs. Simmons, Mankin, and Zarins. MGH HCORP Archives.

ABOS, three other members were added from the AAOS. This newly organized orthopaedic RRC met for the first time on May 17 and 18, 1973. Its purpose was to review and accredit residency programs and develop special requirements for the educational programs of orthopaedic residencies.

It wasn't long before conflicts developed between the LCGME and the RRCs, essentially because the LCGME tried to control the RRCs but lacked knowledge of the particular specialties.

In 1977 or 1978…the RRC for Orthopaedic Surgery proposed changes in the special

requirements…which had been unchanged from 1964: "Surgical and orthopedic facilities must be satisfactory and clinical material sufficient to afford residents adequate experience in the correction of congenital and acquired deformities and in the treatment of fractures and other acute and chronic disorders that interfere with the proper function of the skeletal system and its associated structures. Residents should become thoroughly familiar with all methods of diagnosis and treatment, corrective exercises, physical medicine, operative procedures, and the use of orthopedic appliances. Instruction in surgical technique should be sufficient to enable residents to undertake operative work on their own responsibility, especially toward the end of the residency program. Clinical instruction should include teaching rounds and departmental conferences. Residencies must be organized in the fields of adult orthopedics, children's orthopedics, fractures, or in combinations of these. As preliminary training, the Council recommends one year of general surgery in addition to the internship. Quantitative Requirements—Both hospital and outpatient facilities are desirable, and institutions offering residency instruction should treat a minimum of 200 patients annually. Applied Basic Science Instruction—Anatomy, bacteriology, biochemistry, embryology, pathology, and physiology are especially desirable and should be closely correlated with clinical experience."

The RRC for Orthopaedic Surgery repeatedly tried to upgrade these special requirements to improve the quality of education in orthopaedic surgery residencies and were repeatedly blocked by the LCGME...Fortunately, other RRCs also had difficulty with the LCGME. This ended in the discontinuance of the LCGME and the creation of the Accreditation Council for Graduate Medical Education (ACGME) in 1981...composed of five member organizations: The American Board of Medical Specialties, the American Hospital Association, the American Medical Association, the Association of American Medical Colleges, and the Council of Medical Specialty Societies. Each member organization has four voting members, a resident representative and two public representatives. Also, two nonvoting representatives are included: one from the federal government and the Chair of the RRC Council. The ACGME approves and publishes the "Essentials of Accredited Residencies." The Essentials include the "Institutional Requirements" and the "Program Requirements." The Program Requirements are developed by the RRC and must be approved by the three parents of the RRC and after that by the ACGME. Typically, the ACGME delegates authority to the RRC to accredit the programs in their specialties...The ACGME approved the Special Requirements for Orthopaedic Surgery that became effective July 1, 1981...[enabling] continued modification and improvement in the educational requirements for orthopaedic residency programs in subsequent years. (D. P. Kettlecamp 2006)

In the 1980s the RRC became more autonomous under the ACGME. As of 2001, the orthopaedic RRC included 10 members—nine appointed by the AAOS, ABOS, and AMA, and one resident chosen from among those recommended by program directors. In 2019, the orthopaedic RRC listed 12 members, including a public member.

Dr. Mankin, with the newly formed executive committee, began to reorganize the combined residency program on the basis of these new guidelines. He was a member of the ABOS at that time (1976–1982). The executive committee began to meet monthly, and around 1976 it officially named the program the Harvard Combined Orthopaedic Residency Program (HCORP), a teaching program of the three major teaching hospitals of Harvard Medical School (MGH, Brigham & Women's Hospital, and Boston Children's Hospital). "I also did something that sometimes people didn't like...I had breakfast with the residents" (H. J. Mankin, pers. comm., Dec. 22, 2008). Dr. Mankin started these daily breakfast meetings in 1973. They were held at 6:30 a.m., and residents at MGH were expected to attend. Residents presented and discussed with Mankin one or more cases, and Mankin essentially quizzed the residents. Residents either thought these sessions were the best conferences, or they feared them (or Dr. Mankin) or disliked them. During my interview with Dr. Mankin, he emphasized that his overriding goal was to "have an excellent teaching program and a competent clinical center" (H. J. Mankin, pers. comm., Dec. 22, 2008).

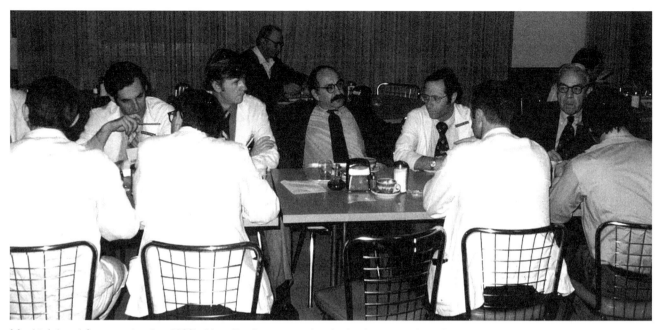

Mankin's breakfast meeting (ca. 1980). Note Dr. Jones seated in the back row on the right. Courtesy of Bertram Zarins.

In Dr. Mankin's first known "Report of the Orthopaedic Service" in 1980, he wrote: "The Ortho Service has led the MGH caretaking units in 2 areas: We were the first to 'privatize' the ward services in an attempt to establish one class of care; and the introduction of 'blocktime' in the operating room so that each individual surgeon is given priority on specific operating times and could book cases as he or she wishes during the sequestered period" (MGH HCORP Archives). He did this by requiring graduating residents to spend an extra six months following completion of their residency to cover all ward cases: "Two chiefs are selected for White 5 Service [at MGH,] extending their training by 6 months" (MGH HCORP Archives). These two chief residents were given staff privileges and ran the ward clinics, cared for the patients on the White 5 ward, and covered trauma cases in the emergency department. They had completed the ACGME residency requirements and could bill for their services.

At that time the HCORP was a three-and-a-half-year program with 12 residents per year (a total of 42 residents at a time). Nineteen were assigned to MGH, where there were eight fellows

(two each for the hand, hip, and laboratory; and one each in trauma and general orthopaedics). By 1981 the program was three-and-a-half or four-years long with a total of 48 residents. Nineteen of these, with two "chiefs," served at MGH. The number of fellows had increased to eleven with the addition of two in sports medicine and one in spine. Half of the residents spent six months in the laboratory. During their additional six months the chiefs were given the titles of assistant in orthopaedics and chief of the teaching service. As noted in Mankin's 1982 "Chiefs of Service Report":

This time [PGY6] is in excess of board requirements. An assistant in orthopaedics operates with minimal supervision and is responsible for private patients, admissions, operating room activities, etc., usually on the trauma team of the participating hospitals.

He adds:

Although the Harvard program is a single program for ease of administration and availability of personal supervision, the program has been divided into two tracts: the MGH-CH-BI [Beth Israel] tract and the Brigham-CH-BIH [Beth Israel Hospital] tract. (MGH HCORP Archives)

Each tract required equal time at Children's Hospital and approximately equal time on specialty services. Twelve residents started at the MGH and four started on the Brigham tract. Assignments were random. The three-year "core" program met ABOS requirements. The pediatric experience included six months of the first year spent on pediatric orthopaedics and three months of the second or third year, both at Children's Hospital. All residents then spent another six months as "chief" or assistant in orthopaedics at one of the teaching hospitals. Other than the addition of a third fellow in the laboratory, no changes occurred to the HCORP in 1983.

Dr. Mankin wrote his final annual report in 1987. The program followed the new ABOS requirements, "shift[ing] to a 4.5 or 5-year program [with 10 residents per year] following one year of preliminary general surgery" (MGH HCORP Archives). One Tufts resident also rotated on the orthopaedic service at MGH. Dr. Mankin wrote about coverage of the ward services, which was "privatized in 1972 and [is] now run as private practices by our former 'chief residents'...now Associates in Orthopaedics" (MGH HCORP Archives). The number of fellows at

MGH had increased to 18 (four in the laboratory; three each for hand, tumors, sports medicine, and hip implantation; and one each for microsurgery and pediatric orthopaedics). Mankin wrote that "The orthopaedic service is by standards of other services in the country and abroad, a successful one" (MGH HCORP Archives).

A core curriculum was started in 1984:

Twelve years ago [1984] the Harvard Combined Orthopaedic Residency Program initiated a weekly program for all house officers and interested personnel which was designed to provide key information regarding major subjects in each of the subdisciplines on a bi- or tri-ennial basis. A subcommittee for each subject area, composed of members representing teaching units in all of the hospitals, were assigned a block of time to introduce to the house officers concepts and principles (including especially research and basic science subjects) regarding a specific 'essential' core of information in the discipline. The goal was to provide not only lectures, but through the use of preassigned reading lists, a syllabus and pre- and post-tests, a format which could be instructive and more responsive to educational needs. (MGH HCORP Archives)

The first RRC-related letter in the residency program director's office is dated April 8, 1987, from Steve Nestler to Dr. Mankin, approving Mankin's "request for a temporary increase in resident complement by three for a total of 48 residents...[to] facilitate the transition from the current two-three [3½ year] program which has a complement of 12 per year to a one-four program with a complement maximum of 10 per year. It is understood that the new program will be initiated July 1, 1987 and the reduced complement of 40 (10-10-10-10) will be achieved July 1, 1991" (MGH HCORP Archives). HCORP requirements changed from two preliminary years (one in surgery) before a resident would be accepted into the

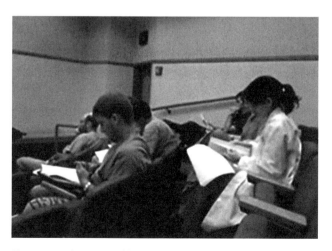

Core curriculum started by Dr. Mankin. Courtesy of Bertram Zarins.

orthopaedic program to one preliminary year to meet new national requirements. The length of the program changed from three-and-a-half years to four years, and the total number of residents in the program changed from 42 to 40. Before Mankin's tenure as program director, only those in their last six months of the three-and-a-half-year program could be designated as chief resident. When changing the program to four years, Dr. Mankin and the executive committee continued the additional six-month requirement for residents after they had completed the formal program, as required by the ABOS. The additional six-month period was called a "chief residency," during which a resident was given a junior staff position with admitting and surgical privileges at the hospital to which he was assigned. Their responsibilities included covering non-private patients in the ward clinics, the ward inpatient service, and orthopaedic cases in the emergency department, especially on nights and weekends. Thus, the total duration of the older program was five-and-a-half years; the new Harvard Combined Orthopaedic Residency Program matched that.

Dr. Mankin and Dr. Crawford Campbell (whom Mankin hired to help teach orthopaedic pathology, now a retired chief of orthopaedics at Albany) added another main element to the program in 1978: the very successful Boston Pathology Course (see chapter 40). The course was open to all orthopaedic residents in the three Boston residency programs. It was held at the Salve Regina College in Newport, Rhode Island, for many years. In 1998, Dr. Mankin turned it over to Dr. Mark Gebhardt (then a staff orthopaedic surgeon at MGH; see chapter 51), and in 2018 had its 40th anniversary.

A core curriculum committee with Dr. Richard Gelberman as chairman was formed at MGH in 1987 (see chapter 39). In September 1987, a new two-year cycle of lectures that included clinical and basic science was held on Saturdays from 8:30 to 10:30 a.m. In a review of the curriculum in 1993, Dr. Gelberman reported to

the curriculum committee that, on average, 12 Harvard and eight Tufts residents attended the lectures each Saturday. After reviewing the residents' concerns, the Core Curriculum lectures were changed from Saturday mornings to Wednesday evenings, from 7:00 to 8:00 p.m.; announcements were improved, now naming speakers as well as the time and place of their presentations; efforts were begun to increase the faculty's commitment to the curriculum; and the syllabus was improved to include topic reviews, more detailed information, and references. In the 1994 review, Gelberman noted that attendance continued to range only from 23% to 30% of the residents. Boston University residents could also now attend. Again, new adjustments were made: a four-year cycle instead of two years, with numerous speakers presenting over two years and the subject matter varying (some subjects were repeated only once). Also, the balance of clinical topics was improved, and visiting professors were added to the program.

Dr. Gelberman left MGH for Washington University in 1995, at which time John Emans took over as head of the Core Curriculum Committee. Attendance varied but would remain low. At that time residents had various concerns. In a January 22, 1996, letter to Drs. Peter Waters, John Wright, and Mark Gebhardt, Emans wrote:

> The Core was not comprehensive enough… the "top" is not committed to optimizing the educational experience, particularly with regard to enforcing protected time, a substantial…[portion] of the senior staff are "absentee landlords" who utilize resident work services, but don't directly contribute to resident education, the core syllabus was missed and should be replaced with a text, protected time was not available to attend existing conferences, Core and other conferences did not occur in a sequential logical fashion…and jumped from subject to subject…there was little opportunity for resident-based hierarchical teaching (senior

to junior resident), [and] there is little account-ability for learning-periodic tests, etc. and no disciplinary consequences for those who would not learn. (MGH HCORP Archives)

The committee planned continued adjust-ments and modifications to the core curriculum. In addition to this curriculum, in the early 1990s a "summer teaching program oriented for the new first-year Orthopaedic Residents [was begun] to provide basic information to aid in the first year Residents being able to function in the Emergency Department, and in the Clinics in a more comfort-able fashion" (MGH HCORP Archives). A new series of presentations, organized by Dr. Fulton Kornack in 1992, were given in the Smith-Petersen Library at MGH on Wednesday evenings in July and August. Topics ranged from fracture reduc-tion, splinting and casting, and introductions to major joints and the spine, to traction pin inser-tion, measurement of compartment pressures, and application of a halo.

Other excellent educational resources were available to residents. Dr. Joseph Barr Jr. orga-nized the Boston Prosthetics Course at the VA Hospital in the late 1990s. The Cave Travel-ing Fellowship at MGH was established in 1972 through the efforts and generosity of Dr. Cave, who established an endowment

to provide funds for the travel of orthopaedic res-idents to meetings and other activities designed to enhance their education; and to finance post-residency travelling fellowships awarded to recent graduates...who are, or expected to become, members of the visiting staff. The funds for travel are awarded by the Board of Trustees upon the recommendation of a com-mittee composed of the Chief of the Ortho-paedic Service acting as chairman, and three other members appointed by the Chief from the Orthopaedic Visiting Staff. It was Dr. Cave's expressed wish...to accomplish two goals: to further the education of the recipients and to

widen the horizons of the Orthopaedic Staff of the Massachusetts General Hospital through the knowledge brought back by the recipients of the fellowship. (MGH HCORP Archives)

One or two fellowships were awarded each year (**Box 11.2**). Since 2001, funds from the Cave endowment have been used occasionally to cover travel—especially travel abroad—by senior residents.

Box 11.2. Recipients of the Cave Traveling Fellowship

Carlton M. Akins (1973)	Timothy Lane (1983)
Sheldon Simon (1974)	Mark Steiner (1984)
Stanley L. Grabias (1975)	Bernard Bock (1985)
Bertram Zarins (1976)	Craig Weston (1985)
Stephen Lipson (1977)	Jonathan Deland (1985)
Jesse Jupiter (1978)	Richard Friedman (1985)
Victor Tseng (1979)	Gary Ackerman (1985)
Stephen Trippel (1980)	and Edward Diao (1985)
Tobin Gerhart (1980)	Jon J.P. Warner (1988)
Michael Joyce (1981)	Paul Re (1997)
John Siliski (1981)	Andrew Yun (1998)
A. Ingrid Erickson (1982)	Eric Giza (2001)
Thomas V. King (1983)	

The first ACGME Orthopaedic RRC Com-mittee review of the HCORP I found in the resi-dency program director's files was dated December 1990. The site visitor was Dr. Michael A. Simon. The program was undergoing the changes (from a three-and-a-half- to a four-year program) approved by the RRC in 1987. All residents were required to complete a year in general surgery before entering the HCORP. In the first year of the program, five residents spent six months at the MGH and five residents spent six months at the BWH; the groups switched hospitals for the sec-ond six months. In the second year, the residents rotated at Children's Hospital for six months and spent the remaining six months on BWH rotations and at Spaulding Rehabilitation Hospital. In the third year, they rotated for six months at the MGH on the Baker service (private adult patients) and spent the other six months at Children's Hospital, the Beth Israel Hospital, and on the tumor service at MGH. In the fourth year, they focused on adult patients, spending six months at MGH and six months at the BWH. The educational program included the core curriculum; clinical conferences at each hospital; grand rounds at both MGH and the Longwood area hospitals; the Boston Pathology Course in February and March; and a course titled "Basic Science in Orthopaedics," held in June. Drs. Gebhardt and Brown led both of the latter courses.

Research was an important part of the program. In their joint report, "The Resident Thesis: An Evaluation," Carole J. and Henry J. Mankin wrote:

> Since 1973 each resident in the Harvard Combined Orthopaedic Program has been asked as a requirement for graduation to present a thesis based on a clinical or basic research project performed during the residency years…half of the residents have a six-month "elective" period during the middle years during which the project is usually carried out. For the other half of the residents, the project is completed in 'spare time' often occurring during the lighter periods (such as they are) in the training program…all but one of the 153 residents completing the program between 1973 and 1986 not only submitted a written thesis but presented it…at formal Thesis Day programs, which occurred twice yearly, in June and December. (MGH HCORP Archives)

Dr. Mankin analyzed the success of the residents' academic productivity on the basis of the number of publications of their theses that appeared in the literature after the program had been in existence for 14 years. The publication rate was 54%.

The initial request to change the existing program of two preliminary years/three years of residency, with twelve residents per year, began in 1987. In July 1991, the RRC approved full accreditation of the "one-four" program, which required only one preliminary year of general surgical training but now would provide four years of residency training, with only 10 residents in each year. A letter to Dr. Mankin on July 10, 1991, from Executive Secretary RRC for Orthopaedic Surgery S. P. Nestler includes one critical comment made by the committee: "Ancillary support at the Massachusetts General Hospital is inadequate to support contemporary resident education. Residents should not regularly be expected to draw blood, start IVs, etc." (MGH HCORP Archives). The response from MGH to this comment is not documented.

RRC representative Dr. William Enneking reviewed the HCORP again five years later, in 1996. Enneking reported various changes on the Program Information Form for the RRC. The pre-orthopaedic year in general surgery (PGY1) now included rotations in trauma, the intensive care unit, plastic surgery, neurosurgery, and other specialties; no changes occurred in PGY2; residents in the third year now spend six months at Children's Hospital and six months at BWH, at the Veterans Administration Hospital, and on the spine service; in the fourth year the residents rotate on the Baker Service for six months and spend the other six months at the Beth Israel Hospital, Salem Hospital, Cambridge City Hospital, and Children's Hospital; no changes were made to PGY5.

In the narrative description of the program on the Program Information Form (PIF) it was stated:

> In 1987–1988 the Harvard Combined Orthopaedic Residency Program began a program designed to reduce the number of house officers entering each year (12 to 10) and according to ABOS policy, increase the duration of the orthopaedic component of the residency from three to four years. This change has in

our opinion enhanced the learning experience without altering the opportunities for specialization or academic pursuit…During the first year [PGY 2], the faculty at the two major adult units [MGH and BWH] and their associated institutions are responsible for providing the assigned residents with a basic education in orthopaedic diagnosis, physical evaluation, imaging technology and interpretation, surgical anatomy, operating room skills, ambulatory management and emergency care. Throughout that first year, residents serve as part of a team and have limited independence or responsibility. In the second year [PGY 3] of the four-year core, each of the residents spend five continuous "program months"…at the Children's Hospital (and MGH pediatric unit for one of the decile months). Drs. Kasser, Zaleski and coworkers are convinced that such continuous exposure at this level is necessary to establish a firm basis for understanding of orthopaedic problems in the pediatric age groups. (MGH HCORP Archives)

At the request of John Hall (then chief of orthopaedics at Children's Hospital) in 1992 (see chapter 26), to whom Mankin wrote the following January 21 letter (MGH HCORP Archives), Mankin finalized the pediatric orthopaedic experience to "include an uninterrupted six months at Children's Hospital in the second orthopaedic year (PGY3)…[and] more senior people (whose status is less well defined) can send a person to the MGH to cover the pediatric unit at that institution."

Enneking's 1996 report said:

In the second 5-program month segment of this year, the house officers spend a portion of the time at the Brigham and Women's Hospital on the Arthritis Service…and are also responsible for the Emergency Service and the Veteran's Administration Hospital caretaking. The responsibility is increased but…[residents] are still part of a team.

In July of the third year five of the ten residents enter their laboratory 'elective' during which they learn principles of research and the scientific method. Selection for the research tract…is entirely…their choice…Dr. Hayes has arranged a system where each of the four hospitals are responsible for supporting one resident…and the fifth is supported by monies contributed by all four…the Cave Fund…and Barr Fund…are very helpful in provided monies for House Officer subsistence during this period… the laboratory elective produces a "stagger" in the program, so that half of the House Staff are now five program months ahead of the other half in their training and hence begin their six month chief residencies in July immediately following completion of their fourth year while the other groups (lab electives) are available to commence their chiefships in January.

The entry into the third year [PGY4] either in July or after the five-program month elective in January marks the beginning of the 'Senior Residency' during which…independence and responsibility for patient care progressively increases…on Services in which he or she has considerably greater responsibility or is the senior person on the team…During the first period of the Senior Residency, the House Officer rotates through the Children's Hospital and Beth Israel…and through Salem Hospital. They then enter the MGH Private Service (named the Baker Service after the building in which it was formerly housed) …responsible for the care of patients on the various anatomical units, such as Sports Medicine, Upper Extremity, Hip and Implant, etc. and are assigned for a period of one program month to the Emergency Ward.

During the fourth year [PGY5], the House Officers are once again assigned to the MGH and BWH Adult Units (but not the same one that they were at as first-year residents) and are appropriately distributed throughout the various Hospital Units…The fourth year is a time of independent action and during this period at least six months is spent as the senior on one of the teaching services (under the guidance of the Staff and the chief resident). The year included significant periods of very busy and intense but well supervised exposure to trauma, adult reconstruction, back, foot, tumors, hand and microvascular surgery…

Each of the Hospitals maintain full clinic sessions in general orthopaedics…trauma… [and other specialty services]. Each of the clinic sessions is attended by one or more consultants (staff and teaching faculty) and the residents, although often considered by the patient to be the "physician of record," are closely supervised…

Following the completion of the four-year core and the presentation of the graduation thesis…the house officer enters a match for a position at one of the chief residency slots at the major hospitals (two at the MGH and one each at the BIH, BWH and CH)…

In keeping with the status of the program as part of a unified effort of all of the teaching hospitals, the Department has no chairperson, but instead is run by an Executive Committee which meets monthly. Current membership includes Drs. Sledge, Lipson, Kasser, Mankin and Hayes. Dr. Clement B. Sledge (BWH) is Secretary of the Committee and is responsible for setting the agenda and for academic affairs (appointments, promotions, etc. and sits on the Dean's Departmental Chairperson Committee), Dr. Stephen Lipson (BIH) is in charge of resident evaluations; and Dr. Henry Mankin (MGH) directs the Residency Program…Dr. Hayes is in charge of the research opportunities for the residents. (MGH HCORP Archives)

In addition to the regular conferences listed in **Table 11.1**, a pathology course was held over a long weekend in February, the Boston Prosthetics Course (covering prosthetics and orthotics) over a weekend in May, a biomechanics course over one weekend in September every other year, an arthroscopy workshop one weekend in May every other year, and the aforementioned Basic Science in Orthopaedics course, held during the last two weeks in June each year in Newport, Rhode Island.

Dr. Mankin acknowledged a few weaknesses in the program during Enneking's 1996 site visit:

> The program is large and by some standards, too large…[that] requires the resident assume considerable responsibility for his or her own education and social life…another minor issue is the possible interference of fellows with resident education and experience. We have been wary of this possibility for a number of years…A third issue is that managed care, capitation, health maintenance organizations, etc. have invaded our educational lives and made it difficult to teach or learn as effectively as in prior years. Care is administered rapidly and many aspects of the relationship between patients and caregivers are lost…In addition federal and state decreases in funding for health care and more particularly education make downsizing of the residency almost mandatory in some settings (including ours where the Partners [Partners HealthCare] have mandated a 20% reduction). (MGH HCORP Archives)

After Dr. Enneking's site visit, the RRC approved the HCORP's continued full accreditation as a five-year program with 10 residents per year; this accreditation applied for five years, although the RRC requested a specialty site visit to occur in 1998. The RRC concluded that the program could strengthen three areas of resident education, spelled out in the August 1, 1996, letter from RRC Committee for Orthopaedic Surgery's executive director, Stephen P. Nestler, to Dr. Mankin:

> 1) It is not clear that there is an educational need for resident assignments at the Veteran's Administration Medical Center, Salem Hospital or Cambridge Hospital…it is not clear that [these] residents…are able to adequately

Table 11.1. Conference Schedule at the Four Main Teaching Hospitals

	MGH	BWH	Children's Hospital	BIH
Daily	Breakfast conference	—	—	—
Weekly	Basic science tumor conference Combined radiology-orthopaedic tumor conference Hand walk rounds Core curriculum Pediatrics conference Hand conference Shoulder rounds Trauma conference Tumor conference Sports conference	Chief resident's conference Knee and foot conference Fracture conference Spine and revision arthroplasty conference Hand conference Core curriculum Combined orthopaedic grand rounds General orthopaedics topic conference	Orthopaedic basic science Clinical pediatric orthopaedic conference Chief's conference Fracture conference Orthopaedic grand rounds Complications conference Fellows conference	Chief's conference Joint replacement conference (Reilly) Joint replacement conference (Murphy) Spine conference Walk rounds
Biweekly	Pathology conference	—	—	—
Monthly	Journal club Mortality & morbidity conference Grand rounds	—	Journal club	Upper extremity conference Sports medicine conference Quality assurance conference

MGH HCORP Archives.

participate in the program's CORR [sic] curriculum courses...2) The interaction among sports medicine fellows and orthopaedic residents must be carefully monitored to ensure that the surgical experience of the residents is not diluted by the fellows. 3) The anticipated downsizing of the resident complement of the program must be carefully monitored to ensure that there are no adverse impacts on the educational experience of the residents. Given the anticipated change in the leadership of orthopaedics and the residency, the next site visit of the program will be in approximately two years. (MGH HCORP Archives)

On February 27, 1996, Dr. Mankin wrote to the MGH Orthopaedic Executive Committee a memorandum concerning the residency schedule and the Partners' planned reduction in the number of orthopaedic residents:

As all of you have heard the MGH has mandated a "right-sizing" for the Orthopaedic Service by a reduction of 30% of our residents over three years. (I have trouble figuring out what's "right" about it!); and similarly, the BWH has been ordered to knock off 20% of their cats as well. This leaves us with some problems in residency distribution...The fun will come next year when Clem and I each have to drop another...but either we'll worry about that then...or it may be an issue for the yet-to-be-named-El Jefe Grandissimo [Partners chairman]! (MGH HCORP Archives)

PROGRAM RESTRUCTURING UNDER DR. JAMES HERNDON

I was that Partners chairman. When offered the position by Partners after a national search, I accepted the position in the Partners Department of Orthopaedic Surgery (at MGH and BWH), and I began the appointment January 1, 1998. Just as Dr. Mankin had required that he be named the orthopaedic residency program director before he accepted the position of chief of orthopaedics at MGH, so I required that I become the residency program director before I accepted the Partners chairmanship. At that time, the orthopaedic residency program was probably the only combined

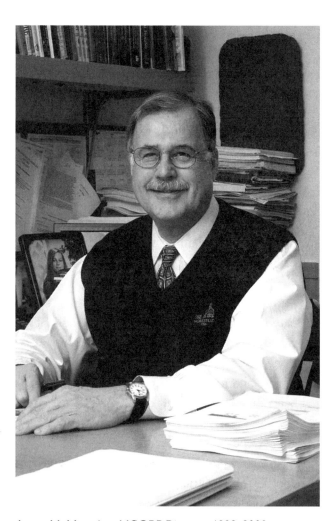

James H. Herndon. HCORP Director: 1998–2009.
MGH HCORP Archives.

and fully integrated residency in the Harvard system. Partners leadership had told Dr. Mankin to reduce the number of residents accepted into the program—from 10 per year to six per year; this reduction was to occur over several years, beginning in 1998. I rejected this. I wanted to maintain the size of the HCORP (10 residents per year, for a total of 50 residents). In an October 1998 letter to the Partners Education Committee, I wrote in defense of maintaining the current numbers of residents in the program:

> The Orthopaedic Residency Program is undergoing significant reorganization…development of Orthopaedic specialty services…at the Massachusetts General Hospital and the Brigham and Women's Hospital. Each service consists of junior and senior residents to insure graduated responsibility and an educational program…[allowing] information to be passed from attending to fellows to senior residents to junior residents in a meaningful way…to provide an extensive surgical educational program as well as outpatient experiences that allow residents to learn how to examine patients, to develop physician/patient interviewing skills as well as decision-making skills and to observe ethical practice. Prior to this reorganization our residents did not have adequate outpatient training. For example, the "Baker" rotation at the Massachusetts General Hospital is a leftover from the Baker [Memorial] building which doesn't exist today…The residents appeared in the operating room each day and scrubbed on different cases. They served as surgical technicians, spent only five weeks on the service, and had no or minimal outpatient experiences. This service was dismantled, and each new sub-specialty service has a responsible service chief, a group of faculty as well as residents, both at the junior and senior levels, fellows and students. The chiefs are responsible for organizing a teaching program in the sub-specialty and significant outpatient as

well as operative experiences. The rotations have been expanded to ten weeks to allow an in-depth experience for each resident...Additionally, we have developed a newly revised core-curriculum...an intense adult educational environment...[which] includes protected educational time on Wednesdays from 7 a.m. until 12 noon. All service obligations except emergencies are suspended. Each resident's obligation is to be at these core conferences. All residents come from each teaching hospital and assemble in one area for this curriculum. These changes are consistent with the mission of the Partners Education Committee...If our services expand and grow [Faulkner Hospital and Dr. Thier's agreement with the Newton-Wellesley Hospital merger to replace their Tufts orthopaedic residents with Harvard's Combined Program's residents], there will be an additional resident[s] requirement[s]...There has been an overall programmatic growth in the HCORP...an increase in outpatient volume; fifteen percent over the past two years [at Children's]...surgical volume...increase...for this fiscal year has been approximately 9%. [at Children's]...At the Brigham and Women's Hospital, the Orthopaedic Service has increased by approximately 3% in 1998...the overall increase in volume of the orthopaedic practice...has been 12.4%...anticipat[ing] increased volume of ambulatory and short stay cases at the Faulkner Hospital... At the Massachusetts General Hospital, the service has grown only modestly over the last three years because of transition of chiefs... staff relocations as well as retirements... growth [is expected] to increase dramatically as new clinicians are being recruited... Dr. Warner in Shoulder Surgery...Dr. Thomas Gill in Sports Medicine and...a Partners Chief of Trauma [Dr. Vrahas]...recruiting another hand/microsurgeon...spine surgeon...an adult reconstructive surgeon...and a foot and ankle surgeon...It is obvious that our resident

numbers can't be decreased without injuring our educational mission and goals...The residency training program of this caliber should not reduce its trainees further. It will dilute our educational experience...[and] harm our outstanding orthopaedic educational program. (MGH HCORP Archives)

Eventually the leadership at Partners agreed: the number of orthopaedic residents in the HCORP would not decrease.

When I arrived in January 1998, residents in the HCORP took the following path: a preliminary year of surgery (PGY1) at either MGH, BWH, or the Beth Israel Deaconess Medical Center (BIDMC). The first orthopaedic year (PGY2) was spent at MGH and BWH; a few residents rotated for about five months at BIDMC. The second

A Clinical Curriculum for Orthopaedic Surgery Residency Programs

Developed at a workshop sponsored by
American Board of Orthopaedic Surgery and
Academic Orthopaedic Society

Neil E. Green, MD ABOS
James H. Herndon, MD AOS
James A. Farmer, Jr. EdD Facilitator

June 14-15, 1990
Boston, Massachusetts

Supported in part by an educational grant from The Upjohn Company

National Orthopaedic Workshop of the ABOS and the Academic Orthopaedic Society held in Boston, June 14–15, 1990. Goal: To develop a clinical curriculum for orthopaedic residency programs. MGH HCORP Archives.

year of orthopaedics (PGY3) comprised rotations through Children's Hospital for six months, about two months at the West Roxbury Veterans Administration Hospital (WRVA), about two months at BWH, and one month at the BIDMC. The third year (PGY4) consisted of about five months at MGH on the Baker service; about five weeks on the pediatric service at MGH; five-week rotations through one of either the BIDMC, WRVA, or Salem Hospital; and about five months in research. The final year of residency (PGY5) was divided between MGH and BWH. The "chief residents" who became assistant or junior staff members at the hospitals spent six months at MGH (two residents), BWH (one resident), Children's Hospital (one resident), or the BIDMC (one resident). Residents were selected, volunteered, or were chosen by lottery for these chief resident positions.

Three months after my arrival, on Saturday, March 28, 1998, I held the first faculty retreat on the residency program; leaders from each hospital attended, with the goal of organizing a restructuring committee for the HCORP. Initially the committee included Drs. Gebhardt, Kasser, Lipson, Rubash, and Wright; I acted as chairman. We planned to enlarge the committee to include additional faculty and two residents from each year of the four-year orthopaedic program.

Newly developed guidelines from the Orthopaedic RRC were to become effective on July 1, 1998. Our restructuring committee planned to use these guidelines—along with clinical curriculum guidelines developed during an ABOS/Academic Orthopaedic Society workshop held in Boston on June 14 and 15, 1990, and the Academic Orthopaedic Society's 1994 document titled "A Curriculum for the Ideal Orthopaedic Residency of 1996, A Standard Setting Exercise Using the Delphi System"—as a foundation for restructuring the HCORP.

As captured in the report of that March 28 meeting, "Initial Committee on Restructuring the HCORP Retreat," this restructuring had numerous goals:

[1.] a) Incorporation of the newly-developed Residency Review Committee (RRC) guidelines;

b) The number of residents per year will remain at ten and all will be in the match [previously, some residents were accepted outside the match program];

c) The Partners' institutions plus Children's Hospital and the Beth Israel Hospital shall be the core institutions of the residency program. In addition to the four core hospitals, the program commitments shall also include Salem Hospital, Newton-Wellesley Hospital and West Roxbury VA Hospital as general orthopaedics rotations for the residents; specialty rotations should be three months in length;

d) An outpatient experience as well as inpatient experience shall be included in the residency program; [the author's stated goal was that every resident spent at least one day in the outpatient clinic each week];

e) The superchief concept will remain intact, although the responsibilities may be modified;

f) There may be teaching and nonteaching services;

g) The PGY-1 curriculum will be enforced as per the RRC guidelines and a committee shall be structured to deal with the PGY-1 year (see #2);

h) The negative impact of the Fellows on the residency training program will decrease;

i) The new residents' services should include a PGY-IV or V level resident with a PGY-1, PGY-II or III level resident, there will be resident responsibilities in teaching, as well as a mentoring process and graduated responsibility.

The attendees at the retreat identified various other changes to the HCORP:

2. A PGY-I committee was established; chair will be John Wright, MD, the committee membership will include Mark Gephardt, MD, Don Riley, MD, Kevin Bozic, MD (resident representative) and Peter Waters, MD.

3. Orthopedic rotations:

   a) Children's Hospital. The Children's Hospital will include a six-month experience at the PGY-III level; there will be an attempt to coordinate the activities of the Children's Hospital and the pediatric service at the MGH; the super chief resident rotation will continue; there will be an attempt to ultimately offer her a three-month chief resident (PGY-V) elective for those interested in pediatric orthopedics. The current 5-week PGY-V rotation will be eliminated. A committee composed of Jim Kasser, Harry Rubash, Jim Herndon and Dave Zaleski will meet to discuss issues concerning coordination of pediatric orthopedics. The question of pediatric orthopedics at Newton Wellesley was discussed but not resolved.

   b) General Orthopedic rotations shall include Salem Hospital, Harvard Community Health Plan, Newton-Wellesley Hospital [NWH] and the VAMC.

      i) Salem Hospital—currently Salem Hospital has one resident (PGY-III). Ideally an attempt should be made to have a PGY-II or III -level resident with a more senior resident for increased resident teaching, but because of work force issues it may not be possible to have two residents at Salem;

      ii) HCHP [Harvard Pilgrim]—currently two residents (consider teaching vs. nonteaching service);

      iii) NWH—currently three orthopedic residents from Tufts; since the Partners' organization will be merging with NWH, the three orthopedic residents (PGY-II, III and IV) will leave the hospital (beginning in 1999?). We will have an obligation to three residents at NWH for one year with a review of the program at the end of the year;

      iv) VAMC—currently co-directed by Drs. Ready and Martin. There are currently two PGY-III level residents. We will ultimately need to again provide a more senior and a more junior level resident for this rotation. Ideally this would be a three-month rotation with a junior and a senior level resident.

4. Rehabilitation—there was a general discussion concerning rehabilitation and its importance in the orthopedic training program. Although there are no specific guidelines for rehabilitation, it is felt that rehabilitation is provided at Children's Hospital with good exposure for cerebral palsy, as well as other children's neurologic disorders, that there is exposure at BWH and MGH for total joint arthroplasty patients; (we will check to see if there is an amputation unit at MGH), and there is also a question about the spinal cord unit at the VAMC; Spaulding Hospital will be eliminated from the resident program, unless a suitable rotation such as a stroke rotation or spinal cord injury could be developed.

5. The adult services at MGH were next discussed; they include a) adult reconstruction, b) tumor, c) sports medicine, d) trauma, e) hand/upper extremity, f) spine, g) foot and ankle/podiatry and h) shoulder.

6. At the BWH rotations include—a) adult reconstruction, b) sports, c) hand, d) spine,

e) shoulder, f) foot and ankle/podiatry, as well as, g) trauma.

7. At the BI there are currently four residents plus a chief resident for 15 attendings; there are generalists which include Drs. Glick, Yett, Gerhart, Levine, Murphy and Davis. Drs. Glick and Yett have a large geriatric practice; spine (Glaser, White and Lipson), joints (Reilly); trauma, chief resident, hand (Skoff), sports (Meeks). The full-time group at the BI include Levine, Davis, Lipson and Don Riley.

8. At the conclusion of the retreat, the general overview of the day's activities was summarized. A major point for conclusion included a three-month rotation concept to include a senior level resident (PGY-IV or PGY-V) as well as junior level residents (PGY-I, PGY-II or PGY–III). Each specialty rotation could be subdivided such that there might be specific rotations within the services (if needed). The faculty will become familiar with the residency review committee requirements. The residents will rotate as both a junior and senior in the same subspecialty for graduated responsibility although the site of rotation (and therefore faculty) may be different. The Pediatric Orthopedics requirement is 6 months (currently established at Children's Hospital). Currently, there is also 6 months of an established rotation in general orthopedics (? change). Therefore, there basically are 2.5–3 years available for specialty rotations (the reason for 2.5 is that half the residents are going to the lab for 6 months).

There was a general feeling that this was an excellent half–day retreat, that several major points were agreed upon by the group, and that a spirit of congeniality and cooperation was developed. The plan is for the expanded committee to be constituted and develop the specific rotation schedule to begin 7/1/1998.

Table 11.2 shows a breakdown of the rotation schedule during each postgraduate year after the restructuring. This schedule was designed to give the residents a junior and a senior level of experience, with graduated responsibility in each of the orthopaedic specialty services. **Table 11.3** lists the distribution of residents and teaching staff among the hospitals. As spelled out in the August 17–20, 1999, site visit by Dr. Joseph Kopta, "Following the completion of the PGY5 year and presentation of the senior thesis, residents are assigned to one of the chief residency slots at the major hospitals (two at the MGH, one each at BWH and BIDMC) [and one at Children's Hospital]. This is an intense 'junior attending' experience primarily in trauma and general/reconstructive orthopaedics at these institutions" (MGH HCORP Archives).

Table 11.2. Organization of Rotations under the Restructured HCORP

PGY	Duration	Content	Location
1	4 months	General surgery	MGH, BWH, or BIDMC
	1 month	Orthopaedics	
	1 month	Each of plastic surgery/ burns, vascular surgery, trauma surgery, neurosurgery, emergency department, intensive care unit and anesthesiology	
2	10 weeks	Adult reconstruction	MGH or BWH
	10 weeks	Trauma	MGH or BWH
	10 weeks	Sports	MGH or BWH
	10 weeks	Spine	MGH or BIDMC
	5 weeks	Each of oncology and hand/upper extremity	MGH
3	6 months	Pediatric orthopaedics	Children's Hospital

	10 weeks	General orthopaedics	WRVA
	5 weeks	Each of trauma/hand/ upper extremity	BWH
4	10 weeks	Adult reconstruction	MGH or BWH
	10 weeks	Trauma	MGH
	10 weeks	General orthopaedics and trauma	BIDMC
	5 weeks	Each of oncology and spine	MGH
	5 weeks	General orthopaedics	Salem Hospital
	5 weeks	General orthopaedics	BWH (Harvard Vanguard Associates)
5	10 weeks	Adult reconstruction	MGH or BWH
	15 weeks	Trauma	MGH or BWH
	10 weeks	Hand/upper extremity	MGH or BWH
	5 weeks	Spine	BWH
	5 weeks	Sports	MGH
	5 weeks	Foot and ankle	BWH

MGH HCORP Archives.

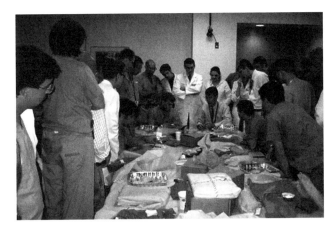

Core curriculum workshop. Residents practice using orthopaedic equipment with saw bones and cadaver specimens. MGH HCORP Archives.

Table 11.3. Distribution of Residents and Teaching Staff after Program Restructuring

Institution	Residents	Teaching Staff
MGH	16	35
BWH	12	19
Children's Hospital	5*	14
BIDMC	4	12
WRVA	2	3
Salem Hospital	1	Varying number of community physicians

*Plus two additional residents who were on 6-month rotations from the Lenox Hill Hospital program.
MGH HCORP Archives.

We changed and strengthened the core curriculum in orthopaedics (including basic science), as described by myself to Dr. Kopta for his site visit report (MGH HCORP Archives):

When Dr. Herndon assumed the Chairmanship and Program Director of the HCORP, a new Core Curriculum was developed with a faculty (clinical and basic science) and resident committee under the Chairmanship of Mark C. Gebhardt, MD. To stress the importance of this educational commitment to the residents, a block of 4 hours free of clinical duties was set aside every Wednesday morning following grand rounds. The Core Curriculum Committee reviewed the prior Core Curriculum, the RRC requirements, the recommendations of the AOS [Academic Orthopaedic Society] and the curriculum at the University of Pittsburgh and Washington University. Dr. Herndon outlined his objectives and vision for this course. Discussion between the faculty and resident members of the committee led to the establishment of the following principles for an "adult" education experience in the Core Curriculum:

Principles:

1. Core should be interactive between faculty and residents ("adult education").

2. Formal lectures should be short (15–20 minutes) and the number of lectures kept to a minimum. "Chalk talks" and overheads used in presentations are preferable.

3. Basic science topics related to the clinical topics of the day should be included as an internal part of the presentations.

4. Core will be a two-year cycle (each resident will partake in two Core Curricula during their residency), and the topics will be taught in teams ("Blocks") composed of faculty from the major Orthopaedic subspecialties (Adult Reconstructive, Trauma, etc.). Each block of subjects will be organized by a chairperson working in concert with a resident and will employ all faculty with expertise in that and related areas (i.e., orthopaedics, radiology, infectious disease, basic scientists, pathology, etc.). Learning objectives for each "block" will be generated and provided to the residents and pre-–and post–tests will be encouraged.

5. Residents will actively participate in the planning of the curriculum and in the presentations, but the faculty will give lectures and be responsible for the program. Fellows and residents may participate in case presentations and presentations of some aspects of the program (such as journal-article discussions, case presentations, etc.).

6. Case scenarios will be provided prior to each "block" which sequentially present a case history, physical examination, radiographic and laboratory findings and treatment options. These cases will provide a basis for more in-depth study of principles discussed in the literature, and each section of the cases will include study questions to be considered prior to the session. A copy of key and/or classical articles will accompany the cases so that the residents have enough background information to partake in the discussions. The complexity of the questions will increase so that all PGY levels will learn. These scenarios can be used to emphasize points relative to ethics, basic science (pharmacology, infectious disease, radiology, etc.), treatment controversies and seminal articles.

7. A syllabus will be generated as the year progresses so that at the end of the 2-year cycle the residents will have a "text" of key articles and lecture handouts. Handout materials will be available to the residents before each "block."

8. Current journal articles may be used to augment the discussions (a "mini" Journal Club).

9. The use of actual patients who illustrate pertinent physical findings is encouraged.

10. All faculty who are part of a particular block are required to be present for their sections to participate in the discussions.

11. Motor skills (Dr. Jupiter and Poss) and pathology (Dr. Rosenberg) will be incorporated into the Core Curriculum.

12. OITE questions are to be used to reinforce points made during the conferences (not as a means to memorize old questions in preparation for the OITE).

I also provided a breakdown of the subspecialty teams (blocks) (**Table 11.4**) and the general format of each case session (**Table 11.5**).

Table 11.4. Specialty Blocks, Associated Faculty and Residents, and Annual Time Allotments as of the 1999 RRC Site Review

Specialty Block	Faculty	Resident	Time (weeks) per Year
Sports Medicine (including the shoulder)	Tammy Martin	Sonu Aluwalia	5
Tumor	John Ready	Valarae Lewis	2
Pediatrics	John Emans	Hieu Ball	4
Trauma (excluding the spine)	William Tomford	Wael Kaawach	5
Adult Reconstruction (including the shoulder)	Richard Scott Arun Shanbhag	Andrew Hecht	4
Spine (including trauma)	Frank Pedlow	Sigurd Berven	4
Hand & Elbow	Jesse Jupiter	Greg Erens	5
Rehab & Prosthetics	Don Pierce	Valarae Lewis	2
Foot & Ankle	Tammy Martin	Shahram Solhpour	3
Ethics	Tammy Martin	—	1

MGH HCORP Archives.

Table 11.5. Breakdown of Case Sessions in the Core Curriculum[a]

Time	Activity	Comments
8:15–9:15 a.m.	Introductory presentations of the topic(s)	Lectures (15–20 min.) on clinical and related basic science
9:15–10:00 a.m.	Discuss case scenarios in small groups	10 residents, 1 or 2 faculty
10:00–10:15 a.m.	Break/coffee	
10:15–11:00 a.m.	Motor skills lab/pathology	Depending on location/topic
11:00 a.m. –12:00 p.m.	Journal club/further discussion or appropriate additional lecture topics	

[a]These sessions could be modified to fit the specific requirements of the particular topic. MGH HCORP Archives.

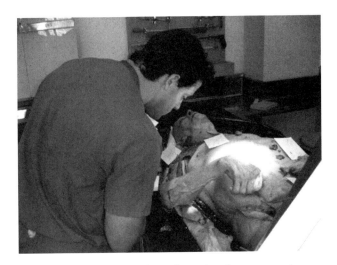

Human anatomy with cadaver dissection for two months (July & August); a major component of the core curriculum. MGH HCORP Archives.

I continued:

An evaluation sheet is filled out by each resident at the completion of each session. Attendance is mandatory except under special circumstances. The Core Curriculum is held at either the MGH or BWH, and one resident (senior) or intern must remain at each hospital to cover emergencies. Because the Core is given twice, this is not felt to be a major problem.

We have successfully completed the first year of Core Curriculum. A copy of the syllabi for the various units is included…Appendix E. It should be noted that topics of rehabilitation and amputation are included as a separate block, but in addition are incorporated into each of the individual subspecialty CORE curricula. In this way, the rehabilitation of the orthopaedic patient is covered as it pertains to daily practice, especially in areas such as sports medicine, pediatrics, oncology, adult reconstruction, foot and ankle, and spine. We are currently in the process of establishing the curriculum for the second year this summer, incorporating ideas and changes based on feedback from the first year. In general, it was a very successful undertaking and the feedback from the residents was nearly uniformly positive.

Basic science education had been incorporated into this program so that the sciences are not viewed as a separate but "unrelated" component to the clinical educational material. (MGH HCORP Archives)

In addition to the core curriculum, subspecialty conferences, indications conferences, daily inpatient rounds, and morbidity and mortality conferences were held at each hospital. Faculty at Children's Hospital taught a pediatric core curriculum every six months to the new group of PGY3 residents. An anatomy course, which included cadaver dissection, was begun at Harvard Medical School every Wednesday during July and August (8:00 a.m. to 12:00 p.m.). Dr. Richard Ozuna initially led this course; Dr. Scott Martin took over after Dr. Ozuna left BWH. PGY3 residents were required to attend the four-day Boston Pathology Course held each year at Tufts Medical School. The two-day Boston Prosthetics Course was held in the spring every other year. HCORP

held a weekend course in biomechanics. A six-month research elective was available for half of the PGY4 residents, and research opportunities were available to residents before starting and after completing the residency program. Journal clubs were held on various services in each hospital. A bioskills (simulation) laboratory was introduced to the residents under the leadership of Dr. Dinesh "Danny" Patel. Sessions included arthroscopy of the knee and shoulder.

I met with the residents for breakfast on Saturday mornings and led a series of discussions on important issues in healthcare for practicing physicians; these issues were not specific to the specialty of orthopaedic surgery. These meetings provided a valuable opportunity for me to keep the residents informed of local and national developments and seek their input and feedback. Later, at the residents' request, this conference was changed to lunch on Wednesdays after CORE. A sample of the topics we covered are listed in **Box 11.3**.

Box 11.3. Topics Discussed During the Weekly Program Director's Conference

1. Practice Decisions	6. Coding and Billing	16. Racial and Ethnic Disparities
• Location	• CPT/ICD-9	17. Communication issues
• Check list for setting up practice	• E&M	18. Outcomes
• Marketing your practice	• Fraud Issues	19. How Residents Are Paid
2. Your First Employment Contract	7. Gain sharing	20. Ethics in Sports Medicine
• How to evaluate/negotiate	8. Pay for Performance (quality)	21. National Data Bank
3. How to Run a Practice	9. Malpractice	22. Clinical Trials
• Private vs. academic	• Subpoenas	23. Physician Profiling
• Services you will need	10. Financial planning	24. Balance Budget Act
• Practice Models	11. Ethics/Conflicts of Interest	• RBRVS
• Revenues/Expenses (margins of operations)	• Professionalism	• RVUs
4. Reimbursements Issues	12. Medical Errors/Patient Safety	25. HCORP Resident Issues
• Medicare	13. Orthopaedic Alphabet Soup	26. Duty Hours
• Medicaid	14. Board Exam (ABOS)	27. Resident Portfolios
5. Starting Salaries/Benefits	15. Physician/Hospital Relationships	28. Leadership issues
	• Specialty Hospitals	
	• ASCs	

Over the years 1994–1998, residents' scores on the Orthopaedic In-Service Training Exam (OITE) were within the 28th to the 50th percentile. With the revised teaching program, MGH HCORP Archives show that in two to three years these scores improved to within the 61st to the 80th percentile (1999–2002). To help residents improve their performance on standardized exams—the ABOS certification examination and OITE—I asked Dr. Karen M. Wulfsberg, an education specialist at Harvard Medical School, for assistance. Although our residents were outstanding, an occasional resident repeatedly stumbled on standardized multiple-choice tests. As an expert on such exams, Dr. Wulfsberg identified two problem areas: (1) content and (2) process. With content-related issues, the examinee may fail if they do not study enough, their study habits are ineffective, or they underestimate the level of detail required. For process-related issues, the examinee misses key details in a question, is often caught by distracters, has difficulties with negatively worded questions, or second-guesses the real question. She consistently found that as many as 25–50% of errors are process related; that is, they are unrelated to content. If a resident performed poorly on the OITE or ABOS examination, I would arrange for them to see Dr. Wulfsberg for a series of meetings during which she would identify which of these issues—content, process, or both—was responsible for their poor performance and advise them how to manage the problem. Over a period of almost 10 years, in almost every case she was able to improve each resident's scores on these important examinations.

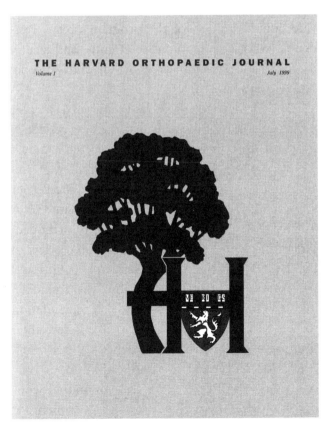

Cover of the original "The Harvard Orthopaedic Journal." MGH HCORP Archives.

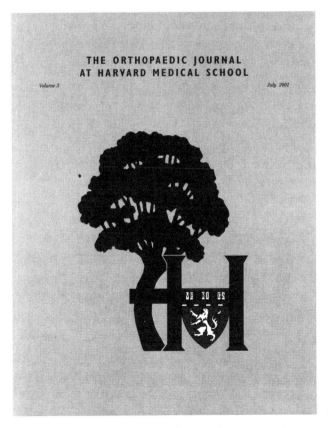

New name of the journal required by the HMS leadership: "The Orthopaedic Journal at Harvard Medical School." MGH HCORP Archives.

I had successfully started the *Pittsburgh Orthopaedic Journal* during my tenure at the University of Pittsburgh. I used the same model to create an orthopaedic publication at Harvard—a journal of scientific articles, yearly status reports from the program director and hospital department chairmen, and alumni news, all produced entirely by the residents with the support of their faculty advisors. The journal would be published yearly and distributed at the senior resident's graduation banquet and to all alumni and medical school deans. The first issue, the *Harvard Orthopaedic Journal*, was published in July 1999. After the second year of publication, the Medical School Dean Joseph Martin told me that the journal title could not include the name "Harvard." I was shocked. My experience was totally opposite that of Dr. Mankin's experience when the residency program was named the Harvard Combined Orthopaedic Residency Program. After several meetings with and required presentations to the dean's committee and finally to the faculty council, I received an "OK" on the use of *Harvard*, but with a slight change: the *Orthopaedic Journal at Harvard Medical School*. The HCORP's annual journal has been continuously published ever since; it is now peer-reviewed and "pursuing the goal of PUBMED/Medline indexing" (Kwon, email to author, Sept. 28, 2016).

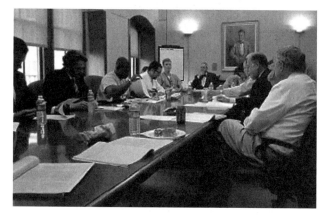

Meeting of the Journal Club. Dr. Heckman is in the foreground on the right. MGH HCORP Archives.

We also modified another main element of the HCORP: combined grand rounds.

> Previously grand rounds were held monthly at MGH and separate weekly grand rounds for the Brigham and Women's, Children's Hospital and Beth Israel Deaconess Medical Center were held in the Longwood area. All of the Harvard Institutions now come together for Grand Rounds [on Wednesdays at 7 a.m.]. The location varies between the MGH and the BWH [and rotate two weeks at each during every month]. Many of the talks are teleconferenced to the other site and to the North Shore [Hospital]. In its first year, this Combined Grand Rounds has attracted a set of speakers that represents a veritable who's who of Orthopaedic Surgery. (Herndon 1999)

The core curriculum followed the combined grand rounds at the same hospital sites. This provided opportunities for the program's many residents—who were required to attend—and faculty to meet and develop professional and personal relationships.

The Orthopaedic RRC had required a site visit within one year of my arrival as the new residency program director. This visit occurred August 17–20, 1999. The status requested was full accreditation for five years with 10 residents per year (total: 50 residents). The specialist site visitor was Dr. Joseph Kopta, the chairman of orthopaedics at the University of Oklahoma. His review of the HCORP, including the core curriculum and the rotation schedule throughout the residents' five years in the program, and his recommendation to the RRC resulted in continued full accreditation for five years for 50 residents (10 per year). The RRC had asked for clarification about only one thing: the PGY6 year. The committee wondered whether the sixth year was a requirement for all residents, or could residents enter a fellowship immediately after completing PGY5. I responded in an April 4 letter to Dr. Steve Nestler, the executive director of the Orthopaedic RRC, that this was indeed a requirement for all residents: "This is a six-month period of time after completion of their residency and as a chief resident are given faculty status and participate in the practice plan at the appropriate hospital...the majority of residents complete the PGY6 requirement prior to entering fellowship programs."

Dr. Nestler wrote to me after the visit regarding the RRC's approval, commending myself and our teaching staff on our development of the HCORP into a truly integrated program, thereby improving both "the structure and organization of resident education" (MGH HCORP Archives). The program developments described above and our ability to successfully recruit outstanding clinicians and scientists to the program led to our success. Another site visit was planned in five years.

Two other significant events occurred in the 2000–2001 academic year. Dr. James Heckman, the new editor of the *Journal of Bone and Joint Surgery*, moved to Boston and joined the Harvard faculty. In his new role, he, along with David Wimberly, a PGY4 in the HCORP, initiated a monthly *Journal of Bone and Joint Surgery* journal club for the residents. This was a wonderful teaching experience that the residents thoroughly enjoyed. While Harvard gained Dr. Heckman's expertise, it lost another's: in December 2000 Steve Lipson was replaced by Ben Bierbaum as the chief of the Orthopaedic Department at the BIDMC. Dr. Bierbaum was the chief of the orthopaedic service at the New England Baptist Hospital. Joseph Martin, the dean of Harvard Medical School, also appointed Bierbaum as a clinical professor of orthopaedic surgery. This latter appointment would prove to be very disruptive for the HCORP.

During a meeting with Dean Martin on October 11, 2000:

[It was] agreed that the Harvard orthopedic residency would continue to include the Beth Israel Deaconess (but not the Baptist) and that Ben Bierbaum would join the Executive Committee as the BID chief certain conditions were agreed on that will help Jim (as chair of the Orthopedic Executive Committee) in his goals to improve orthopedics Harvard-wide, and could form the basis for changes in the future if that is necessary...these conditions are:

1. Bierbaum has a 3-year term and the search for a full-time academic successor will begin at the end of year 2.

2. Bierbaum will spend 60% of his time at BID as a teacher and supervisor (with a small amount of surgery).

3. All faculty hired at BID will be full time. Part time faculty at the Baptist will not be given Harvard appointments.

4. There was an acknowledgement that teaching, supervision and conferences in orthopedics at BID have been deficient and need to improve.

5. The number of residents at each site is appropriately subject to review based on caseload and other programmatic issues. Any reallocation should be the decision of the Executive Committee with input from all the program participants.

6. The search for the Mueller Chair will be renewed with a commitment by BID to support academic orthopedics.

7. The group that met with the Dean will meet again in approximately 8 months to review compliance with this agreement.
(MGH HCORP Archives)

In addition to becoming chief of the orthopaedic service at BIDMC, Dr. Bierbaum remained in a leadership position at the New England Baptist Hospital, where he had a large private practice, and as a member of the CareGroup Board of Trustees. This proved to be a difficult situation:

He had committed to spend 60% of his time as a teacher and supervisor at BIDMC, but apparently it was difficult, if not impossible, for him to maintain those commitments. I began to receive complaints from the residents at BIDMC, especially the chief resident, that very little elective orthopaedic surgery was occurring, except in sports medicine. The chief resident did little other than cover the emergency department and clinics. During a retreat held June 2, 2001, the BIDMC residents shared with me various issues: the PGY2 and PGY3 residents were on first call every other night for the emergency department, the two PGY4 residents were on call at home or on call in the hospital with the PGY1 every other night, and the chief resident was on call all the time. Dr. Reilly, who had a large private total joint practice, "at the request of the CareGroup Board of Directors...moved his adult reconstructive practice to the New England Baptist Hospital [away from the BIDMC]" (B. E. Bierbaum 2002). Other staff also left.

Therefore, although Dean Martin objected, I removed from the BIDMC all orthopaedic residents except those on the sports service (where teaching was reported to be excellent); this removal would remain in effect until the orthopaedic leadership changed and resident education became a priority. In June 2002, Dr. Josef E. Fisher, chairman of the department of surgery at the BIDMC, became the acting chief of orthopaedic surgery. He was charged with leading the search for a new orthopaedic department chair. The search committee selected a new chairman in September 2002: Dr. Mark Gebhardt (see chapter 40).

In January 2001, I and the executive committee invited two outstanding leaders in orthopaedic education—Drs. C. M. "Mac" Evarts and Reginald Cooper—to independently review the HCORP. They were charged with providing to the program's leadership an extensive review of the complete orthopaedic program. We asked them to concentrate on various issues

such as "the quality of our teaching program, the service to education ratio, effectiveness of the PGY1 year rotation schedule, graduated responsibility, integration of research into our resident program, the ever increasing demands on our residents and faculty for service and how to balance that with academic productivity, the value of the Chief Residency, the role of fellows[,] and our overall residents' program role and value in each of our teaching hospitals" (MGH HCORP Archives).

Evarts and Cooper visited our facilities and interviewed faculty, administrators, and residents on January 31 and February 1, 2001. They stated the following in their report:

EDUCATIONAL PROGRAMS

RESIDENT EDUCATION: During PGY1, there are several rotations that do not meet the requirements for resident education in orthopaedic surgery...A major concern of the entire combined program is the lack of continuity of care during the residency experience. This theme was mentioned by all of the residents at every level from PGY1 to V and by the chiefs...[a] person stated that in practice the goals of the residency were one, two, and three service; education was four. The residents receive less than broad education as regards the pre-op indications for surgery. Residents state they have no graded responsibilities and lack resident-to-resident teaching...During the Children's Hospital rotations, there is greater continuity of care for the residents. The educational experiences from PGY-II through PGY-V indicate an imbalance between service and education. Part of the imbalance rests with the number of attendings vs. the total number of residents...there is an 'entitlement' mentality amongst the attendings in regards resident coverage...it is important that the resident complement be sufficient in numbers to sustain an educational environment. This is not true under the current system in the HCORP. There is little funding available for the resident's educational experiences…The board exam record of the HCORP is improving but is not at the level of the very top programs in the United States in regards the board exam pass rate. There are several excellent features of the Combined Program including excellent patient volume; a variety of patients and the core curriculum; the program at Children's is outstanding; and there are committed faculty members at all four institutions.

THE QUALITY OF FACULTY: Several excellent faculty members are devoted to teaching and superb patient care…There is a wide variation in the quality of the faculty and the commitment to education…one approach taken in other large programs, would be to create teaching and nonteaching services…[allowing] a redistribution of resident coverage…providing greater continuity of care.

INCREASE IN NUMBER OF RESIDENTS: Clinical material exists to support two additional residents per year. However, given the wide learning experiences by the residents, as well as the lack of physician extenders by all the hospitals…an increase of residents should occur only after the institution of faculty-teaching services. A new pattern of block assignments should be developed with…major services…[to] include a senior, and a junior resident…

RESEARCH: Under the leadership of Dr. James Herndon, considerable attention is being given to scholarly activities, including both clinical and bench research. Research volume has grown at the MGH and research efforts are being strengthened at the BWH… Obviously, there is great value in having a rich research presence in any department…However, the mandatory assignment of residents

to research is not a valuable experience for the great majority of residents. Therefore, it is our opinion that research should be on a voluntary basis and lasting for at least one year…opportunity…available for all residents on a voluntary basis. The funding…provided by either federally funded research grants…or by seed money coming from the various institutions in the HCORP.

CHIEF RESIDENCY: After discussing this year with the residents as well as the attendings, it is the majority opinion…that the educational value of the six-month experience does not warrant continuation of this program. The chief's year is a de facto additional year in the residency program…With the growth of the Trauma Program and the strengthening of the orthopaedic trauma rotations for PGY-IV and V under the leadership of Mark Vrahas and others at both MGH and BWH, there is not a necessity for further trauma education…

FELLOWSHIPS: In our discussions with residents and fellows, fellowships were not thought to interfere with the resident's experience… The fellowship programs should be examined carefully…to make certain that a loss of continuity of responsibility by the residents because of the presence of fellows does not occur. It might be possible to create services that contained only fellows and medical students in contrast to services with residents, fellows and medical students…

CLINICAL PROGRAMS

Throughout the HCORP clinical program integration has not fully occurred. To some extent trauma Care under the leadership of Mark Vrahas has been integrated…Competition between the affiliated hospitals [MGH and BWH] is viewed as important and is actually encouraged by more than one senior leader.

The statement was made that the arrangement creating Partners is not really a true merger of equals, but rather the creation of two holding companies. It has been very difficult to develop major programs under single leadership with common missions between the BWH and the MGH. The cultural differences are great and any real collaboration between the partners in regards clinical care is missing. The two institutions have not integrated.

THE BETH ISRAEL DEACONESS HOSPITAL:

Without question, there were universal concerns expressed in regards to the educational experience for orthopaedic residents at the BIDH...Over the past few years, there has been a loss of attending anesthesiologists as well as attending general surgeons...This exodus has been significant and has affected the teaching and learning environment...The PGY-II and PGY-III residents were...vocal in their concerns...and listed [for us] some very serious allegations about the quality of care and educational shortfalls. This rotation is referred to as the "penalty box"...Dramatic changes must occur in the next few weeks/months in order to bring this program back on line and up to the caliber of the programs at MGH, BWH and Children's Hospital. This seems highly unlikely in view of the timing and the past and present association of the Chair [Ben Bierbaum] with the New England Baptist Hospital. He has indicated that he will move joint reconstructive and spine surgery to the New England Baptist and leave trauma at the BIDH. In the final analysis, this rotation adds little to the educational program with little promise, if any, of change.

CLINICAL PROGRAMS IN THE PARTNERS HOSPITALS:

Clinical programs at the Partners Hospitals remain rich in content... The caseload volumes are heavy at both hospitals and there is ample clinical material for the residency education. The general criticisms and suggestions for change apply to these hospitals as well as others with the Combined Program.

LEADERSHIP:

Since his arrival, Dr. James H. Herndon, MD, MBA, has made major contributions to education and research in the HCORP. There was no question and no doubt in the minds of many individuals we interviewed that the educational environment has markedly improved at both sites. The Saturday morning meetings, the core curriculum, the attention to grand rounds, the emphasis on research and scholarly activities have been emphasized since the arrival of Dr. Herndon. He is given the highest marks by many faculty and residents who span the time interval prior to his arrival and afterward. They have nothing but the strongest praise for his influence upon their educational experiences. Tangible evidence exists in the improvement of orthopaedic in-training exam scores, the certifying board pass/fail rate, the publication of the Harvard Orthopaedic Journal, as well as the improving caliber of residents in the HCORP. Many mentioned the "impossible" nature of Dr. Herndon's position as Chair of the Partners Department of Orthopaedic Surgery given the long-standing traditions and different cultures between the BWH and the MGH. Some stated that he has been given significant responsibilities with little authority insofar as the actual directions of the program at both institutions. Obviously, the appointment of Dr. Thornhill, prior to his arrival and without significant input from him is of concern as well as the manner in which Dr. B. Bierbaum was appointed to the post at BIDH [by Dean Joseph Martin]. There is implication of micro-management of orthopaedics by the Harvard Medical School. These factors have made continuing leadership of both the department as well as the combined residency by Dr. Herndon quite difficult.

RECOMMENDATIONS

EDUCATION:

Correction of the PGY1 rotations.

Institution of continuity of care for PGY-II to PGY V residents

Creation of teaching and nonteaching services

Creation of a fellowship service without residents

Greater emphasis on faculty development

Improvement of resident benefits

Elimination of the 6th year chief resident rotation

Elimination of the Beth Israel Deaconess Hospital resident rotation

Creation of salary incentives for teaching

RESEARCH:

A commitment to support unfunded research by each of the HCORP hospitals

A commitment of funding of the Mueller Professorship and laboratory efforts by the BIDMC. Recruitment of a new professor to fill the professorship.

A consolidation of molecular and biomechanical research at the same site.

The recruitment of a full research complement at BWH, MGH, and Children's Hospital.

Develop opportunities for resident research at all of the Harvard Combined Orthopaedic Residency Programs

Creation of salary incentives for research.

CLINICAL:

Creation of combined centers of excellence across subspecialty services

Consolidation of subspecialty services at one site

Recruitment of residents and faculty of the highest caliber to the Combined Residency Program

FINAL COMMENTS

The Partners Department of Orthopaedic Surgery must be considered an experiment. Progress has been made...but much remains to be done on the clinical side in regard to collaboration (which will ultimately help to strengthen the Harvard Combined Orthopaedic Residency Program). A discontinuance of the Partners Department might well result in a return to a bunker mentality between the Partner's hospitals as well as the other members of the Combined Residency Program in regard to clinical care, residency programs and research. More of the old cultures will surface. The entitlement mentality might well carry the day and true educational, research and clinical progress will not be made. The residency program will not ascend to the highest level. It is our own belief that much can be accomplished at the Harvard Combined Orthopaedic Residency Program, as there is more than ample talent to restore the program to greater national prominence. However, the continuing leadership of Dr. James Herndon is critical to this equation.
(MGH HCORP Archives)

In response to this review, faculty and residents in the HCORP made efforts to continuously improve the residency program. I monitored and collected data annually through private interviews with each resident, discussions during the Saturday breakfast meetings, reviews of the confidential annual ACGME resident surveys, and reviews of each resident's performance evaluations from the services, hospitals, and faculty. These data included resident and faculty evaluations; OITE

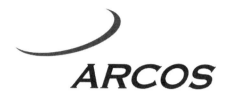

Association of Residency Coordinators in Orthopaedic Surgery. A national organization formed to allow coordinators to meet and share ideas, provide continuing education and support as well as advocacy.
Association of Residency Coordinators in Orthopaedic Surgery (arcosonline.org.)

scores; ABOS certification examination scores (parts I and II); resident scores of the faculty and services regarding teaching quality, teaching in the clinics, and the amount of scut work required; the resident's operating room experience (teaching and individual responsibility) and operative logs; and the residents' work hours.

We began implementing 360-degree evaluations for each resident in the program in 2003. I evaluated each resident every six months. During a private meeting, I asked residents to answer one of five questions dealing with ethical issues, difficult patient care or operating room decisions, and other challenging real-life situations, and we would discuss the issue.

The ACGME's 2002 Outcome Project, which was designed to improve the quality and assessment of residents' education, required six core competencies: medical knowledge, patient care, professionalism, interpersonal communication skills, practice-based learning: personal improvement, and system-based practice. The ACGME required these competencies so "[Residents could] communicate effectively and demonstrate caring and respectful behaviors when interacting with patients and their families; perform competently all medical and invasive procedures considered essential for the area of practice; and work effectively with others as a member or leader of a healthcare team or other professional group" (MGH HCORP Archives). After these core competencies were introduced, the HCORP leadership monitored each resident's compliance through a

"portfolio," a folder that contained descriptions of the resident's experiences with each of the competencies and the relevant outcomes.

I used additional tools to evaluate the outcomes and effectiveness of the program's overall curriculum. These included new evaluation forms, case logs, residents' self-assessments, anatomy examinations, and a patient safety examination. Each hospital described the goals, objectives, educational methods, and evaluation procedures for each level of resident on each service. Some of the services administered objective examinations that aimed to measure a resident's knowledge about their subspecialty; others used questions from the OITE, the self-assessment examinations of the American Academy of Orthopaedic Surgeons, or both.

Around the time the ACGME was beginning to require core competencies, it became obvious within the orthopaedic specialty's educational programs that the role of both the program director and the program coordinator were changing and greatly expanding. As a result, the Association of Residency Coordinators in Orthopaedic Surgery (ARCOS) organized in 2003. This group followed the lead of the Association of Residency Administrators in Surgery in supporting a certifying examination, to be administered through the National Board for Certification for Training Administrators of Graduate Medical Education

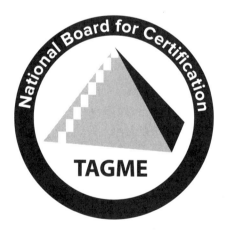

Training Administrators of Graduate Medical Education. A National Board for Certification of residency coordinators.
Training Administrators of Graduate Medical Education logo (tagme.org.)

Programs (TAGME). Diane Sheehan, who had been HCORP's coordinator since 1998, became board certified as a training administrator of graduate medical education in orthopaedic surgery in 2007—she was one of the first in orthopaedics to do so in the Boston area.

The HCORP has had a long-standing tradition of supporting diversity in the program itself and in Harvard's teaching hospitals. As early as 1850, Harvard faculty debated granting admission to two "young men of color," as the Committee of the Colonization of Society and one Charles Brooks had written letters to the faculty on the men's behalf (Beecher and Altschule 1977). On November 4 of that year, the faculty accepted them both as students and allowed them to attend lectures.

To my knowledge, Miriam Katzeff, an assistant surgeon in the orthopaedic department at Children's Hospital in 1926 (see chapter 23), was the first female orthopaedic surgeon in the Harvard system. She had graduated from the Boston University School of Medicine in 1925. I could not find the site where she completed her internship.

Women were accepted to Harvard Medical School, and received equal standing with men, in September 1945. Maureen K. Molloy seems to be the first female orthopaedic resident in the HCORP. Dr. Molloy trained under Dr. Green and Dr. Barr, graduating in June 1963. Dr. Malloy informed me that, according to Dr. Green, she "was the second woman to go through the program, the first having preceded [her] by twenty years" (M. K. Malloy, letter to author, January 2, 2003 [MGH HCORP Archives]). I could not identify the other woman to whom Dr. Malloy was referring.

Women on staff at MGH sometimes performed surgeries, but no women were instated as house officers until mid-1973. Beecher and Altschule (1977) interviewed women at MGH and reported that none had experienced sexual discrimination.

Carolyn Rogers (2000) notes that during Dr. Mankin's 27 years with the HCORP, the leadership accepted five "diverse" candidates (women, blacks, or Hispanics) each year. Mankin and other faculty considered such residents as essential to HCORP's success. Rogers interviewed me in 2000, while I was chair of the HCORP, and I assured her that I would continue this legacy.

In a 1999/2000 survey by the AAOS Diversity Committee, Harvard Medical School was first on a list of schools most frequently attended by minority respondents. The HCORP, tied with the Division of Orthopaedics at Howard University for the largest number of minority residents.

Beginning around 2000, Partners performed internal reviews of its residency programs before each RRC site visit. By 2003 the clinical faculty had gained 26 new physicians (22 at Partners and four at Children's Hospital). New subspecialty services had been developed. In July 2003, a two- to three-month-long required research rotation replaced the six-month elective research rotation, and the six-month chief residency was discontinued. In addition, a night float system was started with PGY2s in order to meet the required ACGME duty hour requirement of a maximum of 80 hours per week. Also, in 2003, a resident council was formed, two representatives of which were assigned to the Executive Committee. In light of these significant changes and in order to maintain the quality of the education program, I requested that the RRC approve an additional two residents per year (10 across all years; 12 in each year), for a total of 60 residents in the program. Simultaneously, I asked the Partners Education Committee to provide funding for these additional residents. Partners agreed to my request on December 15, 2003, and the RRC for Orthopaedic Surgery (ACGME) approved the increase in July 2004.

The next ACGME site visit of the residency program was April 7, 2004. The ACGME had begun a requirement that residents complete a confidential online survey in order to monitor their clinical education. HCORP residents completed the survey in January and February 2004. Two

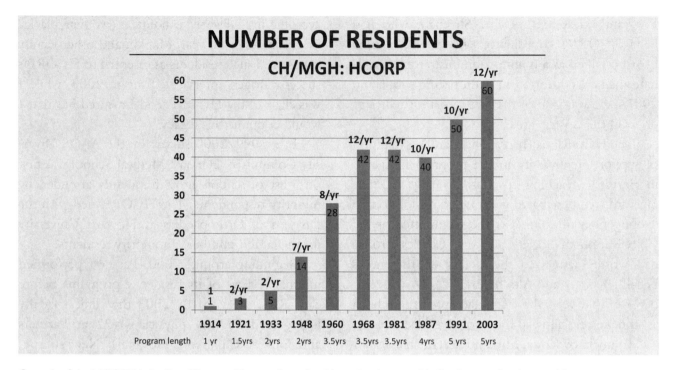

Growth of the HCORP in its first 82 years. The number of residents has been stable for the past for the past 18 years.
Data and chart provided by the author.

problem areas were cited on the basis of their survey responses: residents performed too much "scut work" (starting IVs, transporting patients, etc.) that should be done by support staff; and the program did not comply with duty hour regulations, as residents worked more than 80 hours per week and had no days completely free from all educational and clinical responsibilities. I requested that the RRC allow us to increase the maximum hours worked per week from 80 to 88 hours, which the committee approved in September 2004.

After the April 2004 site visit, the RRC requested additional information:

1. During the site visit, it was noted that fellows have an adverse impact on resident experience on the MGH sports and shoulder services. What steps can be taken to improve the interaction of residents and fellows on these services?

2. How does the program comply with accreditation requirements regarding a

final written evaluation of all graduating residents?

3. The committee would like additional information on the proposed 2-month research rotation. What will residents be expected to accomplish during this time? Will there be any involvement in basic research?
(MGH HCORP Archives)

I responded:

1. I thought we had resolved all our fellow versus resident issues. None of the orthopaedic hospital chiefs (Executive Committee)…nor myself want the fellows to have an adverse impact on resident experience…the chiefs of each service have made a firm commitment to insure the fellows do not adversely impact the residents' experience. They have reorganized the schedule so that each resident will have specific time assigned to one of the attendings…when no fellow is present…

2. Beginning this year, the Program Director has provided a final written evaluation of all graduating residents…This was done in the past informally and with a written summary evaluation usually given to the resident two or three months prior to graduation…

3. The residents are expected to accomplish the completion of their research project that is required during the residency program. Basic research is included…the residents are given a teaching curriculum… regarding research [that includes] seminars on epidemiology, statistics, scientific method, how to establish and conduct clinical trials, hypothesis testing, etc. In addition, the residents will be expected to attend the research seminars that are held weekly. (MGH HCORP Archives)

In July 2004, HCORP received continued full accreditation for five years, with 12 residents per year (a maximum of 60 residents). The issue of fellowships interfering with residents' education and experience continued, however. By 2007, both MGH and BWH had more fellows than residents.

The RRC for Orthopaedic Surgery Program Information Form (PIF) of 2004 included an

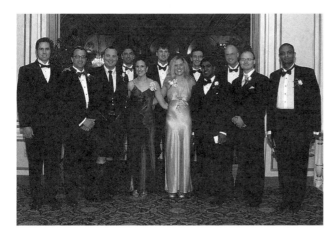

HCORP graduating class (12 residents) of 2005.
MGH HCORP Archives.

overview of the HCORP, which briefly described the purpose of the core curriculum and the other educational resources in the program:

All rotations are guided by a curriculum document prepared by the service chiefs for each rotation. The documents include goals and objectives for each level of resident on their service, the relationship of residents to fellows, a daily schedule for each resident, and an outline of how residents would be evaluated…the foundation of the Program's didactic activities and basic science program is the Core Curriculum…attendance is mandatory…Responsibility for planning and organizing the weekly curriculum is shared by faculty and residents under the direction of the Core Curriculum Committee…The curriculum is designed on a two-year cycle…The curriculum is organized around each of the subspecialty areas with particular emphasis on basic science, biomechanics and current research issues, as well as the clinical aspects of the subspecialty and skills courses as needed…During July and August the core curriculum time is devoted to anatomy dissection…at HMS…In addition to Grand Rounds and the Core, there has been an effort to strengthen subspecialty conferences…local courses in…advanced life-saving techniques, pathology/basic science and Partners GME sponsored courses in communications, ethics and diversity…All residents are required to complete a research project by their senior year…presented at the Program's annual Thesis Day. (MGH HCORP Archives)

The Program Information Form (PIF), also included a brief description of major changes in the program since the last review, which had been in 1999.

There have been several changes in required rotations over the last three years. The most significant changes have involved moving residents from required rotations at the BIDMC to rotations at the other participating hospitals…These steps were taken in response to changes in the leadership and teaching staff in orthopaedic surgery at BIDMC that jeopardized the quality of resident education and supervision in several key rotations [including the chief residency]…In addition to these changes, the program stopped the six-month research rotation required of five residents… in the PGY 4 year. Because this rotation was outside of the approved residency, the salaries were not funded and difficult to support. (MGH HCORP Archives)

Regarding the PGY1 year; which as of July 1, 2000, was under my direction; I sent to the surgery program directors at the MGH, BWH, and BIDMC (where the HCORP had placed orthopaedic interns) annual letters outlining the orthopaedic RRC requirements. In spite of those directors' best efforts, however, the orthopaedic residents often rotated to nonessential services that were low on the list of priority rotations, and they sometimes barely completed the minimum required rotations. I met yearly with some of the surgery program directors to discuss problems and resident complaints, but the outcomes were never fully satisfactory. Several years later, after I had retired as program director, the PGY1 year was removed from general surgery and fully taken over by the new orthopaedic program director (Dempsey Springfield), who assigned specific clinical rotations to all orthopaedic PGY1 residents.

Changes continued in the HCORP. Residents returned to the BIDMC after Dr. Gebhardt became chairman and had hired additional faculty. Thesis day was combined with the graduation events for seniors who completed the program, projected to occur in June of each year, and included a celebratory graduation banquet on a Friday night. I hoped this special day would eventually be combined with an alumni event on the following Saturday, at which alumni would present papers, possibly participate in an afternoon of sporting or social events, followed by a dinner for faculty, residents, and alumni. Other social events for the residents and faculty were encouraged, including an annual Partner's Orthopaedic Department Christmas party and an annual golf tournament.

To quote the new dean, Dr. Jeffrey Flier (2007), "Any organization needs to step back periodically and evaluate whether its culture and organizational structure contributes to or impedes its success" (MGH HCORP Archives). The last retreat during my tenure as program director of HCORP was held on January 5, 2008. I wanted to have another serious discussion about HCORP's educational program, its successes, and areas of needed change. I reminded everyone that the residents were HCORP's customers—not the faculty and staff, the program director, the hospital chiefs,

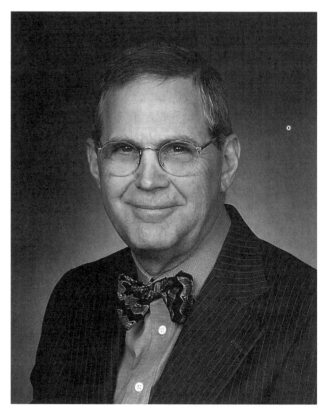

Dempsey Springfield. HCORP Director: 2009–2012.
MGH HCORP Archives.

or the service chiefs. I outlined my concerns about the program:

1. Rotations were too short…providing residents with limited contact with the faculty and therefore decreased experience in the operating room and preventing residents from learning about the total care of patients including outcomes of care;

2. Perceptions by the residents that surgical volume and responsibility in the operating room were decreasing;

3. Continued increase in the number of fellows and lack of understanding the impact on resident education;

4. Expansion of the program with BIDMC requesting additional residents;

5. Continued growth of the faculty;

6. Changes in the CORE…insufficient faculty participation from each hospital on the core curriculum committee and increased difficulty in getting faculty to speak about certain issues and a decline in the amount of basic science included in CORE;

7. Insufficient participation in service requirements of patients by NP/PAs (discharge planning, chart work, dictation, etc.);

8. Continued issues of duty hour violations, lack of resident and faculty completing evaluation forms, residents not logging duty hours, resident not keeping accurate and timely surgical logs, faculty and residents not reviewing the goals and objectives at the beginning of each clinical rotation, lack of open and frank evaluations of residents at the middle and end of their rotations and a decrease in teaching conferences on many services;

9. Insufficient attention, discussion and evaluation of core competencies on each clinical service. (MGH HCORP Archives)

I then provided detailed analyses of the residents' surgical volume, by postgraduate year, over the preceding four years (this included specific types of cases), residents' anonymous evaluations of the faculty and clinical rotations (including their experiences in the operating room, the teaching they received in the clinics, and their estimations of cases on which they were given operative experience and responsibility and the amount of scut work required). This retreat achieved mixed results. Each hospital chief successfully obtained institutional support for more physician assistants or nurse practitioners to reduce the scut work residents had to do. All residents responded positively to the night float system. Residents' operating volume increased when they began being assigned to the ambulatory surgery centers on specific services. I had, however, raised some suggestions that were not accepted: establishing fellow- or resident-only services, dropping residents from services with poor educational evaluations, and—the ultimate change—establishing teaching and nonteaching services.

I retired as program director on December 31, 2008, and was succeeded by Dr. Dempsey Springfield. **Box 11.4** lists all HCORP directors since the beginning of the program.

Box 11.4. HCORP Directors

Robert B. Osgood	1921–1930
Frank R. Ober	1930–1946
William T. Green	1946–1968
Melvin J. Glimcher	1968–1972
Henry J. Mankin	1972–1998
James H. Herndon	1998–2009
Dempsey S. Springfield	2009–2012
George S.M. Dyer	2012–

CHAPTER 12

Harvard Sports Medicine

Three major sports—baseball, basketball, and football—had significant developments in New England during their early history of play in the United States. Baseball was introduced before the Civil War, a game similar to the British game "rounders" (*Wikipedia*, n.d., under "Baseball"). The game is first mentioned in Springfield, Massachusetts, in 1791 in a city ordinance that banned the game within 80 yards of the town meeting house. Basketball was first played in Springfield in 1891. Football began in the 1820s; the first organized football club was in Boston, and the first at Harvard College was in 1827—though then it was not football as we know it but more like a game called "shinny" (A. J. Thorndike 1948).

At Harvard, freshman faced off against sophomores on the first Monday of the fall semester, and they usually lost. Because of the number of injuries, the day of the game has been remembered as "Bloody Monday" (Paisner 1968). The game—played on a triangular area of land where Memorial Hall is now located—was immortalized in a poem in the *Harvard Registry* in 1828:

The Battle of the Delta

The Freshmen's wrath, to Sophs the direful spring

Of shins unnumbered bruised, great goddess sing;

Let fire and music in my song be mated,

Pure fire and music unsophisticated.

The college clock struck twelve - that awful hour

When Sophs met Fresh, power met opposing power;

To brave the dangers of approaching fight,

Each army stood of literary might;

With warlike ardor for a deathless fame

Impatient stood—until the football came;

When lo! Appearing at the college gate,

A four-foot hero bears the ball of fate;

His step was majesty, his look was fire –

O how I wish he'd been six inches higher!

His eye around triumphantly he throws,

The battle ground surveys, surveys his foes;

Then with a look—O what a look profound!

The well-blown ball he casts upon the ground.

How stern the hero looked, how high the ball did bound!

"Let none," he says, "my valour tried impeach,

Should I delay the fight—to make a speech" –

"Let it be warned," a youthful Stentor cries,

No speeches here, - but let the football rise."

Through warlike crowds a devious way it wins,

And shins advancing meet advancing shins;

"Over the fence!" from rank to rank resounds,

Across the rampart many a hero bounds;

But sing, Apollo! I can sing no more,

For Mars advancing threw the dust before.

Meantime the Seniors, on the ladder raised,

Upon the strife sublime, intentive gazed;

Secured from blows by elevation high,

The fight they viewed with philosophic eye,

Save here and there a veteran soldier stood,

A noble darer for the Freshmen's good.

But ah! I vainly strive—I could not tell

What mighty heroes on the greensward fell,

Who lost, who won the honors of that day,

Or limped alas! ingloriously away –

I could not tell—such task might well require

A Milton's grandeur and a Homer's Fire;

A ream of foolscap, bunch of goosequills too,

Would scarce suffice to sing the battle through;

How many moons would wax, how many
    wane,

While still the bard might ply his song in vain;

Yet minstrel's purse and brain but ill affords

Such waste of paper, and such waste of words.

But see! Where yonder Freshman Hector
    stands,

Fire in his eye, and football in his hands;

Ye muses, tell me who, - and whence he came;

From Stonington—and Peter is his name;

That coat, which erst upon the field he wore,

Was once a coat—but ah! A coat no more;

For coat and cap have joined the days of yore.

So when some tempest rages in the sky,

Shakes the Gymnasium mast, erected high,

That mast so sacred to Alcides' cause,

Which oft has made the country people pause,

Or wonder, as they pass at slower speed,

What can a college of a gallows need?

As when the aforesaid storm its tackling rends,

Rope ladders this, and wooden that way, sends;

Still stands the mast majestical in might,

So Peter stood, though coatless in the fight.

At length advancing to the neutral space,

He proudly waved his hand, and wiped his
    face;

Then with a voice as many waters loud,

He broke the silence, and bespake the crowd.

So oft when stilly, starry eve invites,

To wander forth and taste her fresh delights,

I've heard the bugle o'er the common sound,

Though all unknown by whom or wherefore
    wound.

"List to my words; from Stonington I came,

In football matchless, and of peerless fame;

Think ye, faint-hearted, scientific fools,

That such as Peter waste away in schools?

No, glorious battle called him from afar,

From Stonington, to hear the din of war;

Then if there be a Soph, who boot to boot,

Dares meet the vengeance of a Peter's foot, -

Let him advance, his shin shall feel the woe

That lives, though sleeping, in a Peter's toe."

He said, and ceased, - Jotham stepped forth to
    view,

A Soph of stature, and of glory too.

"Vain-boasting Peter, does though think thy
    hand

Can Mars and Jotham in the strife withstand?

Minerva aids thee? vaunter, learn to fear,

Mars in the van, and Jotham in the rear?"

He said, and furious rushed upon the foe,

As when two cows to deadly combat to;

Fate interfered, and stopped the impending
   blow;

For hark! The summons of the Commons-bell,

That music every hero knows so well;

All sympathetic started at the sound,

And ran for dinner from the battle ground.

In the 1820s and 1830s—the early days of football—the sport had few rules, and serious injuries were not uncommon. The game consisted of running and carrying the ball—much like rugby—and kicking, similar to soccer. The forward pass was not part of the game. Because of the frequent, often serious injuries, Yale banned football in 1860; Harvard banned it in 1861.

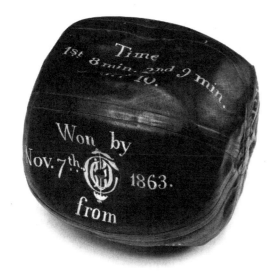

Early designed football. Padded or inflatable. Published in "Remembering the First High School Football games," by Robert Holmes, *Boston Globe*, November 21, 2012.
Courtesy of Historic New England. Gift from the Oneida Team, 1922.768.

In 1862, during the Civil War, a group of high school students in Boston formed the first organized football club in America, the Oneida Football Club. The club included players from Dixwell, Boston English, and Boston Latin schools. Their

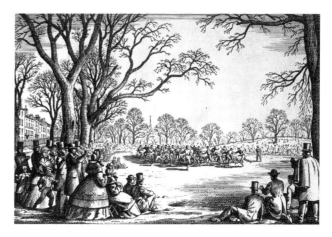

Drawing: Oneida Football Club playing on the Common, ca. 1862-1865. Published in "Remembering the First High School Football games," by Robert Holmes, *Boston Globe*, November 21, 2012. Noble and Greenough School.

game became known as the "Boston Game," and they played on the Boston Common for four years. They played a hybrid game—part rugby, part soccer, with elements of today's baseball and football. Records of an 1863 game might include the first mention of a concussion in the sport: "Like a flash [Edward Lincoln] Arnold shot one heel into the turf, came to a dead stop, ducked, and crouching low, covered his head just as the fellow came on, struck something, capitulated and landed 6 feet further on. Whether, if submitted to modern tests, he could then have given his correct name or age, is open to doubt" (quoted in B. Holmes 2012).

> Harvard's experience with athletes has shown that study of them is valuable to the physician who must treat them and that to return an injured athlete to "normal" is to achieve much more than enable him to regain a basic function.
> —Beecher and Altschule, *Medicine at Harvard: The First 300 Years*

College football resumed play in the late 1870s. During the next two decades, efforts were made to establish rules. Representatives from Columbia, Princeton, Yale, and Rutgers met in 1873 to formalize rules that were based on soccer. Harvard, preferring the rugby type game, refused to

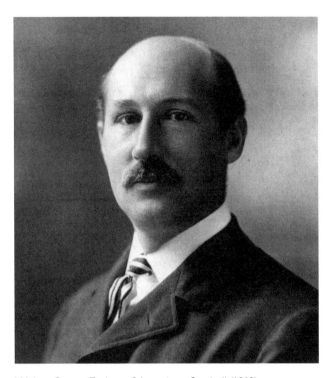

Walter Camp. Father of American football (1910).

Images of Yale individuals (RU 684). Manuscripts and Archives, Yale University Library.

participate, eventually forcing the other programs to join them in creating new rules. These five universities met at the Massasoit Convention and created new rules that were based largely on the Rugby Football Union code. Walter Camp—who played football at Yale from 1877 to 1882—led another series of changes. His efforts led to reducing the number of players from 15 to 11; defining the line of scrimmage, establishing that the beginning of every play began when the ball was snapped to the quarterback; and determining a team retained possession of the ball if they advanced it five yards in three plays. Because of a continued large number of serious injuries and even deaths, President Theodore Roosevelt called for further reform from Harvard, Yale, and Princeton in 1905. In 1906—a memorable year for football—these universities established the National Collegiate Athletic Association (NCAA) and new rules for football, including approval of the forward pass.

These early developments in sports in the United States had a profound impact on the evolution of the orthopaedic surgeon, who was vital in providing care to sports teams. They had a critical role in preventing, resolving, and researching sports-related injuries.

WILLIAM M. CONANT, MD

Physician Snapshot

William M. Conant
BIRTH: 1856
DEATH: 1937
SIGNIFICANT CONTRIBUTIONS: First physician to work with the Harvard University football team; initiated the first use of a training facility; promoted exercise for athletes

Sports teams now practice and play under the medical supervision of team physicians and therapists. This was not, however, the case until 1890, when Dr. William M. Conant became the first medical doctor to work with the Harvard University football team. In addition to the coach, Harvard led the way in athletic training, hiring James Robinson in October of 1881 as the first athletic trainer in the United States. Robinson was hired to improve conditioning of the football team. A graduate of Harvard in 1879 and a former Harvard football player himself, Dr. Conant was an instructor of anatomy at Harvard Medical School and a surgeon in the outpatient department at the Massachusetts General Hospital (MGH). In a striking innovation, Conant created a so-called training room at Hampden Park; there, he could treat players onsite during a game. In a lecture to the Boston Society for Medical Improvement in 1894, Conant declared: "Exercise…has for its aims the promotion of health and the acquisition of correct habits of action. The first is hygenic [sic]; the second is educational…the principles of all forms of physical training, however various, are based upon the power of the nervous system to receive impressions and to note them on their effects" (R. J. Park 1987).

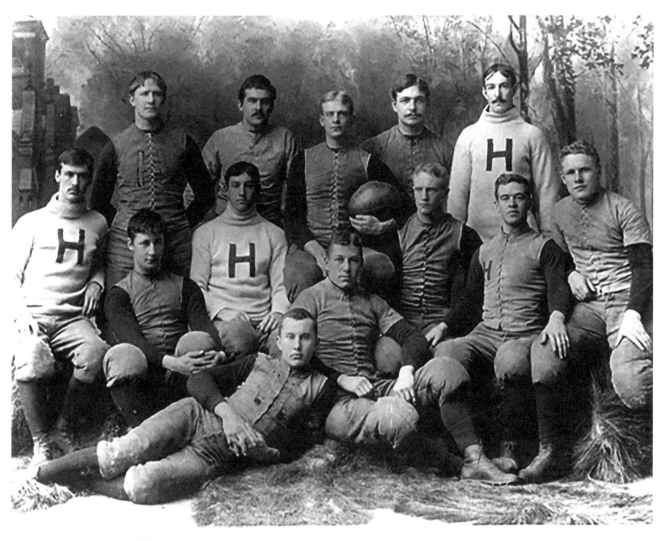

Harvard football team, 1890. Photo by Pach Brothers. Wikimedia Commons.

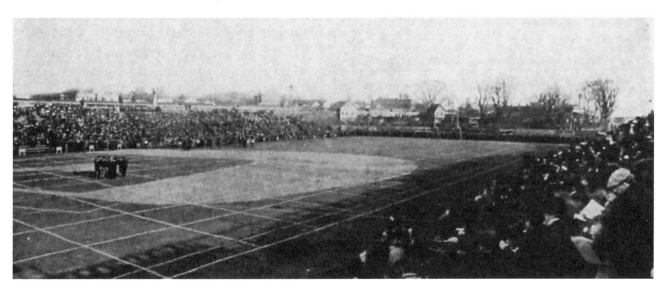

Hampden Park, Springfield, Mass. (ca. 1905). Published in *Springfield: Present and Prospective*, by James Eaton Tower and E.C. Gardner, 1905. The Library of Congress/Internet Archive.

EUGENE A. DARLING, MD

Physician Snapshot

Eugene A. Darling
BIRTH: 1868
DEATH: 1934
SIGNIFICANT CONTRIBUTIONS: Published the first scientific paper on the training of athletes, which addressed the pathophysiological effects of competitive sports (e.g., rowing and football)

The first two scientific papers on the training of athletes were published in 1899. The first was published by Dr. Eugene A. Darling, an assistant in bacteriology at Harvard Medical School; the other was co-written by Harold Williams and Horace D. Arnold about marathon runners in the second year (1898) of the American marathon's existence (the American marathon was later called the Boston Marathon). Darling, a fellow of the American College of Surgeons, was also an instructor in hygiene and an instructor in physiology who later was promoted to assistant professor of physiology at Harvard University. The Harvard Athletic Committee invited Dr. Darling "to investigate physiologic responses of the varsity crew in the hope of shedding light on the much debated question of 'over-training'" because little was known about

Vol. CXLI, No. 9.]   *BOSTON MEDICAL AND SURGICAL JOURNAL.*

Original Articles.   August 31, 1899.

THE EFFECTS OF TRAINING.
A Study of the Harvard University Crews.
BY EUGENE A. DARLING, M.D., CAMBRIDGE.

Vol. CXLIV, No. 23   June 6, 1901

THE EFFECTS OF TRAINING ; SECOND
PAPER.
BY EUGENE A. DARLING, M.D., CAMBRIDGE, MASS.

Two publications by Darling on the physiological effects of training (including the heart).
New England Journal of Medicine (formerly the *Boston Medical and Surgical Journal*): 1899 (pg. 205) & 1901 (pg. 556.)

the physiologic changes that occurred during vigorous athletic training (A. Flint 1878).

Darling studied the Harvard crew teams in May and June, "the more strenuous part of the training period" (E. A. Darling 1899), and the Harvard football team in the fall. He observed them rowing five-to-eight miles daily on the Charles and recorded their sleep duration, bathing routines (general plunge baths were prohibited), and exercise program. He noted that "besides rowing, the men indulged in very little exercise…a five minute walk before breakfast, an occasional game of quoits…or baseball were the only other form of exercise indulged in" (E. A. Darling 1899). Darling (1899) carefully recorded their diet:

A hearty breakfast at 7:30, lunch at one and dinner after the evening row. For breakfast the fare consisted of fruit, oatmeal or shredded wheat, eggs…meat, bread and butter, potato and milk. At noon there was cold meat, potato, bread and butter, marmalade, preserved fruit and milk. Dinner comprised soup, occasionally fish, roast beef or some other hot meat, several vegetables, bread and butter and a simple dessert. No tea or coffee was allowed, but ale or claret was permitted at dinner, also water in small amounts as desired. During the last week before the race, each man received a dish of calves'-foot jelly with sherry wine after the morning row, and a light lunch of oatmeal, milk and bread was served at four o'clock in the afternoon.

He also measured the effects of training on the following: weight, temperature, circulatory system and size of the heart, the kidneys, the blood, and the digestive system. At the time, he had limited available methods to assess the athletes during physical exams, but he determined:

There was a progressive enlargement affecting both sides of the heart…[corresponding] to the period of the most arduous work, late in May and early in June…How much…was due to hypertrophy and how much to dilatation is difficult to say. Probably there were both…The changes in the size of the heart corresponding to the changes in sounds [decreased or absent murmur] and action [slower pulse]…[or] gradual improvement of the heart was one of the most instructive points in the entire investigation…The chief deduction to be made from this study…is that the heart is a muscular organ and that it shows…the increase in size and power due to proper exercise and nutrition. (E. A. Darling 1899)

He found albuminuria—along with large numbers of hyaline casts, red blood cells, and leukocytes—in the athletes immediately after rowing activities. He noted "the sediment in many cases was exactly that of the first stage of acute nephritis, and if examined without a knowledge of the conditions [it] might easily have caused anxiety" (E. A. Darling 1899). Regarding over-training, he mentioned the common symptoms: "a loss of strength and endurance, so that a man previously strong becomes incapable of prolonged effort… [it] may be accompanied by a general nervous restlessness, by listlessness, by a loss of weight, by insomnia and by various digestive disturbances, such as anorexia and diarrhea" (E. A. Darling 1899). He suggested four possible causative factors for over-training:

First…a "'broken-winded" athlete is probably one with a dilated, flabby heart;…second… nutrition…[is] disturbed…by an improper diet…or by disturbed digestion…the third factor may be simple overwork…The fourth factor which suggests a nervous one…more intangible…unquestionably an important one… It may be anxiety about a coming contest… mental strain of mastering the technicalities of such a difficult art as rowing or such a complicated game as football [leading] to a condition of nervous exhaustion. (E. A. Darling 1899)

He concluded by stating:

Finally, this investigation has demonstrated that the physiologic effects of training, on the heart and kidneys in particular, may approach unpleasantly near to pathologic conditions, and that there should be some competent supervision to ensure that the safe limits, when those are determined, shall not be passed. (E. A. Darling 1899)

Darling reported similar findings in his paper on Harvard football players in 1901. He examined 17 men and reported that their hearts were larger than normal, and urine tests revealed albuminuria, increased hyaline casts, and hematuria. "In summary, it may be said that no ill effects, which could reasonably be attributed to training, were to be discovered nine months after stopping the training" (E. A. Darling 1901). Harvard University responded to Darling's research by hiring professional trainers to work with athletes along with the coaches, and eventually they included a team physician who was made available to athletes.

EDWARD H. NICHOLS, MD

Physician Snapshot

Edward H. Nichols
BIRTH: 1864
DEATH: 1922
SIGNIFICANT CONTRIBUTIONS: Published the first article on football injuries and a seminal work on osteomyelitis; required the first use of pads and helmets in football as well as a medical record for each athlete's injury; developed the first concussion protocol

Edward Hall Nichols, a general surgeon, was born in Reading, Massachusetts. He graduated from Harvard College in 1886 and Harvard Medical School in 1892. During his four years as an undergraduate he played baseball for Harvard, and fifteen years later he coached the team. He was a star player; he set a record of striking out 14 players in

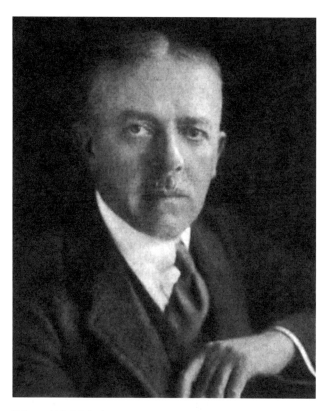

Edward H. Nichols.

A History of Boston City Hospital, 1905–1964, John J. Byrne (ed.),
Boston: The Sheldon Press, 1964.

one game against Yale. After receiving his medical degree, he spent two years at Boston City Hospital, where he trained in surgery first as an assistant and then as an executive assistant. He remained on staff at Boston City Hospital, eventually becoming head of a service; he was also on the staff of Children's Hospital. In 1897, he was appointed demonstrator of surgical pathology and taught the elementary course to second year students. Dr. Nichols was placed in charge of a new laboratory of surgical pathology in 1901 at Harvard Medical School. It was in this lab that his research led to his classic publication on osteomyelitis in which he showed that radical removal of the entire diseased part of the shaft of the bone would heal with new bone regenerated from the periosteum. He was an instructor in surgical pathology, promoted to assistant professor in 1904. Rising in academic rank, he was promoted to associate professor and in 1915 to clinical professor.

In 1904 Dr. Nichols, "one of Boston's well known surgeons" (*Boston Daily Globe* 1918), was appointed football team surgeon. Always with a "warm interest in the college teams from the period of his own participation" (*Boston Daily Globe* 1922b), he had served on the Committee on Athletics at Harvard. In 1905 he was one of the faculty members appointed to the committee on the regulation of athletic sports. It was also in 1905 that Bill Reid (age 26), a Harvard graduate and former athlete, returned as the first paid head football coach. His salary was one of the highest paid to any faculty or administrator. Reid had played football and was the captain of the baseball team in 1901; his coach was Dr. Nichols.

Bill Reid's goals included writing a detailed daily diary with the plan of eventually writing a "how-to manual" for coaches. He documented historical and contemporary unethical practices in football, including failing to keep injured players from game play and even neglecting to notify them of their injuries. He and Dr. Nichols had a long-term friendship, first as player and coach and then for several years as coach and team physician. Throughout his diary, Reid frequently mentions Dr. Nichols and their conversations, often asking his advice about strategy, rules, players' positions, and political issues as well as injuries and player fitness. Nichols often attended the coaches' meetings. At one dinner with coaches Reid and William H. Lewis, Nichols joined a discussion of football tactics, including the use of a tackle back, questions of defense, line's blocking on kicks, how to strategically use the ends, and who should play full back.

Dr. Nichols' main role, however, was team physician. He often emphasized to Coach Reid to avoid injuries by decreasing both the number and the length of scrimmages and to focus instead on precision and speed. Nichols argued that pushing players to their limits with extended practices a few days before a game was not worth the risk of injury, especially since they were unlikely to improve fitness or technique within just a few days. Other coaches argued for long scrimmages, but coach Reid was greatly swayed by Dr. Nichols. After questioning candidates who were seeking the trainer position on the track team, Dr. Nichols commented on their answers:

> To sum up, then, there was no practical agreement upon the amount of work, the length of time during which men could be kept in top condition, or the character of the food to be given to men in training. The whole thing comes down to a very indefinite general impression, plus the indication shown accurately by the weighing scales, and all this seems to show that the science of training is a very indefinite and crude one, and that the most valuable trainer is in all probability the man who knows human nature, especially the nature of young men best. But if it is permitted to me who is neither trainer nor doctor to say it, the last clause saves the whole statement of the Harvard man. The personal education of the athlete is what counts in training. It is the best psychologist who is the best trainer. (*Washington Post* 1907)

One very important event occurred during Dr. Nichols' and coach Reid's time together with the Harvard football team. In 1905, Harvard was considering whether to drop football; some major universities had already done so. The president of Harvard, Charles W. Eliot, strongly opposed football and tried unsuccessfully to abolish the game at Harvard. He described football as "a fight whose strategy and ethics are those of war... that the weaker man is considered the legitimate prey of the stronger" (C. W. Eliot 1904). There were many serious injuries to the head and spine playing football; between 1900 and 1905, 45 players had died from various injuries. After the death of a Union College player, President Theodore Roosevelt called a meeting of representatives from Harvard, Yale, and Princeton at the White House on October 19, 1905, to discuss ethical and clean play in collegiate football. Dr. Nichols

was the only physician present at the meeting. All the participants signed a letter agreeing to show good sportsmanship and to avoid foul play. Reid, as expected, was quite concerned about the future of football given that President Eliot's stated position had long been:

> The game of foot-ball grows worse and worse as regards foul and violent play, and the number and gravity of injuries which the players suffer. It has become perfectly clear that the game as now played is unfit for college use. (C. W. Eliot 1894)

Reid called for the formation of a committee to reform football at Harvard. The Harvard Athletic Association Committee to reform football was announced two months later on December 9, 1905, with Coach Reid as chairman. A movement was also started at the national level to reform football. A National Intercollegiate Football conference—including 68 institutions—met in New York City to form a new football rules committee. The outcome of these efforts by all the participants led to the eventual formation of the National Collegiate Athletic Association (NCAA) in March 1906.

Dr. Nichols, as team surgeon, kept detailed records of the players' injuries. In 1906 he and his colleague Dr. Homer B. Smith, a house officer at Boston City Hospital, condemned such injuries

NCAA logo. © 2021 National Collegiate Athletic Association.

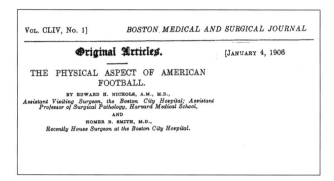

Vol. CLIV, No. 1]   *BOSTON MEDICAL AND SURGICAL JOURNAL*

𝕺riginal 𝕬rticles.   [January 4, 1906

THE PHYSICAL ASPECT OF AMERICAN
FOOTBALL.
BY EDWARD H. NICHOLS, A.M., M.D.,
Assistant Visiting Surgeon, the Boston City Hospital; Assistant
Professor of Surgical Pathology, Harvard Medical School,
AND
HOMER B. SMITH, M.D.,
Recently House Surgeon at the Boston City Hospital.

First original article on football injuries. (Nichols and Smith 1906).
Nichols and Smith. *Boston Medical and Surgical Journal*, 1906; 154: 1.

in an article titled "The Physical Aspect of American Football," which was published in the *Boston Medical and Surgical Journal*. This article seems to be the first report documenting football injuries. As Nichols and Smith wrote, "It has been claimed that the number of injuries this year was unusually great and more numerous than in any preceding season. In this absence of any available records of other seasons, this point cannot be determined accurately, but in our opinion, it is probable that this season is not markedly worse than preceding ones" (Nichols and Smith 1906). They went on: "[I]t must be stated that the position of the surgeon is rather a trying one. Football players are quite unlike ordinary private patients. Their disregard for pain is marked and their great desire is to be sufficiently recovered from injury to be able to play" (Nichols and Smith 1906). Injuries reported in 1905 numbered 145; the most common injuries were concussions (19), followed by sprained ankles (13), acromial clavicle dislocations (11), and dislocated semilunar cartilage (10). "The injuries were received in various ways: some in open play, some in the mechanical drill of 'tackling the dummy,' but a very great proportion occurred in the 'bunch' or 'pile' which forms after a player running the ball is tackled" (Nichols and Smith 1906).

They noted a high frequency of concussions; in only two games during the entire season did no concussions occur. "Concussion was treated by the players in general as a trivial injury and rather

regarded as a joke" (Nichols and Smith 1906). However, Nichols recognized the seriousness of concussions and discussed the problem with neurologists. He carefully examined each player, concerned with a possible middle meningeal artery hemorrhage. After experiencing one case, he sent all players with a concussion to the infirmary for observation overnight. Nichols and Smith concluded:

1) The number, severity and permanence of the injuries…playing football are very much greater than generally is credited or believed.

2) The greater number of injuries come in the "pile "and not in the open plays, although serious injuries are received in the open.

3) The number of injuries is inherent in the game itself.

4) A large percentage of the injuries is unavoidable.

5) The percentage of injuries is incomparably greater in football than in any other of the major sports.

6) The game does not develop the best type of men physically, because too great prominence is given to weight without corresponding nervous energy.

7) Constant medical supervision of the game where large numbers of men are engaged is a necessity and not a luxury.

8) The percentage of injury is much too great for any mere sport.

9) Leaving out all other objections to the game, ethical and practical, the conditions under which the game is played should be so modified as to diminish to a very great degree the number of injuries. (Nichols and Smith 1906)

New revised rules for football had gone into effect for the 1906 football season. In 1909, Dr.

Nichols published his second paper on football injuries, with Dr. Frank Richardson as co-author. "This report presents the statistic results of football injuries received by members of the Harvard Varsity squad during the seasons of 1906, 1907, and 1908. All of the games played during this time were played under the revised rules, which very much lessened the old-fashioned "mass plays" and made open plays [with the introduction of the forward pass] much more profitable" (Nichols and Richardson 1909). Over those three years, 113 total injuries occurred—down from 145 that occurred in 1905 alone, before the rules had changed (**Table 12.1**). This reduction was "the result of preliminary exercise and of slow development of the men. Proper padding…also prevents many of the injuries" (Nichols and Richardson 1909). All players now were required to wear padding on the shoulders, back, thigh, and knees, as well as helmets and special shoes.

Table 12.1. Football-related injuries during 1905–1908

Year	Total Injuries	Concussions	Quadriceps Rupture ("Poop")
1905	145	19	6
1906	34	5	7
1907	45	5	7
1908	34	3	3a

aThis number continued to decrease; no quadriceps ruptures occurred in 1909.

(Nichols and Richardson 1909.) Data are the number of injuries. New rules for football took effect in 1906.

After Nichols had spent 15 years as team surgeon, coach Reid was succeeded by Bob Fisher. Dr. Nichols warned Fisher "against [the candidates for the football team] taking off weight during the Summer, which will cause them to go stale before the big games are played" (*New York Times* 1919). Harvard football management sent two letters to the candidates, the first by coach Fisher and the second by Dr. Nichols which stated:

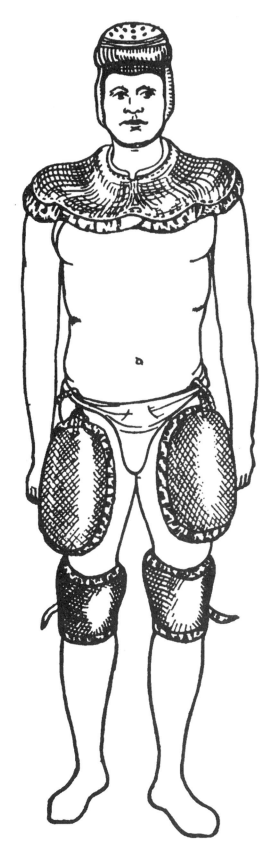

Line drawing from a photograph of protective pads and helmet worn by the Harvard football team in 1909.

Nichols and Richardson. *New England Journal of Medicine*, 1909; 160: 37.

1. Do not try to reduce your weight during the summer. Players often return in the Fall boasting that they are "down to weight." This is very undesirable. Men should come back well above playing weight, so that the coaches may have weight to take off during the preliminary work. Do not worry. Your weight will be taken off...Heavy linesmen should be from 12 to 15 pounds over weight. Light backs and end from 7 to 10 pounds. Do not try especially to regulate your diet. Food as provided in families is better.

2. Exercises. Any exercise which increases speed and co-ordination is desirable, such as handball, fives, tennis and baseball. Do not, however, overdo...Swimming is one of the very best conditioning sports...Golf is a good game for general condition.

3. Special exercise. All bacgfield [sic] men should practice passing the ball. All punters and drop kickers should have enough practice kicking so they do not strain muscles when they first come back. All men should practice quick starts daily for the last three weeks of vacation...from a football crouch. The point of all special exercise is to get the muscles that you will use in football hard enough so that we don't have a lot of charley horse and sprains at the beginning of the season. Come back over weight, eager to exercise and not tired.

(*New York Times* 1919)

The number of injuries reported by Dr. Nichols reinforced his belief that the players required medical supervision. Over his career, Dr. Nichols published over 20 papers: two on football injuries, three on head injuries, six on surgery, and the rest on orthopaedic problems. He co-authored a paper with Dr. Edward H. Bradford on surgical anatomy of the hip joint in congenital dislocations and a classic, oft-cited paper on osteomyelitis. He served for five years as secretary of the original Harvard Cancer Commission, writing in one report that "nothing avails except early and radical operation" (T. B. Quigley 1959c).

Two years before the United States entered WWI, the British government asked Harvard Medical School for a voluntary unit of surgeons and nurses to staff a British base hospital in France. Dr. Nichols organized this unit, consisting of 32 surgeons and 75 nurses. They staffed the hospital for three months, returning to Boston in August 1915. When asked by the press upon his return, Dr. Nichols recalled examples of atrocities committed by the Germans—leaving the wounded on the battlefield for 24 hours without water; offering water, but when the wounded reached for the drink, pouring the water on the ground; and one soldier who had an open leg fracture reporting that a German officer stomped on his injured leg. Dr. Nichols predicted that the Allies would win the war, but it would take three-to-five years. Later, after the United States entered the war, Dr. Nichols, a major at the time, was part of the 2000 bed Base Hospital Unit No. 7, Tours, France, which was organized at Boston City Hospital and left Camp Devens in July 1918. He was promoted to lieutenant colonel in December 1918.

After completing a serious operation on a patient in a Brookline hospital on June 6, 1922, Dr. Nichols suffered a stroke and died. He was 58 years old. Nichols was lauded in an obituary published in the *Boston Daily Globe* (1922a):

Dr. Nichols was in a great measure the architect of his own fortunes and certainly the author of his own fame. Great ability, amounting to almost genius, was his birthright; an interest in anything that came within his view so intense as to make the most distant things seem personal matters, a temperament that would not for an instant...anything that seemed wrong, and new; into indignant action at the site of misdoing; a love of beauty; a human sympathy that led him into extraordinary efforts for people of whom he knew nothing except that they needed a friend or a surgeon—these were the same attributes of one of Boston's really great surgeons.

At his funeral, "a throng of mourners which included many prominent surgeons, physicians, and ex-Harvard athletes paid [him] great tribute" (*Boston Daily Globe* 1922b).

Nichols' contributions have had a lasting influence. Dr. Thomas B. Quigley—in a speech at an Alumni Day symposium in 1959—recalled one story about Dr. Nichols:

On one occasion Dr. Edward H. Nichols '86, surgeon from 1905 to 1921, noted that a player had suffered a blow on the head and seemed to get to his feet rather slowly. The Harvard captain called a time out, and Dr. Nichols ran out on the field. He had previously worked out a simple set of questions which, together with a good look at the player, would help him determine whether a blow on the head had resulted in confusion, disorientation or lack of judgment. These questions concerned the date, the score of the game, the time of day and other simple subjects. The injured player knew this full well and knew if he failed to answer these questions accurately, Dr. Nichols would certainly remove him from the game. As Dr. Nichols ran onto the field, the player ran toward him shouting in a clear voice, "It is Saturday afternoon; we are playing Dartmouth, the score is 7-0, and I feel fine." Dr. Nichols promptly did a neat curve in his run and returned to the bench without further ado. (T. B. Quigley 1959c)

His tireless work continues to influence the present, and his work will not be forgotten in the annals of history.

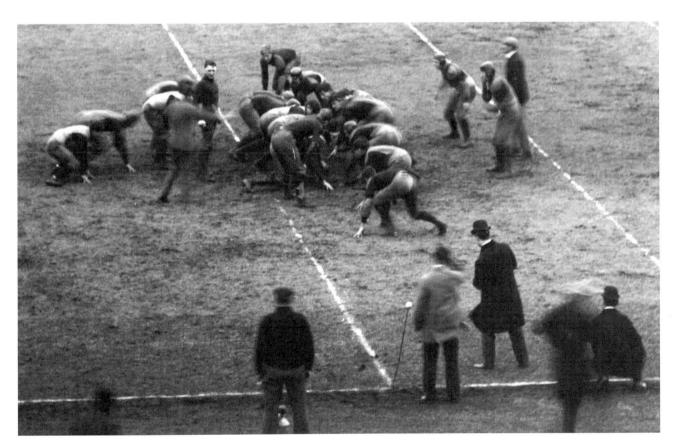

Harvard football game, ca. 1906. HUPSF Football (209), olvwork376381. Harvard University Archives.

THOMAS K. RICHARDS, MD

Physician Snapshot

Thomas K. Richards

BIRTH: 1892

DEATH: 1965

SIGNIFICANT CONTRIBUTIONS: Manager of the Harvard football club; provided oversight of a new field house; required physicians and assistants on the field every day during football practice; required physical therapists in the field house on every game day; initiated policy that a dietician join the team of health care providers for athletes

Thomas Kinsman Richards, known as "Tommy" to some, "TK" to others, graduated from Harvard's undergraduate program in 1915 before attending the medical school. He was manager of the Harvard football club as an undergraduate beginning in 1914. "He specialized in orthopedic work after completing a special course in Liverpool, England [circa 1920] under Dr. [Robert] Jones" (*Boston Daily Globe* 1923). He graduated from HMS in 1919, was a surgical intern at Boston City Hospital, and for more than five years he assisted Dr. Nichols in treating the players. During Richards's first year as assistant to Dr. Nichols in 1920, Dr. Nichols was ill at the time Harvard was to play Oregon in the Rose Bowl (Harvard's only Bowl appearance), and Richards had to manage the team's health alone.

In 1920, he became chairman of the football committee. Richards was an assistant visiting surgeon at Boston City Hospital, where he worked with Dr. E. H. Nichols. He was also team physician for the Boston Red Sox. On one occasion he was asked to see Ted Williams, who sustained a chip fracture in an ankle when sliding into second base playing against Newark of the International League. He told Williams he would be out for about six weeks.

After Nichols' death in 1922, Richards succeeded him as the team physician and as chief surgeon of the Harvard Athletic Association. Richards

made many changes and introduced new developments in the care of athletes at Harvard. He and his two assistants were available at Soldier's Field every day (except Sundays) from 2:00 to 6:00 p.m. A new medical room was built in the field house; it was equipped with radiography equipment, massage tables, diathermy, whirlpool tubs, and staffed by physical therapists. Football players were not the only athletes to receive care here; the medical team treated players from lacrosse, soccer, track, tennis, hockey, boxing, wrestling, and baseball. According to White:

> The medical feature of Harvard's athletic policy is [one of the most] outstanding of its kind in the world, and during the football season an average of 350 men a day report for treatment at the locker building. As great a variety of cases is handled as the average out-patient department of many hospitals in the city. (D. White 1928)

Richards added another significant member to the sports program: a dietician. Under the supervision of the dietician, players avoided all gastrointestinal issues and controlled their weight. This change also led to the discovery that football players and crew members required almost twice the caloric intake of those participating in other sports.

Richards was exceptionally attuned to his athletes' needs. He implemented a follow-up system, requiring the recording of all injuries sustained over time by a player. All injured players had to report each day for treatment until they were discharged. He was unflagging in covering 11 football players at a time on the field, keeping an attentive eye to any injuries warranting removal from a game. No player could successfully hide their injuries from him. He was both skillful in getting players back to necessary fitness levels while also adamant in not allowing players to return if they might injure themselves further in the process.

In 1928, with Dr. T. K. Richards in charge of the medical department, the staff of the medical

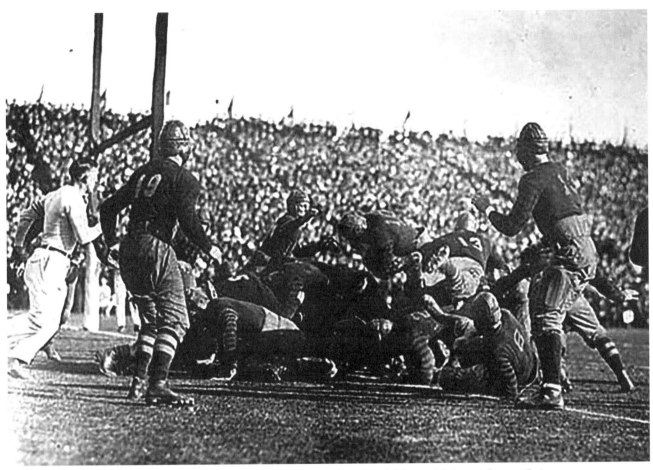

Sixth Annual Rose Bowl, 1920. Only appearance by Harvard in a Rose Bowl. Harvard defeated Oregon 7–6.
James Vautravers/Tiptop25.com.

room and Dr. Richards were under the supervision of Dr. Alfred Worcester, the professor of hygiene, and supported by the Harvard Athletic Association. Richards had two assistants: Drs. A. Thorndike Jr. and N. C. Browder. Although little information remains available about the man, he made a lasting contribution to sports medicine when he courageously stood—as a relatively unknown physician—before an annual conference of football coaches in New York in 1928 and declared that physicians, not coaches, should determine a player's readiness to return to play. At the time—and even in some ways still today—athletic coaches earned more and had more power than college presidents and team surgeons. He argued that an empowered doctor was "an asset, not a liability" (M. E. Webb 1928). In his speech, Richards stated:

I see it from another angle than you fellows. When a fellow gets through college you do not see him again, in all probability. A man gets a bad knee playing football. He finishes his college course and the knee is still bad. I have to explain why his knee is bad, whether anything could have been done to prevent the injury and I must try to straighten it out afterward to the satisfaction of the boy's people. The family never forgets that football injured this fellow.

The doctor's game is something more than going out on the field Saturday to make $10 or $13 or $25 and have a fine afternoon. If he is a good doctor, he will have a mightily poor time in the football game, because he won't see any football. He is watching 11 individuals.

He is counting 22 legs and 22 arms to see if they are all moving every time they get up.

Every year when the season is over, I like to see the Army and Navy play and sit in the stand, and I don't.

Football is a rough, tough game. That is why we like it. A doctor's job is preventing injuries, showing how he can utilize men who are injured to the best advantage, if by so doing he is not going to injure that man further.

To be a doctor with a football team, the doctor has to know a whole lot of it, and the coach has to consider him as much a member of his coaching staff as anybody else. There should be no conflict between your trainer and your doctor.

The man who owns racehorses hires a trainer to get the horses into condition for the race. If something goes wrong with Man o' War the trainer isn't the fellow that he calls on; he sends for the veterinary.

The same thing is true in football. Your trainer is in charge of their physical condition, guided to a certain extent by the doctor if the doctor knows anything about training, and the doctor is in charge of the physical condition, saying when they shall play.

It is the doctor's job to know how to utilize a man who is injured without further endangering the man.

The present style of offences in the last few years has been bringing men out and sending them out to be interference. Take, for example, a balanced line. You have a player going around the left. You have a right guard who has a bad cartilage in his right knee. He is no good for the left side. Every time he turns to the left that cartilage is going wrong. Put him as his left guard and him around the right side of the line and he will never have any trouble.

You have a nearsighted man. (There isn't a trainer in the country who can spot how much vision a man has. And is up to the foot ball doctor to find out how much vision that squad has). He may have a blind spot in his eye where a ball at a given plane won't appear at all.

It would be perfectly foolhardy to put a man who has a blind spot down on the field to play forward position. Train him to backup a line of scrimmage or don't use him. Make the most of what you have.

It is the same way with hearing. You wouldn't put a man who is deaf in the left ear at your right hand if you wished to talk to him at dinner. If he is an end, put him on the left end where he can hear the signals.

The coach must be made to feel that the doctor is just as interested in turning out a first-class football team as he is. I personally take a great deal of pride, when the Yale game comes along, and I go to the head coach and say: 'You have 100 percent men on your field.' And I have done it repeatedly.

Briefly, how are you going to prevent injuries? To prevent injuries, you have to know when they occur and how. If there is any one way to prevent injuries, it is to avoid playing men who are tired.

I know of an instance a few years ago in a game between two colleges where one team had a doctor and the other didn't.

The team that did not have a doctor was playing a man who was very tired. He couldn't protect himself. The doctor of the other team protested to the player's coach and told him to take that man out before he got hurt. It wasn't done. It was a disgrace in those days to be removed from a football game because you were tired. About three plays later the fellow was dead with a broken neck, and it was the doctor of the visiting team who had to explain to the family why that happened.

An unrecognized injury may cost a game. Don't think that I feel that a doctor is infallible, because he isn't and the first instance I shall give you will be a mistake that I made. I went out to see a boy who was poked in the eye. He fooled me to the extent that I thought he could see out of that eye. He was watched carefully. He was playing second defense on the right-hand side.

It was his left eye that had been hurt. The play went through the middle of the line and the ball went right by him. He never saw it at all. I lost that game; no question about it.

I shall mention a few games because I don't think the individuals will care especially. When we played in Pasadena a few years ago at the very end of the game Arnie Horween was pretty nearly done. He told me his legs wouldn't work.

After watching him for a minute it was perfectly evident that they wouldn't work. I told Fisher to take him out. Horween was given the ball in the next play and he made a good gain. Bob said, "What do you think of that?"

I said, "Take him out." Arnie was still left in and he continued to gain. He got down to the three-yard line and by this time I was having a fit. He had gone 56 yards or thereabouts with a pair of legs that I knew he shouldn't be running on. There was a half minute to play and Horween stood still in the line with the ball in his arms.

The game ended right there. When he came in he said, "I am sorry, but my legs just wouldn't work."

There was a substitute that could have scored that touchdown.

Five years ago we evolved a strapping for ankles in Cambridge which we thought was effective. Since then I have never seen a sprained ankle on Soldiers Field on an ankle that has been strapped. In my time I also have seen the convalescence from so-called water on the knee cut down from six weeks to ten days.

At Harvard perhaps we do things a good deal differently than in other colleges. In a brief way I will outline to you our scheme. My word is law as to whether a man shall play or not. That isn't decided from minute to minute, right during a game, before a game, at practice or any other time. I give in writing to Horween before each practice the name of the men that he cannot play, men who are slightly injured, who may do a certain amount of work but can't do it all. On that same slip is given the date when those men will be ready to play and I try to best that date every time.

Second, no man is allowed to decide for himself whether or not he is injured seriously enough to stop playing. All injuries have to be reported. Any man that reports to Horween for practice is 100 percent. In other words, Horween is free to do with him as he sees fit. The man has no alibis.

We try to keep an accurate record of injuries so that when the football season is over the man isn't merely dropped with nobody looking after him. He is followed right straight through until the end; I don't care whether it takes 10 days or 10 weeks or a year. He is followed until he is as well as medical knowledge can make him. Operations may be necessary. If so, they are done.

Why do I speak as I do about a doctor's being necessary? More and more I am seen parents of boys who have been hurt, not only from Harvard but schools throughout New England and many other colleges throughout the country. The parents say, 'because something had been done for this fellow in the beginning?' Of course, it could. If I said it could, then a reflection is cast on the men who have been taking care of them in the past.

So, you coaches, I think, are taking a responsibility which is not yours. It is a good thing to pass the buck occasionally to someone who has been trained to take it.

Perhaps I am radical but I think there is a storm brewing there is going to be an upheaval, perhaps on the part of the colleges, the families of the fellows who are playing football and whatnot, so that it may be not unlike the situation in this country where the United States refused to clean out the saloon and they had prohibition wished on them.

None of us want to see that happen to football. What I want to see you fellows do is to have an intelligent care for your men. We will have better physical specimens and you won't be playing injured men at all.

Let me say that I have never seen a star who was injured that could play football one, two, three, with a second string man who is physically right. (M. E. Webb 1928)

Richards published seven papers throughout his career: a description of a splint for treatment of clavicle fractures that allowed full use of the arms; use of antero-posterior wooden splints in the treatment of distal radius fractures; a case report of a posterior cruciate injury with a locked knee that he successfully treated with manipulation and a cast; a report of three cases of acute bursitis; and two physiology papers about athletes. In the first he reported a study where he measured the diameter of athletes' hearts before and after exercise in an attempt to understand why some athletes collapsed at the end of a race. He took x-rays of the chest from seven feet in varsity and freshman cross country teams, visiting cross country teams and internationally famous distance runners. He was able to report on only 20 athletes because the other athletes' films and data were lost in a fire.

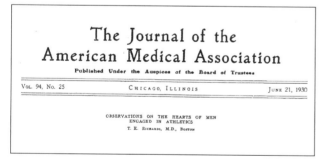

Title page of Richards's article on changes in heart diameter with exercise (T. K. Richards 1930).

Richards. *Journal of the American Medical Association*, 1930; 94: 1988.

He stated:

However these figures are typical of the whole series...the hearts after racing were consistently smaller than those at rest...The

following is offered as a partial explanation of the conditions noted...so-called cramps of striated muscle are due to an excess of lactic acid in the affected muscle...Cannot the contracted hearts of athletes...be explained as some form of muscle cramp which results in a smaller or contracted heart, the clinical collapse accordingly being due to a cerebral anemia...? (T. K. Richards 1930)

In the second paper, he measured the blood sugar, urine sugar, and urine protein of 13 graduate students while they exercised on a treadmill as well as in Harvard football players. He concluded that hyperglycemia is common as a reaction to emotional stress on the football field and that protein appeared in the players' urine in increasing amounts during the game; however, he found it to be an insignificant finding in reaction to general exercise.

In 1931, Dr. Richards announced his resignation as surgeon in charge of athletics. He continued to work through the end of the Harvard baseball season in 1932. Officials at Harvard denied that there was any dissension between Dr. Richards and the university. Dr. Worcester informed the press that Richards resigned in response to the needs of his private practice. Richards was remembered as having a larger than life persona at Harvard, having often rode onto Soldier's Field at 75 miles per hour on his motorcycle or rowed 1,000 miles across the ocean, including at one point from Boston to Miami. He was particularly well known for his ability to treat "bum" knees, and his unwavering attention to the athletes in his care. At one point, he saved a player's life when the player ruptured his spleen; most others at the time had believed the player's injury insignificant. The *Boston Globe* summarized Richards' career with the following tribute: "After his year is out, Dr. Richards will go, but not without the great regret of Harvard men. His will be a great loss to Harvard athletics" (*Daily Boston Globe* 1931).

AUGUSTUS THORNDIKE JR.

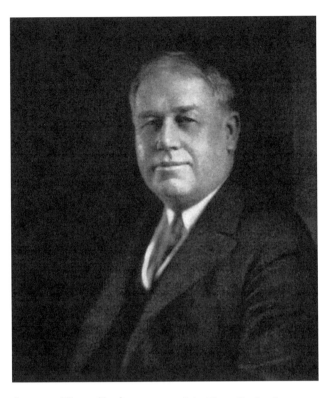

Augustus Thorndike Jr. Courtesy of the Thorndike family.

Physician Snapshot

Augustus Thorndike Jr.

BIRTH: 1896

DEATH: 1986

SIGNIFICANT CONTRIBUTIONS: Authority in rehabilitation; first team physician in hockey; first to require hockey players to wear helmets; designed improved padding and helmets for football players; required all athletes to have a physical exam before the season started; added the first onsite x-ray machine in the Dillon Field House; established the "three knockout" rule. Stressed cold (instead of heat) and compression to treat acute injuries; required a physician attend each game in contact sports, and authored two seminal books on treating injury among athletes

Following Dr. T. K. Richards' retirement, Dr. Alfred Worcester (Oliver Professor of Hygiene) named Augustus "Gus" Thorndike Jr. the next head team physician in 1932. Dr. Thorndike was a friend of Dr. Richards and his assistant for a couple of years. He had also previously worked for the Harvard Athletic Association, whose physicians had been providing care to athletes until that role was assigned to the department of hygiene. With his new appointment, Thorndike worked under Dr. Worcester in the department of hygiene; he was responsible not only for athletes but all students who needed medical care.

Thorndike was born in Boston, attended the Country Day School in Newton, and entered Harvard in the class of 1919. He played football in 1915 and 1916. After two years at Harvard, he quit (March 1917) and "joined the US Navy as Seaman, 1st class, and was assigned to the patrol boat, Wild Goose. He was discharged with a medical disability on August 10, 1917" (MGH HCORP Archives); the reason is unknown. On September 15, 1917, he married Olivia Lowell in what was described as a "notably brilliant wedding" (*Boston Daily Globe* 1917). That same month he also entered Harvard Medical School, graduating in 1921.

He completed two years of surgical training at the Massachusetts General Hospital on the West Surgical Service, where his father had trained some 32 years previously in 1889. Following the advice of Dr. Harvey Cushing, he spent the next year (1923) as an assistant to Professor Einer Key, surgeon-in-chief at the Karolinska Institute. He published his first paper in 1924, a review of 47 cases of spinal fractures from the surgical service at the Maria Hospital in Stockholm. Eighty-one percent of the patients treated at the Maria Hospital were industrial accidents. That same year, he also published a paper from MGH with Dr. Seth M. Fitchet on an improved aeroplane splint for treating fractures of the proximal humerus.

Next, Thorndike spent six weeks (October and November 1923) in Europe doing postgraduate work in the clinics at the University of Vienna. In 1925 he published a report of his experiences in the *Boston Medical and Surgical Journal*, describing the huge outpatient clinics, a lecture he attended about scoliosis, and the large number of autopsies he observed. He also shared details about the exceptional postgraduate teaching in anatomy and mentioned the high-caliber surgeons working there, such as Anton Eiselsberg and Hans Lorenz. However, Thorndike found flaws in the surgical program, noting a lack of materials and supplies and many mistakes. Overall, though, he recommended the university to postgraduates wanting to study further.

Upon returning to Boston, Thorndike was an assistant to William F. Ladd for three years at Children's Hospital. Dr. Ladd became known as the father of pediatric surgery. Ladd also worked at Milton Hospital; Thorndike was on the staff of both hospitals, Children's Hospital and Milton Hospital. Thorndike also had an office with Ladd at 66 Commonwealth Avenue. Shortly after Thorndike left his assistantship, Ladd became surgeon-in-chief at Children's Hospital in 1927; Thorndike went into private practice. Thorndike "and five other physicians purchased land from Children's Hospital and founded the Longwood Medical Building Trust" (MGH HCORP Archives). He moved his office there—319 Longwood Avenue—in 1929. Thorndike practiced general and pediatric surgery, presenting papers to the New England Pediatric Society. He was a junior assistant surgeon at Children's Hospital and active early in his career in the Harvard Medical Alumni Association, serving as treasurer in 1929 through at least 1932. On the faculty at Harvard Medical School, he wrote in his 50th reunion class notes: "clinical surgery was my first slot, not the academic field, although I did some teaching at Harvard before WWII and advanced on the faculty from assistant in surgery to lecturer in surgery, where I remained until I retired" (MGH HCORP Archives).

From his first publication in 1924 until 1927, Thorndike published 11 papers; nine were on fracture treatment, including two with Dr. Charles Scudder and Dr. Tom Harmer in which they described their fracture exhibit shown at the annual meeting of the Massachusetts Medical Society. The exhibit was modeled after those of the Fracture Committee of the American Medical Association who purpose was to convey basic principles to those in practice. He also published a paper on fractures in the newborn with Dr. F. Richard Pierce in 1936. They reviewed 6000 fracture cases at Children's Hospital. Their article detailed current statistics for birth fractures and issued a plea for adequate treatment. In their conclusions they wrote:

1. The incidence of birth fractures to all fractures as seen in a review of 6000 cases... reveals 113:6000 or approximately 1:60.

2. Birth fractures are, in the large majority of cases, accidents occurring in difficult obstetric manipulations.

3. Birth fractures in this series occurred in most cases in large babies.

4. Not one instance of true intrauterine fracture was found in this review. The disease entities of osteogenesis imperfect, fragilitas ossium and the dysostoses should be considered as included in true birth fractures.

5. The pleas for more adequate treatment in fractures of the newborn consist in (1) early diagnosis; (2) early manipulative alignment of the fragments involved; and (3) proper fixation.

6. An outline for methods of fixation with illustrations is presented.

(A. Thorndike and F. R. Pierce 1936)

At the time of that publication, he was listed as associate surgeon at Children's Hospital.

In addition to his research on fractures, he also worked to combat fatigue among Harvard athletes. According to the *New England Journal of Medicine*, Thorndike instituted policy so that:

All competitors are given a thorough physical examination, and a history is taken to insure

[sic] their physical capability of performing adequately under physical stress. They are required to eat at the training table, and diets adequate in caloric requirements and of proper balance are provided. Before competitions, extra carbohydrate is supplied to establish a reserve within the body. Since the loss of chlorides is a factor in the production of fatigue, and since there is no store of chloride in the body, this substance is supplied before, and during the game. This last measure has prevented the occurrence of muscle cramps and has decreased the amount of weight loss during competition...Dr. Thorndike emphasized the fact that the phenomenon of 'overtraining' in athletes is a reality. It is a fatigue of the central nervous system rather than a physical fatigue and may be so severe as to cause loss of co-ordination, insomnia, and loss of weight...
(*New England Journal of Medicine* 1936)

During this time, Thorndike was active in the Massachusetts Medical Society, the American Medical Association and the American College of Surgeons; he served on many committees, including as secretary for both the New England Regional Committee on Fractures of the American College of Surgeons and the Massachusetts Medical Society in 1936. He was a strong advocate of athletic participation and its benefits while acknowledging that injuries are going to happen. He believed most injuries are minor, including sprained ankles, twisted knees, and bruises. He also disagreed with the assumption that injuries follow athletes later in life. Nevertheless, he was a proponent of following the course of an athlete's injury history throughout their career and providing continued support to prevent reoccurrence.

During the next decade, before the US entered World War II, Dr. Thorndike remained very committed to athletes, their care and the care of all students in the university health service which he oversaw. He stressed the importance of prevention of injuries with sports, particularly as participation

was increasing. He often spoke at local and regional meetings about sports injuries and even recommended training lay persons in first aid for recreational sporting activities. He published four papers on sports injuries—one in 1938 and three in 1940–as well as two books. In his 1938 paper, "Trauma Incident to Sports and Recreation," he stated:

> If there is one thought I can leave with you, I should like it to be an emphasis on the importance of early, appropriate and adequate treatment for the control of internal hemorrhage in these minor injuries. The smaller the hemorrhage, the smaller is the hematoma to be absorbed, the smaller the fibroblastic scarring and the shorter the disability period. A good end result depends on a prompt return to function with a minimum of scarring. (A. Thorndike 1938)

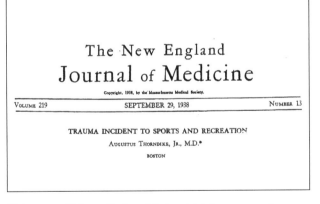

Title page of Thorndike's article in which he stresses the importance of controlling bleeding after injury.
A. Thorndike. *New England Journal of Medicine*, 1938; 219: 457.

In the same year, Thorndike published his classic book, *Athletic Injuries. Prevention, Diagnosis and Treatment.* In it he described his experience with college sports injuries, outlining types and pathology of injury and how to prevent, diagnose, and treat them. In the foreword, Arlie V. Bock, Professor of Hygiene at Harvard, wrote:

ATHLETIC INJURIES

Prevention, Diagnosis and Treatment

BY

AUGUSTUS THORNDIKE, M.D.

Chief Surgeon to the Department of Hygiene, and to the Harvard
Athletic Association, Harvard University; Associate in Surgery,
Harvard Medical School

Title page of Thorndike's book, *Athletic Injuries. Prevention, Diagnosis and Treatment*. Possibly the first book on athletic injuries. This is the first edition of Thorndike's book. The book went through numerous subsequent editions.

Athletic Injuries. Prevention, Diagnosis and Treatment. Philadelphia: Lea and Febiger, 1938.

The occurrence of injuries incident to sport is to be deplored. Fortunately, as the reader will see, few of them are serious. The necessity of competent coaching and medical supervision of all organized athletics is recognized by most of the colleges and many of the schools of the country...The problem of living aptly and well requires the development of the whole personality of a man, and to this end the playing fields make their great contribution. (A. V. Bock 1941)

In chapter 1 of the book, Thorndike described his work with athletes in the department of hygiene. Surgeons, trainers, and physical therapists attended all games and treated all sports injuries, and this oeuvre was expanding to include conditions among all students—graduates and undergraduates, athletes and nonathletes. Their department had grown so much that it now included nine surgeons and one roentgenologist (all part-time), four physical therapists (also part-time), and two trainers (both full-time). He further discussed the important issues of training, physical fitness, fatigue, and even the use of "pep pills."

A favorable review of his book was published in the *New England Journal of Medicine* after its release:

He has possibly used too much of his text for presenting his findings at Harvard University... however his experiences...have given to the book that well recognized touch which is only the product of one who knows by having seen and done. His ingenious treatment for sprains—cold—is revolutionary; it upsets the long-taught adage that one should use alternative hot and cold soaks...The idea of compression with sponge rubber is a good tip for us all...The book will prove a boon to the athletic groups of colleges, factories and camps and to the general practitioner. (*New England Journal of Medicine* 1938)

The book sold for $3 and was republished several times.

VOL. XXII, NO. 2   APRIL, 1940   Old Series Vol. XXXVIII, No. 2

The Journal of Bone and Joint Surgery

MYOSITIS OSSIFICANS TRAUMATICA *

BY AUGUSTUS THORNDIKE, JR., M.D., F.A.C.S., BOSTON, MASSACHUSETTS

From the Department of Hygiene, Harvard University

Thorndike's article describing his method of treating traumatic myositis ossificans.

A. Thorndike. *The Journal of Bone and Joint Surgery*, 1940; 22: 315.

In 1940, Thorndike reported in an article on his personal experience with 25 cases of myositis ossificans, which he observed for over a year and up to five years; all from school or college sports. He concluded:

1. Myositis ossificans traumatica is an inflammatory process of muscle in its early stage

and before ossification is actually demonstrated by the roentgen ray. "Tumor," "dolor," and "calor" are all present at this stage.

2. This inflammatory process gradually subsides as ossification takes place.

3. The ossification is gradually absorbed in part and sometimes in full, depending on its size and location. The muscle function returns to normal, except in those instances where the ossification occurs near a joint.

4. Treatment necessitates the immediate application of cold and a compression bandage to control hemorrhage, and later heat to aid in the absorption of the hematoma. Of great importance is the avoidance of massage on all severe and tender muscle contusions.

5. Operative removal of the ossification is indicated only in those cases in which it occurs near a joint in the original or the insertion of a muscle, where joint function is permanently impaired, and then only from twelve to twenty-four months after injury. (A. Thorndike 1940)

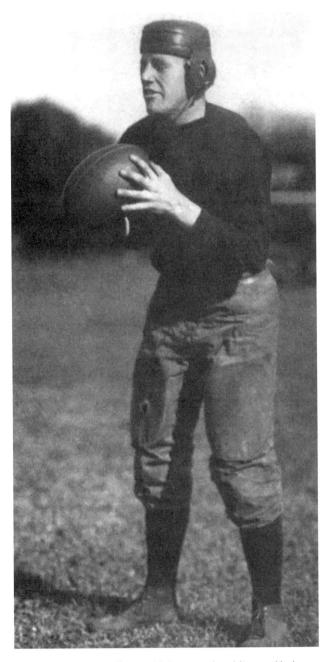

Football player in uniform with improved padding and helmet during Thorndike's era. Courtesy of Bertram Zarins.

That same year, in a paper titled "Athletic and Related Injuries," published in the *New England Journal of Medicine*, Thorndike reported on progress in sports medicine, which *Time* magazine referred to as "gory" (*Time* 1940). Thorndike's article reviewed the existing literature on athletic injuries and briefly reviewed the effects of exercise on the kidneys and cardiovascular symptoms. Interestingly, he did not refer to the studies on the heart and changes in the urine of athletes after exercise, previously published by both Dr. Darling and Dr. Richards.

In another paper published in 1940, Thorndike and Garrey reported on knee joint injuries (exclusive of laceration) in organized sports at Harvard over a seven-year period (**Table 12.2**).

He listed the incident of sprains to each of the specific knee ligaments. Over the seven-year period, the total number of knee sprains reduced from 54 to 12 per year. In his conclusion he wrote:

1. The adequate treatment of knee injuries… requires the institution of early and prompt diagnosis, and immediate application of

cold, compression bandage, and rest, to control hemorrhage and protect the injured tissues.

2. During the convalescent treatment, measures are instituted to promote the absorption of waste products of hemorrhage, and to stimulate tissue repair.

3. All former sprains should be protected by adhesive strapping to prevent a recurrence of such injuries in sports...where stress and strain are expected.

4. The steady decline in the ratio of serious internal derangements of the knee among knee sprains in organized athletics is proof that this treatment is of value.

(A. Thorndike and W. E. Garrey 1940)

Table 12.2. Knee Joint Injuries in Harvard Sports

Injury	Number
Sprained ligament	203
Contusion	
Joint	145
Muscle	78
Bursa	8
Superficial	6
Internal derangements	43
Total	483

Includes all injuries to the meniscus and crucial ligaments.
Thorndike and Garrey 1940.

A MANUAL OF
BANDAGING, STRAPPING AND SPLINTING

Title page of Thorndike's book, *A Manual of Bandaging, Strapping and Splinting*.
A. Thorndike. *A Manual of Bandaging, Strapping and Splinting*. Philadelphia: Lea and Febiger, 1941.

Thorndike wrote a second book, *A Manual of Bandaging, Strapping and Splinting* in 1941. He wrote the book to follow a related course for second-year medical students at Harvard. In the preface he described it as a manual to explain the basics of wrapping injuries, with many illustrations, for inexperienced physicians and nonphysicians. In the foreword, Dr. Elliott C. Cutler, the Moseley Professor of Surgery at both BWH and Harvard, stated that Thorndike achieved his goal—the manual expounds on basic principles, acting as a guide to caring for athletic injuries for those with little or no training in the art. A review of the book in the *Journal of the American Medical Association* also recommended it for practicing physicians. See **Case Report 12.1** for an example of his work.

Case Report 12.1: Acromioclavicular Joint Dislocation in Football

W.B. consulted one of us (A.T., Jr.) sixteen days after sustaining an injury to the right shoulder in a semiprofessional football game. An x-ray had been taken elsewhere and cold applications had been prescribed. After a week of marked discomfort, an osteopath was consulted who strapped the shoulder. Pain and discomfort continued despite the strapping which was removed by the patient after another week.

Upon examination there was found a typical severe dislocation of the right acromioclavicular joint. The clavicle lay on the top of the acromion.

The dislocation was easily reduced without an anesthetic and held with strapping across the joint. Immediately after the strapping was applied the patient stated that he was comfortable for the first time since the occurrence of the injury, sixteen days before. X-rays taken before and after reduction and taping showed normal realignment of the gross displacement of the bones.

Three weeks later the strapping was removed and displacement did not recur. Three and one-half weeks later he resumed football as a blocking back, with protective strapping to the joint. He has played through two seasons since without trouble from the shoulder.

(A. Thorndike and T. B. Quigley 1942)

From 1941 until 1955, Thorndike was on staff at MGH as a consultant in trauma; he was later listed as a consultant in surgery after 1955. With the war expanding in Europe, President Roosevelt had activated the Council of National Defense in the spring of 1940. State organizations of civilian defense were formed, including in Massachusetts. Dr. Elliott C. Cutler, chief of surgery at the Peter

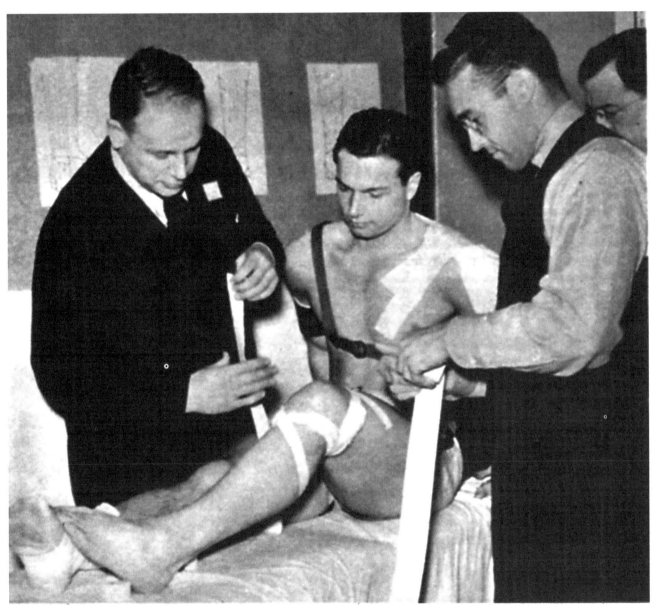

Football Taping Relieves Sufferers from Chronic Strains

Preventive strappings which have drastically reduced the number of recurring ankle and knee injuries among Harvard football players were demonstrated before the American Academy of Orthopedic Surgeons by Dr. Augustus Thorndike (center), squad physician.

Wide World

Collegiate Digest, vol. XIII, issue 15. February 28, 1940.

Dr. Thorndike taping an athlete's knee. Wide World Photos. Courtesy of Bertram Zarins.

Bent Brigham Hospital, was named medical director; Dr. Thorndike assumed an additional role as deputy medical director during this time period. The organization would be activated if the US were attacked, caring for those who are injured. Cutler, Thorndike, and the others on the team were tasked with organizing emergency response throughout the regional divisions and collaborating with other national organizations such as the American Red Cross. In January 1942, Thorndike had to resign as deputy medical director of the Medical Division of the Massachusetts Committee on Public Safety because he was called to active duty in the US Army.

Harvard Medical School, about that same time, had organized General Hospital No. 5, which extended the work of Base Hospital No. 5 that had operated during World War I (see chapter 61). Thorndike was given the rank of major and named the assistant chief of the Surgical Service. Other surgeons serving with Major Thorndike included Major Edwin F. Cave, Captain T. B. Quigley, and Captain Richard Warren. With Thorndike went 372 soldiers to deploy.

Of those originally expected to join General Hospital No. 5, 289—including majors Thorndike and Cave—were routed instead to man the 105th General Hospital in the Southwest Pacific. Few Harvard alumni were sent to the Pacific; most served in

Europe during WWII. They landed in Queensland, Australia; eventually arriving at the US Army 105th General Hospital which opened in July 1942 on the campus of the University of Queensland in Gaston. The hospital had 1,000 beds, was the largest army hospital overseas, and over 20,000 patients were treated there from throughout the Pacific. Thorndike led the Harvard Unit there for almost two years. In addition to Dr. Cave (major) assigned to the 105th General Hospital, Captain Carter Rowe also joined the Harvard Unit. In 1944, after the American forces defeated the Japanese on Biak Island (August 1949), the 105th General Hospital moved to Biak Island for the remainder of the war. A stone memorial remains in Gaston commemorating the occupation of Queensland Agricultural College by the 105th General Hospital, Harvard Medical School USA, July 1942–July 1944.

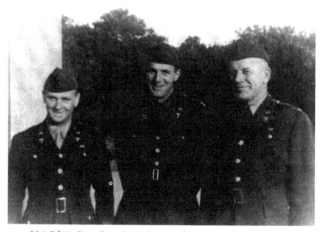

40: Maj. Edwin Cave, Capt. Carter Rowe, Col. Augustus Thorndike, shortly after landing, Queensland, Australia, 1942, with 105th General Hospital.

Major Cave, Captain Rowe, and Colonel Thorndike shortly after arriving in Queensland, Australia, 1942. From Carter Rowe, *Lest We Forget*. Dublin, NH: Bauhan Publishing, LLC, 1996. Bauhan Publishing, LLC.

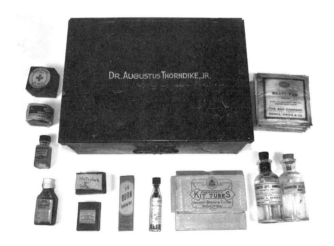

Augustus Thorndike Jr's first aid kit.
Massachusetts General Hospital, Archives and Special Collections.

Thorndike was promoted to lieutenant colonel on November 20, 1942, and later to colonel. In late 1943, he was transferred to Washington, DC, under the Office of the Surgeon General where he was later appointed director of the new reconditioning division of the Army Medical Department in early 1944. Major Cave replaced him as commander of the 105th General Hospital. Thorndike was selected because of the success of his rehabilitation program for wounded soldiers at the 105th General Hospital. Patient rehabilitation—focusing on light exercises while in bed—started immediately after they entered the hospital; it ended when they could make a 15-mile hike carrying a full military back pack. Thorndike, "an authority on rapid restoration of athletic injuries[,] reported: 'In one general hospital, where I witnessed the new program the period of convalescence was cut from an average of 35 days to 24.4 days—roughly a third less time—and 1500 patients went back to full duty in 5 months, 300…from a general hospital of 1,000 beds. And I'm confident that when we really get this thing going, the convalescent time can be cut much more in all Army hospitals'" (F. Carey 1944). He included "grass drills, such as football players do, gymnasium work, obstacle course drills, wall-climbing and scores of other tougheners" (F. Carey 1944).

As chief, Thorndike led the reconditioning program across all Army hospitals, organizing care for both those who could eventually return to service and those whose injuries would not allow it (Harvard Alumni Bulletin 1944). The following interview of Colonel Thorndike was given at the US Army's Schick General Hospital in Clinton, Iowa during a two-day conference announcing the Surgeon General's new reconditioning program headed by Colonel Thorndike:

Reconditioning, though not a new concept to physicians, has been carefully planned to include all phases of the problem…Col. Augustus Thorndike, m.c.…formerly physician to Harvard, where he had practical experience with athletes…the author of a well known book dealing with injuries of athletes…is singularly fitted for the new post. Training for men to be returned to duty as the result of the reconditioning program includes physical reconditioning, educational reconditioning and emotional

reconditioning. Physical exercises are begun at the earliest possible time. In many instances they are done while the patient is still in bed… prescribed by the medical officer in charge of the ward. Strict supervision of the program is maintained by medical officers…responsible for the care of the soldiers. Much of the physical training program is carried out by nonprofessional officers and enlisted men under the direction of medical officers. A graduated system of calisthenics, drills, games and military training is the basis of physical reconditioning. Concurrently, equally well planned programs for educational and emotional reconditioning are carried out by competent personnel. Not only is the disabled soldier to be returned to duty whenever possible physically, but…return him 'a tough, seasoned soldier with an aggressive combat spirit.' Here is a challenge to the medical profession, to restore as many of the nations' sick and wounded soldiers to duty as early as possible…[with] each soldier's welfare…[resting] on accepted scientific principles.
(*Journal of the American Medical Association* 1944)

The American Journal of Surgery
Volume 67, Issue 2, February 1945, Pages 302-318

RECONDITIONING FOR THE WAR WOUNDED
THE UNITED STATES ARMY SERVICE FORCES' PROGRAM
COLONEL AUGUSTUS THORNDIKE
MEDICAL CORPS, ARMY OF THE UNITED STATES

Cover of Thorndike's article, "Reconditioning for the War Wounded." A program initiated by Thorndike for the United States Army.
A. Thorndike. *The American Journal of Surgery*, 1945; 67: 302.

Dr. Harry Mock (1945), from Chicago, Illinois, in discussing Dr. Thorndike's paper, titled "Reconditioning for the War Wounded: The

United States Army Service Forces' Program," lauded Thorndike's plans for rehabilitating soldiers despite naysaying and lack of cooperation from both other military physicians and the army itself.

On May 22, 1944, at the 163rd meeting of the Massachusetts Medical Society in Boston, Colonel Thorndike presented a paper entitled "Surgical Experiences with Wounded in the Papuan [New Guinean] Campaign" (A. Thorndike 1944). At a press conference during the meeting, Colonel Thorndike described the high-level treatment soldiers receive when undergoing surgery in field hospitals. In WWI, the wounded had been moved back from the front to the hospital, whereas in WWII the hospitals were moved closer to the soldiers in the front. He emphasized the dedication of the military surgeons—working for days without rest and handling every injury that presents—and the surgical education they received as they operated in the field.

Dr. Thorndike was awarded the Legion of Merit in 1945 for his major contributions to soldiers' reconditioning during WWII. After the war ended in the summer of 1945, Thorndike returned to Boston and to his position at Harvard as chief surgeon in the department of hygiene. With the development of residency training programs in the Veterans Administration Hospitals, Dean's Committees at the medical schools were established to provide council for the education and training of residents. The deans of Harvard, Tufts, and Boston University led the Dean's Committee for the Massachusetts Veterans' Hospitals. Each dean selected an advisor in medicine and an advisor in surgery. Thorndike was selected by Dean C. Sidney Burwell as Harvard's representative in surgery.

In 1947, plans were beginning for a New England Rehabilitation Center, a joint effort of the Office of Vocational Rehabilitation, the State Department of Education, Bay State Society for the Crippled and Handicapped and the State Commission for the Infantile Paralysis Foundation.

Thorndike was named to head the more than twelve-member planning committee. It consisted of physicians and industrialists. Drs. William T. Green, Joseph S. Barr, and Marius Smith-Petersen also served as orthopaedists on the committee. In February 1947, Thorndike submitted, at the business meeting of the Massachusetts Medical Society, a resolution to study whether a community rehabilitation center would be of benefit to the veterans throughout Boston communities:

> Whereas, the Fracture Committee of the American College of Surgeons has recommended the establishment of community rehabilitation centers in all states, and
>
> Whereas, the National Service Fund of the Disabled American Veterans is sponsoring the establishment of a nonprofit organization in Boston to be called the Rehabilitation Center, on an outpatient service basis for patients in the terminal stages of convalescence, to which may be referred by doctors, by hospitals and by governmental and private agencies veteran and patients with disabilities requiring medical evaluation and treatment, including physical therapy and occupational therapy, as well as evaluation for proper placement at time of release; be it therefore Resolved, that the Council authorize the president to refer to the appropriate committee or committees for study, with a report and a recommendation to be represented at the next meeting of the Council, the question whether there is need for such a community rehabilitation center and service in Boston, organized in accordance with the Report of the Baruch Committee on Physical Medicine. (*New England Journal of Medicine* 1947)

The Baruch Committee was founded during WWII by the millionaire philanthropist Mr. Bernard M. Baruch with objectives to provide facilities to train physicians in physical medicine as well as to provide clinical care, education, and research in the methods of physical medicine. The committee included participants from different medical schools; the representatives from Harvard were Dr. Frank Ober and Dr. Arthur L. Watkins. They achieved their objectives with the development of residency programs in physical medicine and rehabilitation and a board to certify qualified specialists, a national professional organization of specialists, increased teaching of physical medicine and rehabilitation in medical schools, development of rehabilitation centers throughout the United States and advances in clinical care of the disabled.

At a subsequent meeting of the Massachusetts Medical Society on May 19, 1947, President Dr. Dwight O'Hara asked Thorndike, as the author of the aforementioned resolution, to discuss the Baruch report. Thorndike described the proposed center as providing outpatient and ambulatory care to disabled patients of all social classes who had been referred to the center. It would be the second supervised clinic in Boston (and New England) at that time.

Despite his efforts, no agreement about a rehabilitation facility was reached by the Massachusetts Medical Society. But Thorndike persisted in his attempts. "I came home to take charge of the large number of wounded and amputee college enrollees" (MGH HCORP Archives). Finally, through his continued efforts, the "Bay State Medical Rehabilitation Clinic" came into being on property owned by MGH in 1950. MGH permitted use of Ward I, its original orthopaedic ward, for the rehabilitation clinic. The clinic was partially funded by the Bay State Society and the Hyams Trust. It opened to patients on June 21, 1951. Dr. Arthur Watkins acted as director of the Rehabilitation Clinic and coordinated services between MGH and the clinic; Dr. Thorndike was president.

During this same period, Thorndike was appointed director of the Veterans Administration Prosthetic and Sensory Aids Service on July 1, 1948. In 1951, he published a paper on the Veterans Administration Experimental Program on the suction socket prosthesis for above knee amputees. The study included 221 patients. Initially,

> only 4 per cent of the patients were classified as failures, whereas when this same series was re-appraised one year later, 17 per cent were actually classified as failures. It is our opinion that one should not appraise the final result until the suction-socket wearer has worn his prosthesis for at least twelve months or until he has had an opportunity to use it through all four seasons and in all climatic conditions. Excessive humidity, with the complication of sweating, has caused some of our successful wearers to abandon this type of prosthesis. (A. Thorndike 1951)

In 1955 Thorndike reported long-term results of suction socket prosthesis for 2,184 above-knee amputees treated in 30 Veterans Administration amputee clinics: he noted failure in only 15.7%; these failures were caused by things like allergic skin reaction, poor fit and alignment of the prosthesis, loss of suction, gain or loss of body weight, excessive perspiration, and the patient's emotional state, such as feelings of insecurity and lack of motivation. Thorndike believed that faiure could be reduced to 5.9% through increased experience and skill when selecting eligible patients.

Dr. Thorndike spoke frequently at local meetings on rehabilitation, the physically disabled and the disabled veterans of WWII. In November 1954, he was elected president of Perkins Institution and the Massachusetts School for the Blind. The next year he was elected president of the Massachusetts Chapter of the National Rehabilitation Association. From 1948 to 1955, he was a member of the Prosthetic Research and Development Committee of the American Academy of Sciences.

During the 10 years following WWII, Thorndike worked part time for Harvard. In 1955, he closed his Boston office and assumed a full-time position in the Harvard University Health Service with the opening of the new Stillman Infirmary. His new office was located at 15 Holyoke Street, Cambridge. He worked at both the Dillon Field House and the surgical clinic at Harvard.

In 1959, Thorndike published a review article on the frequency and nature of sports injuries (A. Thorndike 1959). He was listed as a lecturer on surgery at Harvard Medical School, a consultant in surgery at both the Massachusetts General Hospital and the Peter Bent Brigham Hospital. He mentioned the significant increase in college students' participation in sports—up to 70%. He advocated for the athlete's Bill of Rights as a response to the increasing frequency of injuries across recreational, high school, and college athletics. Using his over 25 years of experience treating athletes, he recommended:

- Avoiding use of hydrocortisone, hyaluronidase, or chymotrypsin when reducing bleeding
- Using procaine hydrochloride during diagnosis only and not as a therapeutic agent
- Relying upon the team physician to determine a player's readiness to return to play

When assessing player readiness, he suggested the team physician should assess for return of normal function and any remaining palpable tenderness. He recommended athletes must pass a functional test that uses progressive resistance exercise and that they return to play using supportive adhesive strapping to prevent reoccurrence. His obituary summed up Thorndike's contribution to athletics with the following:

> He inaugurated many policies governing athletes during his long tenure. They included the rule that every contact sport must have a doctor in attendance at all games. He instituted practice and game taping of old sprains, corrective exercising, quick treatment and the

rule that doctors determine if a young man should play. He also put into effect the "three knockout" rule barring any player from a contact sport who had three concussions with "unconsciousness." Dr. Thorndike…design[ed] improved protective gear for football players and the first to insist on helmets for hockey players. (E. J. Driscoll 1986)

In 1953 the AMA named Thorndike chairman of the Committee on the Medical Aspects of Sports, tasked with educating physicians about athletic injuries. At the annual Harvard football dinner at the Harvard Club on November 25, 1958, Thorndike was surprised with a varsity letter "H" award in recognition of his years of service to athletes, students, and Harvard. At the time he was also president of the Harvard Club (1956–1959), and his portrait hangs there, given in March 1960. Thorndike's additional volunteer activities included serving as a trustee for more than 30 years on the Northfield and Mount Herman Schools and a trustee of the Dexter and Chestnut Hill Schools. In 1969, Mount Herman dedicated its football field to him. In 1961 the American College of Sports Medicine recognized Dr. Thorndike's many contributions with a Citation Award. After almost 50 years of service as chief of surgery and Harvard's head team surgeon, Thorndike retired in June 1962. His colleagues

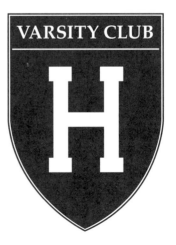

Logo: Harvard Varsity Club. Harvard Varsity Club.

lauded his care for the players and his interest in their well-being, and Coach John Yovicsin touchingly gave Thorndike a football autographed by the 1961 football team, co-champions of the Ivy League. In 1963, Harvard awarded him an honorary degree. His obituary recorded that "Jack Fadden, Harvard's senior trainer at the time of the doctor's retirement in 1962, said [Thorndike] was, 'A man with a healthy interest in sports, an enormous interest in the rehabilitation of athletic injuries and a fatherly interest in the player. By keeping him out of a game on Saturday, he has saved many a boy instead of losing him for the season'" (E. J. Driscoll 1986).

Thorndike died on January 29, 1986, at the age of 89. He was survived by four children, 13 grandchildren, and 10 great-grandchildren. He elevated the care of athletes—especially their rehabilitation from injury—and improved protective gear they wore, including being the first to insist that hockey players wear helmets. He also initiated the "three knockout" rule, which prevented any player from resuming play in a contact sport who had experienced three concussions significant enough to result in unconsciousness. Besides his national reputation, "he was characterized by the student athletes at Harvard as kind and thoughtful, yet thorough, firm and decisive. He was highly respected by the players, parents, coaches and administrators, a true leader in sports medicine" (MGH HCORP Archives). In September 2006, Harvard Medical School and Massachusetts General Hospital established the Augustus Thorndike Jr., MD Professorship in Orthopaedic Surgery.

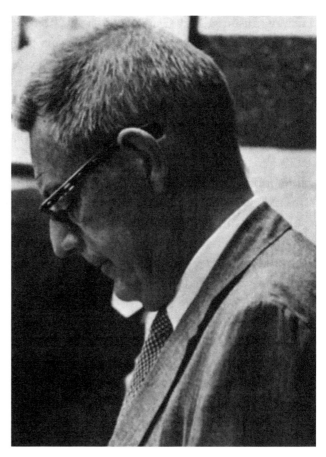

Thomas B. Quigley, "Team Physician."
The Second H Book of Harvard Athletics. 1923–1963. By Geoffrey H. Movius. Harvard Varsity Club, 1964.

Physician Snapshot

Thomas B. Quigley
BIRTH: 1908
DEATH: 1982
SIGNIFICANT CONTRIBUTIONS: Doctor of football; advocate for the college athletes' Bill of Rights; established a new treatment for frozen shoulder; advocate of early knee ligament repair; and coined the term "neuromuscular genius"

THOMAS B. QUIGLEY

Thomas Bartlett Quigley, known by some as "Bart" and others as "Quigs," was born in North Platte, Nebraska, on May 24, 1908. His father, Daniel Thomas Quigley, a surgeon and Rush Medical College graduate, went abroad for his postgraduate work, during which time he became interested in radium therapy. He was one of the founders of the American College of Surgeons and helped to create the American Radium Society. In 1929 he published the book *The Conquest of Cancer by Radium and Other Methods*, which received a critical review in the *Annals of Internal Medicine* (1930). He was friends with William Osler,

Harvey Cushing, and Clarence Darrow. Retiring in 1966, at the age of 90, he was the last surviving charter member of the American Radium Society.

Thomas Quigley was an undergraduate student at Harvard College. He participated in varsity swimming and theater, even performing with James Stewart and Henry Fonda. He graduated in 1929 and immediately applied to Harvard Medical School. Dr. Henry Banks, who worked at the Brigham with Dr. Quigley for years, noted that Quigley was almost not accepted there. At the time of Quigley's admission's interview, he was wearing clothing to usher at a formal wedding later that same day, and the dean mistook his appearance, stereotyping him as a "playboy" (Atkins, n.d.).

After graduating in 1933, he completed both his internship and his residency at Willard Parker Hospital in New York City. The hospital was well-known for treating infectious diseases. Quigley, a prolific writer during his career, wrote his first paper there, entitled "Second Attacks of Poliomyelitis. Review of the Literature and Report of a Case" (1934). He reviewed the 14 cases of second attacks of poliomyelitis that had been reported in the literature and reported a similar case of a second attack of polio, but the first reported case in which the second attack proved fatal. The case was a seven-year-old girl admitted to Willard Parker on August 15, 1931, during the height of an epidemic in New York. She had mild involvement in her legs that resolved but had persistent paralysis of the left deltoid. She was admitted two years later, on July 31, 1933, following a respiratory infection but died from respiratory failure shortly after admission. An autopsy "marked nerve cell degeneration, neuronophagia, congestion and edema were found at every level of the cord" (T. B. Quigley 1934).

After a year of residency in pathology in New York, Quigley returned to Boston, to the Peter Bent Brigham Hospital, as a resident in surgery, along with Elliot C. Cutler, David Cheever, John Homans and Robert Zollinger. He received three fellowships during his tenure there: the Harvey

Cushing Fellowship, the George Gorham Peters Traveling Fellowship, and the Arthur Tracy Cabot Fellowship. Four years later, in 1938, he became resident surgeon at Doctor's Hospital in New York City, 170 East End Avenue, between 87th and 88th streets. The hospital was acquired by Beth Israel Medical Center in 1987 and closed in 2004. That same year, he married Ruth Elizabeth Pearson, a nurse at the Peter Bent Brigham Hospital. After a brief period in New York. he returned to Peter Bent Brigham Hospital; becoming a fellow of the Massachusetts Medical Society in 1939.

Over the next three years, as surgeon (junior associate) on the staff of the Peter Bent Brigham Hospital and an instructor of surgery at Harvard Medical School, he published three more papers, all on general surgery: "Biliary Surgery in the Aged," "Inguinal Herniorrhaphy in the Aged," and "The Differential Diagnosis of Acute Appendicitis and Acute Gastroenteritis in College Men." Early on, he also worked with both the department of hygiene and the athletics department at Harvard University as a surgeon. According to Henry Banks:

> He once stated that "the care of these young men [in Harvard's athletics program] occupy one-third of my time and constituted both an absorbing hobby and a fascinating opportunity to study injuries under ideal circumstances." The other two-thirds of his time were devoted to the teaching of medical students, and to private practice and the ever increasing administrative demands of committees and professional societies…Early in his professional career, he succumbed to an incurable "disease," Cacoethes Scribendi, first described by Oliver Wendell Holmes and literally meaning the "itch to write." This "disease" led to the production of more than 172 publications during his career [although I could find only 75] mainly devoted to the surgery of trauma. His writings have always been clear and precise.
> (H. H. Banks 1982)

> Too many men walk about with what they call a "football knee" or a "baseball shoulder" as though it were a badge of honor. Actually, they are wearing only a badge of ignorant, careless or non-existent medical care.
> —Thomas B. Quigley (quoted in G. H. Movius 1964)

In 1939 he was appointed assistant surgeon to Dr. Augustus Thorndike Jr. in the Harvard University Health Services. His early work with Thorndike treating Harvard athletes influenced him to move into a career in sports medicine, for which he seemed to have a great aptitude, and Thorndike recommended Quigley to many patients throughout their time together. He was one of the first surgeons to recommend early surgical repair of acute ligament injuries of the knee.

His first publication in sports medicine was coauthored with Dr. Thorndike Jr. in 1942. They reviewed 173 cases of acromioclavicular joint injuries, commonly seen in football, lacrosse, soccer, rugby and hockey. They recognized a trend at the time to treat these injuries with rigid fixation of the acromioclavicular joint with pins or screws. They disagreed with this approach, advocating instead simply strapping the arm or placing it in a sling for several days. They applied this intervention immediately for 138 such injuries over six years, and the athletes were barred from returning to play until they were able to function normally, usually about 11 days.

During World War II, Dr. Quigley served in England as chief of orthopaedics in Harvard's 5th General Hospital for two-and-a-half years, beginning in early 1942. Over three-and-a-half years, he cared for innumerable soldiers with fractures; he eventually was appointed chief of the Surgical Service at the 22nd General Hospital. He had begun as a captain in the army and was eventually promoted to lieutenant colonel. While in the army, Quigley published a book, *Plaster-of-Paris Technique in the Treatment of Fractures*, in 1945. It was a manual that described most casts used in practice but only considered one method of treatment.

After the war, Quigley returned to Boston as a junior associate surgeon, eventually becoming visiting surgeon at the Peter Bent Brigham Hospital; and instructor in surgery at Harvard Medical School, eventually promoted to clinical professor of surgery. His office was located at 319 Longwood Avenue. He was certified by the American Board of Surgery. He was still interested in athletic injuries, and he immediately returned to care for athletes at Harvard under Thorndike. "For more than 30 years he revived, mended, and befriended countless Harvard athletes, thus earning the nickname 'Doctor of Football'" (H. H. Banks 1982). In 1963 Dr. Thorndike Jr. retired, and Dr. Dana Farnsworth (director of the Harvard University Health Service) appointed Dr. Quigley to succeed him as chief surgeon to the Harvard Athletic Department.

Quigley was a frequent presenter on trauma and most aspects of different sports injuries at regional meetings: the postgraduate lecture courses of the Massachusetts Medical Society, clinical meetings of the American Medical Association, annual meetings of the Massachusetts Medical Society, the Regional Committee on Trauma of the American College of Surgeons and others. Throughout his career, he continued to contribute frequently to the literature about sports injuries. Banks stated in his 1982 biographical note in a special tribute to Quigley in *Clinical Orthopaedics and Related Research* that "his approach to the management of the frozen shoulder and the development of a procedure to stabilize the knee utilizing the popliteal muscle deserve special attention" (H. H. Banks 1982).

Quigley wrote the first of several papers on the clinical problem of frozen shoulder and its treatment with ACTH in 1952. Treatment at the time included gradual stretching exercises and heat; "manipulation under anesthesia has been almost universally condemned as dangerous and futile" (T. B. Quigley 1954). In order to suppress pain and reaction after manipulation, he preferred ACTH administered one day before manipulation and tapering the dosage for the following seven-to-ten days; or 300 mgs of cortisone administered orally one day before manipulation, continued for the next three or four days, and then tapered off over the next three or four days. He found that patients treated with hydrocortisone injections into the shoulder joint at the time of manipulation had significant pain afterwards requiring treatment with ACTH. He was very specific regarding the manipulation; he instructed that it

> cannot be considered lightly. It is a blind procedure, fraught with considerable potential danger...Gentleness in the application of force is essential. The patient's arm should not be used as a lever. The humerus should be grasped just distal to the axilla...the operator's forearm should press equally at all points against its length. The other hand depresses the shoulder and restricts rotation of the scapula...When free passive abduction has been achieved, external rotation will usually be found to be restored to normal...The procedure requires no more than three or four minutes. Pentothal anesthesia is used in all cases. An intensive program of active motion begins as soon as the patient recovers from the anesthetic...Experience with treatment of twenty "frozen' shoulders...is presented. Ten patients regained normal painless shoulder motion; 13 were improved, and 6 unimproved." (T. B. Quigley 1954)

In 1956, he reported his results after five years of treating 50 frozen shoulders. Approximately 66% achieved full range of motion. The only severe complication occurred when Quigley broke the anatomic neck of the humerus during a manipulation for a patient.

In his 1959 publication "Knee Injuries Incurred in Sport," Quigley introduced his work by noting that knee injuries cause the most issues over time and that athletes can avoid these long-term effects

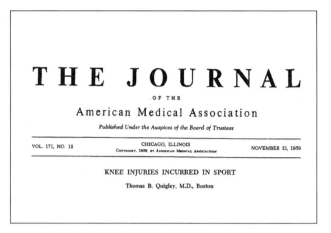

Article in which Quigley introduced his method to treat knee injuries.
Quigley. "Knee Injuries Incurred in Sport." *Journal of the American Medical Association*, 1959; 171: 1666.)

by receiving immediate treatment. He advocated avoiding immobilization, continuing exercise while healing, and taping sprains even after the injuries have healed. He wrote:

> The most frequent injuries encountered are, in descending order of incidence, contusion, ligament sprain, meniscus injury, ligament rupture, and fracture or epiphyseal displacement. Most meniscus injuries are accompanied by sprain, which should be allowed to heal before meniscectomy is advised. Immobilization produces muscle atrophy and should be kept to a minimum. Ligament rupture should be repaired promptly. Progressive resistance exercise is essential in convalescence. Protective taping to support the collateral and cruciate ligaments should be worn at each practice session and game for at least a year after any sprain. (T. B. Quigley 1959b)

For a ligament rupture he recommended immediate repair, and for a torn meniscus he recommended total removal as advocated by Smillie. He further "advised that no college student should indulge in a contact sport unless he can sit at a table and extend his knee from 90 deg. to 180 deg. with a 50-lb weight fastened to his foot 10

times within 40 seconds" (J. Smith 1959). According to Blazina, "almost all the orthopaedists in the
United States attempted to follow" Quigley's recommendations through the next decade (M. E.
Blazina et al. 1982). Eventually, however, a partial meniscectomy, especially with arthroscopy, was
advocated instead.

In this same article he coined the term "neuromusculoskeletal genius" when he commented
that "the gifted athlete or 'neuromusculoskeletal
genius' is rarely injured, and then only under freak
circumstances" (T. B. Quigley 1959b). Essentially, some athletes achieve tremendous skill and
strength without having to work as hard as others,
and these athletes are not injured as often (except
for those in contact sports like football). Other
athletes are more easily injured in their attempts to
rise above their physiological limits.

In 1968, Slocum and Larson reported on the
pes anserinus transplant as an effective treatment
for anteromedial rotator instability of the knee;
this gained national and international acceptance
for over a decade. Quigley developed a new procedure to stabilize the knee in athletes utilizing the
popliteus muscle:

> The meniscus is removed, and the popliteus
> tendon is dissected free and detached from its
> femoral insertion. The floor of the popliteus
> groove in the femur is then freshened to can-
> cellous bone with a curved osteotome. The
> tibia is firmly, internally rotated on the femur
> at about 30° of flexion, advancing the popliteus
> tendon up to 1.5 cm. The tendon is then reat-
> tached to the femur with a staple…stability…
> produced by passive tenodesis, but primar-
> ily by improvement of its [popliteus] dynamic
> function…In all eight patients, gratifying stabil-
> ity of the knee has been achieved and return
> to full function adequate for full participation
> in sports in four months or less. In all but one,
> stability at four months after operation has
> been both static and dynamic. (W. Southmayd and
> T. B. Quigley 1982)

Case Report 12.2 describes the outcome of
a pes anserinus transplant performed by Quigley.

Case Report 12.2: Lateral Meniscectomy and
Advancement of the Popliteus Muscle for Knee
Instability.

> H.H., a 6-foot, 5-inch, 250-pound, professional football
> player, was struck while moving rapidly backward. His
> extended left leg was externally rotated and abducted
> on the thigh. He was treated by the usual cold, com-
> pression bandage, and crutches and later, heat and
> resistance exercise. Pain on the lateral side of the joint
> and 'giving way' on stress persisted. A medial menis-
> cectomy four years previously had left no functional
> deficit. When first seen three months after injury, there
> was moderate effusion, lateral joint line tenderness and
> moderate to fairly marked anteromedial rotator instabil-
> ity corrected by internal rotation of the leg on the thigh
> with the knee at 90°.
>
> Arthroscopy disclosed mild chondromalacia patellae,
> an old rupture of the anterior cruciate ligament, a tear of
> the lateral meniscus extending throughout its length and
> an intact regenerated medial meniscus. Lateral menis-
> cectomy was carried out. After one month of immobili-
> zation and three months of rehabilitation, the knee was
> stable with muscles relaxed and contracted and was fit
> for full participation in professional football…stability
> was restored as well as by a pes anserinus transplant.
>
> (W. Southmayd and T. B. Quigley, 1982)

Physicians working with Harvard athletes
focused much energy on preventing injuries and
evaluating treatments. The Harvard Medical
Alumni Bulletin noted that "The concept of 'athletics for all' is rapidly spreading, and the growing problems of medical care of athletes in high
schools and colleges can perhaps best be expressed
from the point of view of the player" (T. B. Quigley 1959c). In 1957, Quigley—along with Thorndike—suggested a proposal for an "Athlete's Bill
of Rights," a document that described the needs
of athletes, including medical care, and advocated

The American Journal of Surgery
Volume 98, Issue 3, September 1959, Pages 325-327

Organized medicine and athletics: The role of the American Medical
Association committee on injury in sports

Allan J. Ryan M.D., F.A.C.S.

THE BILL OF RIGHTS FOR THE
COLLEGE ATHLETE

Athletes' Bill of Rights proposed by the AMA Committee on
Injury in Sports.
A. J. Ryan. *The American Journal of Surgery*, 1959; 98: 325.

for rights they could expect from their team and
college. At the time, Quigley was a member of
the American Medical Association's Committee
on the Medical Aspects of Sports. Thorndike had
been chairman of the committee, and Quigley
would later become chairman from 1962–1965.
The committee's final document required specific
things from both athletes and their school. Athletes must play fair, train, and behave well. In turn,
the school will provide high-quality coaches and
officiants, equipment and facilities, and medical
care. Read the complete "Bill of Rights for the
College Athlete" in **Box 12.1**.

Box 12.1. The Bill of Rights for the College Athlete

Participation in college athletics is a privilege involving both responsibilities and rights. The athlete has
the responsibility to play fair, to give his best, to keep
in training, and to conduct himself with credit to his
sport and his school in turn he has the right to opti-
mal protection against injury as this may be assured
through good technical instruction, proper regulation
and conditions of play, and adequate health supervision. Included are:

Good coaching: The importance of good coaching in
protecting the health and safety of athletes cannot be
minimized. Technical instruction leading to skillful performance is a significant factor in lowering the incidence

and decreasing the severity of injuries. Also, good
coaching includes the discouragement of tactics, outside either the rules or the spirit of the rules, which may
increase the hazard and thus the incidence of injuries.

Good officiating: The rules and regulations governing
athletic competition are made to protect Players as well
as to promote enjoyment of the game. To serve these
ends effectively the rule of the game must be thoroughly understood by players as well as coaches and
be properly interpreted and enforced by impartial and
technically qualified officials.

Good equipment and facilities: There can be no questions about the protection afforded by proper equipment
and right facilities. Good equipment is now available and
is being improved continually; the problem lies in the
false economy of using cheap, worn-out, out-moded
or ill-fitting gear. Provision of proper areas for play and
their careful maintenance are equally important.

Good medical care including: (1) A thorough pre-
season history and physical examination. Many of the
sports tragedies which occur each year are due to unrecognized health problems. Medical contraindications to
participation in contact sports must be respected. (2)
A physician present at all contests and readily available
during practice sessions. It is unfair to leave to a trainer
or coach decision as to whether an athlete should return
to play or be removed from the game following injury. In
serious injuries the availability of a physician may make
the difference in preventing disability or even death.
(3) medical control of the health aspects of athletics.
In medical matters the physician's authority should be
absolute and unquestioned. Today's coaches and trainers are happy to leave medical decisions to the medical
profession. They also assist in interpreting this principle
to students and the public. (A. J. Ryan 1959)

A similar program was later outlined for high
school athletes. In June 1958, the committee
presented a symposium on athletic injuries, their
prevention and treatment at the annual meeting
of the American Medical Association. Thorndike
presented a paper entitled "Prevention of Injuries

in College Athletics." He reviewed the records of 14,375 Harvard athletes (over a period of 17 years) and found 3,453 injuries that kept a player out of one or more games or practice sessions, an incidence of 24%. Using this data, he argued for colleges to support the player's "Bill of Rights" and included its three major requirements in his paper.

In 1959, Quigley also presented a paper titled "Management of Ankle Injuries Sustained in Sports." Because a possible error in diagnosis and/or inappropriate treatment of these injuries may lead to major problems for the athlete, he argued for reducing a fracture immediately and advocated for using simple noninvasive methods, e.g., cold, compression, rest, and elevation, to care for minor injuries. In his paper, he wrote:

> Decisions regarding them [ankle injuries] should be left to a physician whose authority should not be questioned…If advantage is taken of the 20 to 30 minutes after injury before edema, hemorrhage, and spasm occur, closed reduction of even grossly displaced fractures can sometimes be accomplished with almost no discomfort…Cold, compression, rest, and elevation are the four basic elements of treatment for minor injuries. (T. B. Quigley 1959a)

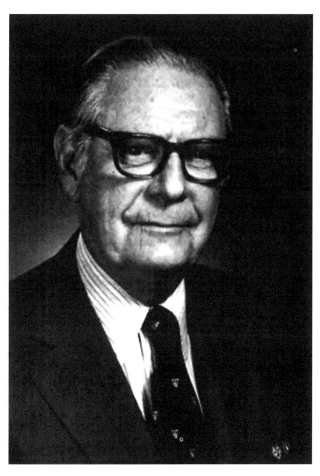

Thomas Bartlett Quigley (J. H. Harrison 1983).

Thomas Bartlett Quigley, 1908–1982. Obituary. *Transaction of the 103rd Meeting of the American Surgical Association*, 1983; 101: 56. Courtesy of the American Surgical Association.

He also recommended avoiding administering procaine in any case, which is in line with his earlier correspondence (1946) to the editor of the *Journal of the American Medical Association*, in which he stated his opposition—based on the treatment of approximately 750 ankle sprains—to using procaine injections in ankle injuries.

In 1959, Quigley was an editor of the *American Journal of Surgery* that published a special edition in sports injuries: After his introduction, the special edition contained 26 papers, including one by Thorndike on the "Frequency and Nature of Sports Injuries" and one by Quigley on "Fractures and Ligament Injuries of the Ankle." The symposium had papers by sports notables at the time: James T. Harkness, Hans Kraus, Mack L. Clayton,

William H. Frackelton, Donald B. Slocum, H. F. Moseley, Marshall R. Urist, Carl E. Badgley, and Don H. O'Donoghue. In his introduction, Quigley explained the rationale for the symposium. He noted the extensive participation in sports at even recreational levels and the inevitable injuries that will occur. He advocated for the inseparability of the mind and the body, and the importance of encouraging this increased healthy participation while simultaneously acknowledging the responsibilities of physicians to properly care for injuries as they emerge.

Thomas Quigley was a contributing member of various national and local surgical and orthopaedic organizations. He served as clinical professor of surgery at Harvard Medical School and as president of the Harvard Medical Alumni Association. He was vice president of the Boston Surgical Society and the Boston Orthopaedic Society. He was also a fellow of the American College of Surgeons as well as a member of the New England Surgical Society and the American Surgical Association. In 1971, he was a recipient of the American College of Sports Medicine's Citation Award. Other numerous honors included: editor of the 1978 Year Book of Sports Medicine, honorary membership in 1976 in the American Orthopaedic Society of Sports Medicine, "Sportsman of the Year" in 1978, and a position serving on the Board of Editors of *Clinical Orthopaedics and Related Research*. He was revered as an educator, and he was a prolific writer and an accomplished surgeon. A stroke in 1979 confined him to a wheelchair, but he continued to practice and lecture, even after he retired. He died in August 1982. His wife Ruth and three children survived him.

In 1982, Dr. Henry Banks, a long-time colleague of Dr. Quigley's at the Peter Bent Brigham Hospital, was guest editor of a special edition of *Clinical Orthopaedics and Related Research*, titled "Major Sports Injuries: Tribute to Thomas B. Quigley, M.D." The special edition contained 14 papers by Drs. Blazina, Grana, Hughston, Feagin, Slocum, Richmond, Pappas, O'Donoghue, Leach, and others; including a "classic" by Dr. Quigley, "Checkrein Shoulder: a Type of Frozen Shoulder:

Diagnosis and Treatment by Manipulation and ACTH or Cortisone." At the end of the article and in the tribute to Quigley, the journal reprinted his poem about the popliteus muscle:

Lines in Praise of the Popliteus Muscle

Behind the knee in shy retreat
Lies a muscle hard to beat
For keeping leg and thigh in
    sync
It is a quintessential link.
In twisting outward femur on tibia
(or inward tibia which is vice versa)
It unlocks the knee from full
    extension
But also (and this has had too little
    mention)
It converts laxity to tension
Correcting instability sagittal
(the cause of which remains a
    riddle)
As well as looseness rotatory,
The subject of many a learned story
In orthopaedic lore.
The glamorous anserinus pes,
    transplanted, does the job
    with style and grace
But there be times when the
    popliteus
From a second incision happily can
    free us
And to cinch up the knee is
    What it's for!

(T. B. Quigley 1978)

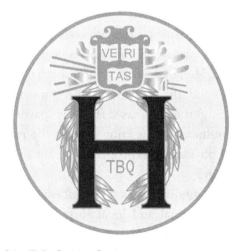

Logo of the T. B. Quigley Society. Harvard Varsity Club.

In 1988, a group of former Harvard football players who had become orthopaedic surgeons honored him—in his role as Harvard's team doctor and for his love of football (Atkins, n.d.)—by forming the Thomas B. Quigley Society. There are over 65 members in the society today, including such notables as Drs. Carlton M. Akins, Peter Asnis, Bernard R. Bach Jr., Donald Bae, Arthur L. Boland Jr., Thomas J. Gill, John S. Gould, William A. Grana, Brian E. Grottkau, Holly Johnson, Bruce S. Miller, Arthur M. Pappas, Lars Richardson, Lawrence T. Shields, William Southmayd, Mark E. Steiner, and others.

ARTHUR L. BOLAND

Arthur Lawrence Boland Jr. was born and raised in Lynn, Massachusetts. Interested early in sports,

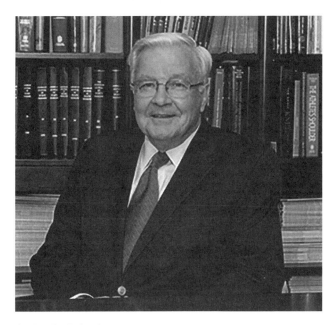

Arthur L. Boland.
Massachusetts General Hospital, Archives and Special Collections.

Physician Snapshot

Arthur L. Boland

BIRTH: 1935

DEATH: N/A

SIGNIFICANT CONTRIBUTIONS: First US-trained board-certified orthopaedic surgeon to head Harvard's athletics program

he participated in football, baseball, and track at Lynn English High School. He attended Cornell University (1952–1957) and played quarterback on the football team there. He was team captain in 1956, and he received various awards, including "Most Outstanding Athlete" in 1957. Other football awards included "first team 'All-Ivy' and 'All-East' accolades. His track career was equally stellar. He was captain of the 1957 team, a winning member of the 4 × 220 event at the prestigious Penn relays, and was the 100 and 200 yard Ivy League champion...in 1980 [he] was elected to the Cornell 'Hall of Fame'" (B. R. Boch 2003). After graduation he remained at Cornell, attending the Cornell University Medical College and graduating in 1961. He interned at the New York Hospital from 1961 to 1962 and completed a junior residency in general surgery from 1962 to 1963. He then "entered military service as a Commanding Officer of the 731 Medical Detachment, 7th Army training area in Germany" (B. R. Bach 2003). Following two years of military service, Dr. Boland entered the Children's Hospital/Massachusetts General Hospital combined program in orthopaedic surgery. His orthopaedic training included research at Children's Hospital; he was

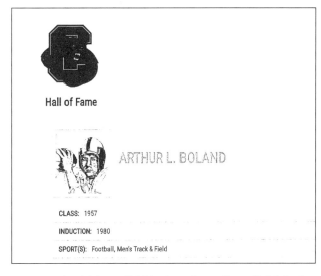

Hall of Fame

ARTHUR L. BOLAND

CLASS: 1957

INDUCTION: 1980

SPORT(S): Football, Men's Track & Field

Arthur Boland (class of 1957) elected into Cornell's Hall of Fame, 1980, in 2 sports: football, men's track & field.
Cornell University Athletics.

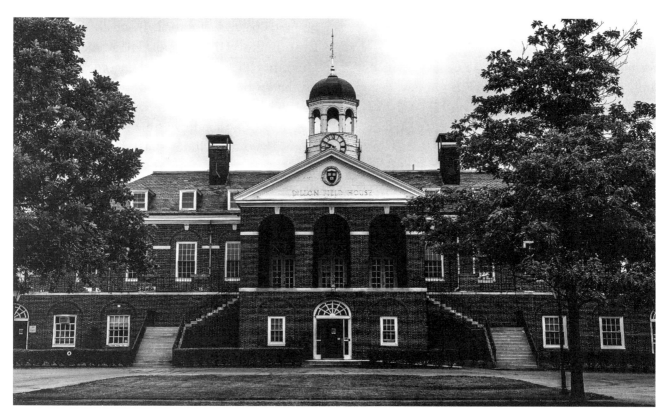

Dillon Field House.   Kael E. Randall/Kael Randall Images.

also a chief resident at the Massachusetts General Hospital. He completed his training in 1969.

Dr. Boland was a clinical instructor at Harvard Medical School from 1969 to 1984; he was later promoted to assistant clinical professor of orthopaedic surgery. With his strong interest in and commitment to sports, he was a natural to become involved in the Harvard University Health Service and the Athletic Department. In 1969, Boland joined as the team physician and orthopaedic surgeon; he was selected for the position not by an orthopaedic chief but instead by the director of the University Health Service, Dr. Farnsworth. He also worked in private practice in Winchester, Massachusetts, with Drs. Bill Kermond and Wendell Pierce for about 10 years.

He was recruited in 1979 to the Brigham and Women's Hospital by Dr. Sledge. At that time, he had been the Head Surgeon for Athletics at Harvard for four years. After Thomas Quigley retired, Boland became chief of orthopaedic surgery at Harvard in 1975. The previous chief surgeons of Harvard Athletics had all been general surgeons, including Dr. Quigley who was a general surgeon with orthopaedic surgery experience. Boland was the first fully trained orthopaedic surgeon to be appointed head surgeon for athletics and the first to be appointed a chief of orthopaedics at the Harvard University Health Service.

Dr. Bernie Bach, chief of sports medicine at Rush Orthopaedics, recalled his one-month elective rotation as a senior medical student with Dr. Boland:

I remember many hours spent with Art down at the Harvard field house, where he stoked my fire for a career in sports medicine. In a one year-time period, he impacted the career direction of Hosea, Stephen O'Brian, David St. Pierre, and me. This elective, initiated in 1977, resulted in six to eight medical students rotating with Art annually. Many of us saw

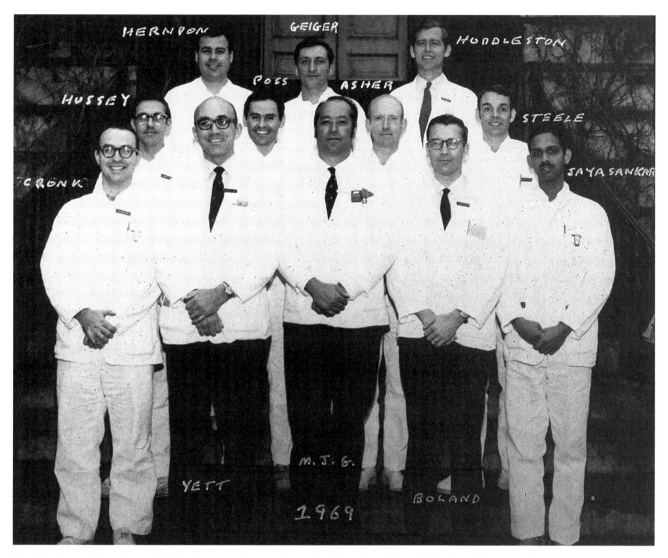

Dr. Glimcher with residents (1969). Front row from left to right: Drs. Cronk, Yett, Glimcher, Boland, and Jayasankar.
MGH HCORP Archives.

firsthand Art's dedication, compassion, and enthusiasm for athletes in the Dillon field house or on the football field…The medical care of Harvard athletes has been nothing short of spectacular [from Dr. Conant, to Dr. Darling, to Dr. Nichols, to Dr. Richards, to Dr. Thorndike, Jr., to Dr. Quigley and then from Dr. Boland]. Dr. Boland has nurtured a team of caring and competent physicians during his 27 years as team orthopaedist. In addition, the complexities of medical care have dramatically changed during the last quarter century. Title IX has resulted in an increase in the number of female

athletes and teams. Currently, Harvard has 41 intercollegiate varsity team sports. Art has co-ordinated and improved care in many arenas; the quality of care provided to the Harvard athletes is superb! (B. R. Bach 2003)

McDonagh and Pappano (2008) described Boland's work with female basketball players at Harvard, the goal of which was to reduce the number of injuries and improve their jumping technique. Boland discovered that although early on women experienced more ACL injuries in basketball than their male counterparts, this difference disappeared when women were trained to land after a jump with flexed—rather than straight—knees. At this point, Boland had noted that women athletes were as well trained and conditioned as men, and thus injuries were better categorized more by sport than by gender. The one exception was ice hockey, and only because the rules differed across gender lines, i.e., the men's game allowed checking and the women's game did not.

During his years as head surgeon for Harvard Athletics, Dr. Boland has given hundreds of presentations and published about 15 articles, several book chapters, and co-authored a book on athletic training for the American Academy of Orthopaedic Surgeons. As chief resident at the Massachusetts General Hospital, he presented two cases in two different articles in the Fracture of the Month series edited by Dr. Aufranc: a traumatic dislocation of the radial head (No. 96) and a case of gas gangrene in a patient with a fractured tibia (No. 97). He has co-authored numerous articles on sports medicine; to name a few, he addressed oxygen levels in tendons and ligaments, team physicians in college athletics, the history of anterior cruciate ligament surgery, motion analysis in ACL deficient knees, rowing in older athletes, and the effect of donor age on the biomechanical properties of bone-patellar tendon-bone allografts and patellofemoral pain.

In December 1997, the American Orthopaedic Society of Sports Medicine (AOSSM) held a Concussion Workshop in Chicago. It was chaired by Edward Wojtys and included 20 members from different professional organizations, including from the National Football League, the National Hockey League, the National Collegiate Athletic Association, the National Trainers Association, as well as physician specialty professions. Dr. Boland was a member, representing the AOSSM. Wojtys et al. (1999) discussed the challenges of treating concussions and the importance of allowing the brain to heal. These were issues Boland's predecessors at Harvard—Drs. Conant, Darling, Nichols, Richards, Thorndike Jr. and Quigley—also

dealt with. All were ahead of their time in their advocacy; we still have inadequate concussion protocols today. The attendees developed nine recommendations for dealing with concussions, including identifying symptoms that require the athlete to avoid returning to play, indicators for neurologic evaluation and imaging, the importance of multiple examinations, and the need for ongoing concussion research:

1. Every athlete with concussion should be evaluated by a physician.

2. Loss of consciousness precludes return to play that day.

3. Persistence of (longer than 15 minutes) or delayed onset of any symptoms such as headache, dizziness, malaise, slowness to respond mentally or physically at rest, or with provocation (supine with legs elevated) or with exercise precludes return to play that day.

4. Any deterioration in physical or mental status after the initial trauma, such as increasing headache, dizziness, or nausea, warrants immediate transport to an emergency facility where neurologic or neurosurgical consultation and neuroimaging are available.

5. When prolonged symptoms (greater than 15 minutes) are experienced after a concussion, great care must be exercised in returning an asymptomatic athlete to practice or competition. Without at least 5 to 7 days of rest, neurofunction may not yet be normal…Repeated examinations of the athlete are needed during a gradual increase in physical exertion to determine if these stresses trigger symptoms. If symptoms recur, the athlete is not ready to return to play…Repeated and thorough evaluations, preferably by the same clinicians, are most helpful in determining readiness to play.

6. Newer tools such as balance testing, cannot be recommended for clinical decision-making after concussion at this time.

7. We recommend further study of the SAC [standardized assessment of concussion] as part of the initial evaluation of an athlete with concussion to gain experience with its use.

8. We recognize the need for continued clinical and basic science research of sports-induced concussions…We recommend that establishment of cooperative studies across athletic organizations at the junior, high school, college and professional levels that would promote the longitudinal study of large groups of athletes.

9. We specifically promote the establishment of data-bases on all athletes with concussions. (Wojtys et al. 1999)

In 2005, a consensus statement on concussion and the role of the team physician was published by a twelve-member expert panel (which included Dr. Boland) representing the American College of Sports Medicine, the American Academy of Family Physicians, the American Academy of Orthopaedic Surgeons, the American Osteopathic Academy of Sports Medicine, the American Medical Society for Sports Medicine and the American Orthopaedic Society for Sports Medicine. The document provided clear guidelines for team physicians regarding game day evaluation and treatment (sideline and on-field), post-game day evaluation and treatment, diagnostic imaging, management principles, return to play decision (same day and post-game day), complications of concussion and prevention of concussion. The experts also listed the signs and symptoms suggestive of concussion, which were categorized as cognitive, somatic, or affective (**Table 12.3**).

In addition to the important contributions on concussions, Dr. Boland also participated with another expert group, a committee of international knee experts (International Knee Documentation Committee) who began in 1997 to revise the original knee ligament evaluation form developed by the original International Knee Documentation Committee (IKDC) that was published in 1993. They intended to develop a reliable and valid measure of results in patients with all manner of knee injuries. In 2006 the same group—and 12 additional members of the IKDC—reported that the group had achieved this goal. Interestingly, Agel and LaPrade reported in 2009 that the IKDC Subjective Form and the Cincinnati Knee Rating System produced similar results.

As his predecessors had done, i.e., maintain a database of athletic injuries, Dr. Boland and his colleagues developed a different database, one

Table 12.3. Signs and Symptoms Suggestive of Concussion

Cognitive	Somatic	Affective
Confusion	Headache	Emotional lability
Posttraumatic amnesia	Fatigue	Irritability
Retrograde amnesia	Disequilibrium, dizziness	
Loss of consciousness	Nausea/vomiting	
Disorientation	Visual disturbances	
Feeling 'in a fog,' 'zoned out'	(photophobia, blurry/double vision)	
Vacant stare	Phonophobia	
Inability to focus		
Delayed verbal and motor responses		
Slurred/incoherent speech		
Excessive drowsiness		

ACRM-MSSE.org 2005.

cataloging the actual clinical work of collegiate team physicians. In summary over a two-year period they reported that almost 75% of players were evaluated for musculoskeletal injuries (4% of which required surgery), whereas only 10% of the overall student body required treatment for musculoskeletal issues. This highlights the prevalence of such injuries among athletes. The other 25% of evaluations were for general medical issues such as concussion or infection. Football players counted for the majority of visits—almost 25%.

Changes in the heart size of athletes also preoccupied Dr. Boland's predecessors at Harvard (Drs. Darling and Richards). Dr. Aaron L. Baggish, associate director of MGH's Cardiovascular Performance Program and cardiologist for Harvard University Athletics, along with Dr. Boland and others, published a paper in 2008 on changes in cardiac structure, size, and function in athletes

J Appl Physiol 104: 1121–1128, 2008.
First published December 20, 2007; doi:10.1152/japplphysiol.01170.2007.

Training-specific changes in cardiac structure and function: a prospective and longitudinal assessment of competitive athletes

Aaron L. Baggish,[1] Francis Wang,[3] Rory B. Weiner,[1] Jason M. Elinoff,[2] Francois Tournoux,[1] Arthur Boland,[3] Michael H. Picard,[1] Adolph M. Hutter, Jr.,[1] and Malissa J. Wood[1]
[1]*Division of Cardiology, Massachusetts General Hospital, Boston;* [2]*Department of Medicine, Massachusetts General Hospital, Boston; and* [3]*University Health Services, Harvard University, Cambridge, Massachusetts*

Boland was the third team physician to publish research on changes in heart size and function in competitive athletes.
Baggish, et al. *Journal of Applied Physiology, 2008*; 104: 1121.

assessed using modern technology. In a prospective study, they studied 40 endurance athletes (male and female long-distance rowers) and 40 strength athletes (male American football players) before and after 90 days of team training. Electrocardiography showed that the endurance athletes had larger hearts and better heart function than strength athletes, who displayed left ventricular hypertrophy, less left ventricular diastolic function, and no change in heart size. They concluded that

particular types of training result in specific levels of cardiac structure and function.

Boland received numerous awards and recognition for his outstanding contributions to the field throughout his career. According to Bach, Boland is

a nationally and internationally recognized figure in sports medicine…[He] commands an incredible amount of respect because of his scholarly, thoughtful, and respectful approach to the specialty. He is a member of the American Academy of Orthopaedic Surgeons, the American Orthopaedic Society for Sports Medicine (AOSSM), the International Society of Arthroscopy, Knee Surgery, and Orthopaedic Sports Medicine (ISAKOS), and a founding member of the Herodicus Society. He is the ultimate 'team' player, working tirelessly on many committees. He has provided yeoman efforts— serving on the Outcomes, International Knee Documentation, Membership Program, Council of Delegates, and Budget and Finance Committees—and has served on the AOSSM 'Concussion' consensus task force. In 2001 he received the prestigious 'Mr. Sports Medicine' award from the AOSSM [awarded for his outstanding service to sports medicine] and served as a 'Godfather' for the AOSSM Pacific Rim Traveling Fellows, mentoring three young sports medicine physicians. While touring Singapore, Malaysia, Hong Kong, and Japan during a very unsettling time—the tragedies of September 11 interrupted the completion of their tour. He has been president of the AOSSM (1994-1995), Herodicus Sports Medicine Society (1981-1982) and…[was] elected as the only non-Harvard alumnus of the Quigley Society to serve as its president. (B. R. Bach 2003)

He has also received the annual Dr. Marion Ropes Award. Dr. Boland has served as assistant team physician for the New England Patriots and the Boston Bruins; team physician for the United

States Hockey Team (1993 World Championships); member of the medical staff for the 1984 Olympic Games; and consultant for the United States Rowing Association. In 2005, he was inducted into the AOSSM Hall of Fame, the society's highest honor. In 2006, he gave the annual Kennedy Lecture at Specialty Day of the AOSSM, entitled "Sports Medicine Societies: Their Origins, Functions and Values." The Massachusetts Orthopaedic Association on April 27, 2016, named Dr. Boland "Orthopaedist of the Year." In 2010, the Harvard Department of Athletics honored Dr. Boland by bestowing annually an eponymous award to a "senior varsity athlete who will be attending medical school who in addition to excellent scholarship, character and leadership, the recipient shall have demonstrated a passion for the field of medicine, a deep commitment and concern for others and a desire to give uncompromising good care" (Harvardvarsityclub.org, n.d.).

Dr. Boland's presidential address to the American Orthopaedic Society for Sports Medicine (June 1996) was entitled, "Our Qualifications as Orthopaedic Surgeons to be Team Physicians." He focused on two issues that the society had been discussing the previous year: (1) whether such physicians should be considered orthopaedic surgeons or team physicians, and (2) whether to

award certificates of added qualification (CAQ). With regard to the first issue, he recognized the value and training of primary care sports medicine specialists, but believed that qualified and highly-trained orthopaedic surgeons already fulfill this need. Regarding the controversial issue of the CAQ, he and the board of the AOSSM would create a CAQ to be implemented at the appropriate time.

As of 2019, Dr. Boland is Team Physician Emeritus at Harvard. In his history of the sports medicine service at Harvard, he wrote about his goal, as Harvard's chief of orthopaedic surgery, of assembling a well-qualified team that could care for any orthopaedic injury. Dr. Boland was followed by Dr. Mark Steiner as head team orthopaedic surgeon and chief of the orthopaedic service at the HUHS in 2003. Steiner completed the HCORP and acted as chief resident at MGH, and he was the first head orthopaedic surgeon for athletics at Harvard to finish a sports medicine–related fellowship.

Boland had married Jane Macknight in medical school, had four children and four grandchildren. Boland has led a rich life with numerous personal and professional contributions.

Bach sums up his character best with the words:

A warm, caring gentleman, a raconteur of Harvard athletic history and sports medicine, a surgeon with superb judgment and technique, a dedicated sports medicine physician…Art is one of the least imposing 'giants' in sports medicine. He is the type of person you can meet for the first time and after fifteen minutes feel you have known him for years. He has no pretensions, is slow to anger, has never in my years demonstrated arrogance (he missed that class in medical school), and I have never heard him say an unkind word about another physician. (B. R. Bach 2003)

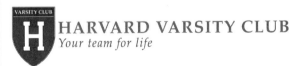

VARSITY CLUB

HARVARD VARSITY CLUB
Your team for life

Arthur L. Boland Award

This award was established in 2010 by the Department of Athletics to honor Arthur Boland, MD in commemoration of his 40 years of dedicated service to Harvard Athletics. The award is presented each year to a senior varsity athlete who will be attending medical school and who best exemplifies those characteristics and qualities which have been the hallmark of Dr. Art Boland's care for Harvard athletes.

Harvard Varsity Club honors Dr. Boland with an annual award in his name to a graduating varsity athlete planning to attend medical school. Harvard Varsity Club.

CHAPTER 13

Murder at Harvard

In 1849, a Massachusetts Medical College (now Harvard Medical School [HMS]) professor murdered Dr. George Parkman. The case triggered one of the most well-known scandals at the college, causing great distress both at the loss of a beloved benefactor of the school and in ensuing division over the guilt of the convicted murderer. On November 7, 1850, Dean Oliver Wendell Holmes began his introductory lecture to the students and faculty at the college with the following words:

> The loss, within the past year, of one to whom this institution is deeply indebted is brought back to us, with all its associations by the nature of the stated period of instruction. One duty remains, which no pang of memory must prevent us from discharging. A friend and benefactor has been taken from us, and we claim, as a mournful privilege, to speak a few words in grateful remembrance of those virtues and good deeds, too little known by the many to whom his name has grown familiar. Let us recall some traits of his character, in connection with subjects and names upon which we are pleased to dwell, which he loved while living, and with which he would have asked that his memory should be associated after his days should be numbered. (Holmes 1850)

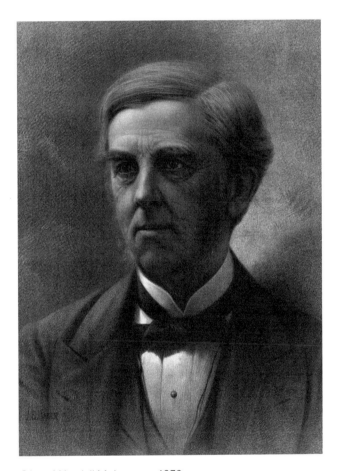

Oliver Wendell Holmes, ca. 1879. Library of Congress.

Although most HMS students today are unfamiliar with the case, it was widely published both nationally and internationally at the time. Both victim and perpetrator alike had close connections to the school, surgeons weighed in on the evidence at the time, and the case continues to be fodder for discussion among historians today.

DR. GEORGE PARKMAN: THE PEDESTRIAN

George Parkman was born in Boston on February 19, 1790. His father, Samuel Parkman, was a very wealthy businessman who had made his fortune in real estate. His father had a total of 11 children, six from his first marriage and five (including George) from his second marriage. Samuel founded and was a part owner of the towns of Parkman, Ohio, and Parkman, Maine. His children married into the well-known Beacon Hill families of Blake, Cabot, Mason, Sturgis, Tilden, and Tuckerman. Samuel eventually chose George to administer the large Parkman estate.

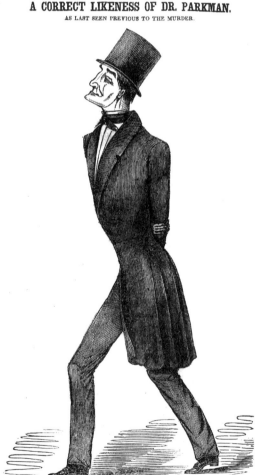

A CORRECT LIKENESS OF DR. PARKMAN.
AS LAST SEEN PREVIOUS TO THE MURDER.

Drawing of George Parkman. U.S. National Library of Medicine.

George Parkman navigated frequent health issues in his early years, and he "learned to value the services of medical art from his own experience; a circumstance which may have probably turned his attention to the profession" (Holmes 1850). He entered Harvard College at age 15 in 1805. Recognized as an intelligent and serious student, he became involved in two established literary societies and was chosen to deliver the salutary oration at graduation, the highest of honors in classical studies. After graduating, Parkman apprenticed with a physician, Dr. John Jeffries, who was "the physician of his father's family… an instructor and a friend…During this time he [Parkman] also attended lectures at the Medical Institution of the University" (Holmes 1850). He probably attended these lectures in the Holden Chapel in Cambridge (closed in 1810) and possibly some lectures in the new medical school building in Boston on Marlborough Street (opened in 1810). Some of the lectures he heard would have been given by Dr. John Warren (professor of anatomy and surgery) and his son, Dr. John Collins Warren, who was appointed adjunct professor of anatomy and surgery in 1809. Holmes wrote: "I can recall the enthusiasm and delight with which he [Parkman] dwelt upon the merits of his early teaching, and I cannot refer to it without being reminded of the immeasurable influence exerted by every instructor, who must stamp his own zeal or apathy, his own high or low relief, upon the plastic minds of his yet unmoulded pupils" (Holmes 1850).

In 1811, Parkman sailed to Europe aboard the frigate *Constitution* (Holmes 1850). He hoped to complete his medical education. He had the advantage of two patrons when he arrived in France: Joel Barlow, the newly appointed US Ambassador to France; and Count Rumford (formerly of Woburn, MA), a friend of his father who lived in Auteuil, four miles from Paris. "With introductions and patrons like these, every thing lay open before him that the great metropolis could offer the student of science and the enlightened observer of men and manners. Mr. Barlow introduced him to the acquaintance of Lafayette; Count Rumford carried him to the sittings of the Institute…welcoming him…to her ample hospitals and vast asylums" (Holmes 1850).

Before he left for Paris, Parkman had developed an interest in the care of the mentally ill, especially their harsh treatment and the horrible state of overcrowded asylums. He was familiar with Benjamin Rush—who was considered the "Father of American Psychiatry"—and his efforts to treat mentally ill patients humanely in a normal hospital setting without restraints, coercion, or physical punishment and overcrowding in a dungeon atmosphere. It was in 1812 that Rush published his classic textbook on mental illness, "Medical Inquiries and Observations Upon Diseases of the Mind." During his travels, Parkman was introduced to Dr. Philippe Pinel, "who was instrumental in the development of a more humane psychological approach to the custody and care of psychiatric patients, referred to today as moral therapy" (*Wikipedia*, n.d., under "Philippe Pinel"). Since 1795, Dr. Pinel had been the chief physician of the Hospice de la Salpâtrière (for mentally ill women), which at one time cared for 7,000 patients. Parkman wrote in a letter that:

My first knowledge of the Salpâtrière was with the high privilege of the guidance of its great physician, Pinel, and of his now illustrious associate, Esquirol. Pinel received me kindly, and inquired with much interest after Dr. Rush, who had lately written his book on "Diseases of the Mind." Pinel was then nearly seventy years old. His mildness, patience, forbearance and encouraging spirit towards the insane women, some hundreds, under his charge…were admirable. As a teacher he excelled…His frequent question was, "How are we to know when, and how far it is advisable to intermeddle with a malady, unless we have learned its natural and ordinary termination, if left to itself?

We do not know enough to be authorized in every case to try to alter or correct its course." (Holmes 1850)

Parkman planned to bring these enlightened approaches to the care of the mentally ill back to Boston and the United States. Before returning home, however, he traveled to England for a few months. He returned to Boston in the fall of 1813, reportedly with a medical degree from the University of Aberdeen, Scotland. It is not clear whether or not he received this degree in Great Britain.

Upon his return home, the United States was engaged in the War of 1812 with Great Britain. While waiting to begin service as a surgeon in the first division of the Massachusetts militia, he continued to study mental illness and also started a medical practice that helped the poor. After he completed his militia duty, Parkman was placed in charge of one of the three districts of the Boston dispensary. The other two physicians in charge included Dr. John Ball Brown (who was six years older than Parkman, and who was also physician/surgeon to the Almshouse on Leverett Street) and Dr. John Revere (who would later become professor of surgery at Jefferson University in Philadelphia). When Revere became ill, John Ball Brown took over his district because "no one would send for Dr. Parkman" (J. B. Brown 1852). At the time, Parkman was involved in the care of patients other than the mentally ill. In a case report published in the *Boston Medical and Surgical Journal*, he is mentioned along with two other physicians who assisted Dr. Josiah Bartlett in the paracentesis of a patient with advanced ascites. They drained nine gallons of fluid weighing 76 pounds.

Parkman surveyed the clergy, postmasters, and others in Boston for the purpose of determining the number of mentally ill in the area. Afterwards, he produced a pamphlet in 1814 titled "Proposals for Establishing a Retreat for the Insane," where he described his general views as to the proper treatment of insanity, which it is needless to say were modeled upon those of his illustrious master, Pinel…"In New England," said Dr. Parkman…"little ingenuity has been exercised to increase the comforts of the insane, or to procure his recovery. He has, in many instances, been left to subsist on bread and water, and to lie on straw, chained in a dark, solitary and loathsome cell, experiencing no solicitude in his fate, and a victim of an idle and sometimes interested maxim that 'Insanity is incurable.' His personal liberty has been taken away from him, perhaps by his nearest relative or dearest friend, whose occasional reproaches have wounded him deeply"…All the proposed arrangements of the Institution were to be ordered on the mild and humane principles which the experience of the Salpâtrière had so remarkably indicated as the only just and successful foundation of treatment in this class of diseases. The character of the house was to resemble, as much as possible, that of a private residence, affording as many enjoyments of social life as circumstances permitted; and the aim of the superintendent was to be, to show himself a "friend, indefatigable in his exertions to render the patients happy, and to restore them to usefulness. (Holmes 1850)

Parkman was anxious to establish a local hospital for the mentally ill as a replica of the Hospice de la Salpâtrière, using the treatment methods of Dr. Pinel. Holmes opined:

Here was a young man, expecting to inherit a princely fortune, choosing voluntarily a branch of the profession which would be sure to require of him the most incessant devotion and the largest sacrifices…Few persons are aware of the degree of credit fairly belonging to him for his agency in fixing public attention on the great object…[but] circumstances…caused the work in which he had interested himself, to be

consigned to other hands for its completion. A Lunatic Hospital had been organized in accordance with his plans, and he had taken his place at the head of the institution. (Holmes 1850)

Parkman rented a location for this hospital at the Shirley Mansion (Magee property) in Roxbury. The mansion was located on 16 acres. In 1816, the leaders of MGH planned to build a branch of the main hospital as an asylum for the mentally ill, and Parkman believed it to be advantageous to have the Magee property become that branch of the MGH. The property was for sale for $16,000. Although Parkman offered to pay the majority of the cost if MGH raised $5,000, the trustees ultimately rejected his offer and did not purchase the Magee property; they instead built the Asylum for the Insane in Charlestown. They initially agreed with the plan, but because Parkman also had his own private institution on the property where he acted as superintendent, they did not want the public to believe Parkman had purchased a position as superintendent physician of their institution as well. The MGH asylum was officially named The Asylum for the Insane in 1826, and then renamed McLean Hospital in 1892.

With the future McLean Hospital in place, Parkman felt there was no need for a second asylum in Boston, and he abandoned his efforts to build his own hospital for the mentally ill. Parkman believed

it proper to resign his office…That this was a great sacrifice we can hardly doubt; but he never allowed it to alienate his affections from his cherished branch of study. (Holmes 1850)

However, "'he was never weaned from his first love, Medicine,' says an old friend, 'and ever afforded an encouraging word and deed to aid all generous endeavors to alleviate human suffering'" (Holmes 1850). He often visited patients in the MGH's Asylum for the Insane, and he said,

"I have ever since continued to attend to insanity and to subjects which are allied to it, and to record observations relative to it" (*Boston Medical and Surgical Journal* 1835). He donated a piano to the hospital for their entertainment, and he even offered his own mansion on Cambridge Street to serve as a hospital during two different epidemics in Boston. The city did not use his home during the first epidemic of cholera, but they did use it during the second, an epidemic of small pox in December of 1839. Records from the report of the committee of the city council state:

> There is at present no public building which can be used for this purpose and the Committee were unable for some time…to find a suitable private one…Dr. George Parkman has kindly offered to the City the gratuitous use of several of his houses, so long as the necessity of the case may require it…the Committee have accordingly accepted two houses, which will be ample for the purpose. (Holmes 1850)

When Parkman's father died in 1835, he fulfilled his father's wish and began to manage his family's fortune. He substantially increased the family fortune through real estate purchases and money lending. He owned a great deal of property around MGH in the west end of Boston. In addition to these enormous responsibilities, however, he continued to treat occasional patients and maintained his interest and knowledge of the treatments of the mentally ill. In 1820, he published a case in which he treated an alcoholic going through withdrawal. Although his dream went unfulfilled, Parkman believed that the Boston community needed an "institution for drunkards [like one he had seen near Edinburgh, Scotland]…separate, or a section of a house for insanity, or of a bridewell [a prison]" (G. Parkman 1820). In addition, he was called on frequently to testify in court as an expert medical witness on the mentally ill, and he was a prolific writer. In 1817, he published

an essay entitled "Management of Lunatics, with Illustrations of Insanity,"…containing… many valuable remarks on the history and treatment of mental disease…In the following year he published "Remarks on Insanity," containing some interesting observations on the analogies of diseased states of mind…The most distinguished writer on Medical Jurisprudence that this country has produced declares that he is greatly indebted to the publications of Dr. Parkman, whom he characterizes as "A learned and diligent examiner of the subject of insanity." (Holmes 1850)

Dr. Parkman was also a generous benefactor. In addition to his many gifts to the Asylum for the Insane, he was

> a generous friend to the Society for Medical Improvement…the cause of Medical Education, and especially its interests as connected with this Institution [Medical School of Harvard University]…The College in Mason Street, erected in the year 1816…was far removed from the Massachusetts General Hospital, where the student must obtain a large part of his most valuable instruction…both Lecture Rooms and Museum were clearly inadequate to the demands for space made upon them… Dr. Parkman proposed to present a lot of land [North Grove Street] for this purpose and the faculty having voted to accept his very liberal offer…In honor of the giver of this donation, the Government [President Edward Everett] of the University bestowed his name [Parkman Professor of Anatomy and Physiology] as the perpetual title of the office [Dean, HMS] which it is my privilege [Oliver Wendell Holmes] for the present to hold. (Holmes 1850)

Parkman's love for medicine and learning never waned. In 1837 he had returned to Europe and revisited Paris hospitals, including the Salpâtrière. Later, in 1847, the illustrious Dr. John

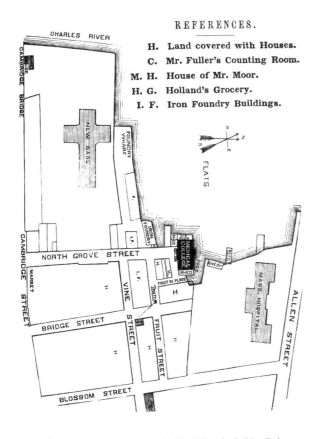

H. Land covered with Houses.
C. Mr. Fuller's Counting Room.
M. H. House of Mr. Moor.
H. G. Holland's Grocery.
I. F. Iron Foundry Buildings.

Map showing the location of the Medical College in the West End

Map of the west end with the medical school located close to MGH. Notice the new jail (cross-shaped building) between the Charles River and the medical school. From *Report of the Case of John W. Webster Before the Supreme Judicial Court of Massachusetts* by George Bemis, Boston: Charles C. Little and James Brown, 1850. U.S. National Library of Medicine.

Collins Warren prepared to resign as a chairperson in the Harvard Medical School, a position he had held for more than 40 years. Parkman attended Warren's final lecture, where many people spoke about Warren's contributions and accomplishments afterward at a reception. Holmes stated that "nothing was said with more graceful propriety and true feeling, than [those] words, spoken with much emotion by Dr. Parkman" (1850). Parkman said;

It was my youthful farewell to Alma Mater: *te pracvideo prospicio rerum pulcherrimam,*

praeclarissimam. I apply it here to this Temple of Minerva Medica our "Latin quarter," its probable improvements and accessories to the Hospital, to the Children's Infirmary, where the sick poor have all that riches can command; and to you, gentlemen, be every happy result. I thank you for the cheering, cordial greeting which you have uttered whenever I have come here to share instruction with you. "*Grata vestra erga me voluntas; nullum praemium insigne monumentum postulo praeter hujus diei memoriam; in animis triumphos ornamenta colloco; hujus temporis memoria, me muro septum arbitrabor.*"

When he spoke from the head of the table, he gave the audience "a feeling of continued interest of that opulent and kind-hearted man [Parkman], in the onward course of literature, science, and broad-cast philanthropy" (*Boston Medical and Surgical Journal* 1847).

When describing the reception, Holmes said, "From this day to the time of his [Parkman's] death, he never lost sight of the interests of this spot, which he had devoted to the cause of medical education, and which was to him, to use his own words, 'A piece of Holy Land'" (Holmes 1850). Parkman knew all the medical faculty at Harvard University, including: John C. Warren (anatomy and the operations of surgery); John W. Webster (chemistry); Walter Channing (midwifery and medical jurisprudence); Jacob Bigelow (*materia medica*); George Hayward (principles of surgery and clinical surgery); and James Jackson and John Ware (theory and practice of physics and clinical medicine). He also knew Dr. John Ball Brown; he was one of 23 physicians (including Harvard Medical faculty) that publicly approved and supported Brown's opening of the Orthopedique Infirmary in the late 1830s. They all agreed to serve as consultants to Dr. Brown whenever he requested their advice. Parkman also generously contributed to the Warren Museum of Anatomical Specimens.

Although Parkman was well loved at Harvard for his generous philanthropy, he was often difficult, and he had an explosive temper. His ruthless money-lending practices also left him disliked by many. His fortune totaled about half a million dollars in 1849—which would have been about $15.7 million in 2015, but he nevertheless had little compassion for his debtors.

"Dr. George Parkman was called '"The Pedestrian"' by a Boston newspaper because it was well-known he took daily walks to collect payments in town" (*Murder by Gaslight* 2010). He would not invest in the cost of owning a horse. His figure was well-known: "He was tall, lean, had a protruding chin, and wore a top hat" (*Wikipedia*, n.d., under "Parkman-Webster Murder Case"). "Oliver Wendell Holmes, Sr. said 'he abstained while others indulged, he walked while others rode, he worked while others slept'" (*Wikipedia*, n.d., under "Parkman-Webster Murder Case"). Frances (Fanny) Longfellow, wife of the poet Henry Wadsworth Longfellow, "called him 'the lean doctor… the good-natured Don-Quixote'" (*Wikipedia*, n.d., under "George Parkman").

He was a man of regular habits. In addition to his daily walks, he had lunch with his wife at 2:00 p.m. each day like clockwork (*Murder by Gaslight* 2010). He never missed that luncheon in their

MASSACHUSETTS MEDICAL COLLEGE.

THE Medical School of Boston is about to re-commence its annual course of instruction, under advantages greatly exceeding those which it has been able to offer in any former period of its history.

A new and elegant Medical College, of ample dimensions, is now in the process of erection, and will be completed in season for the coming course of lectures. It is situated in Grove Street, on the land, liberally given by Dr. GEORGE PARKMAN, near the Hospital, in a quarter of the city highly convenient for the lodgings of students. Its museum and collections for illustrating the different courses, is most ample, and in some respects unequalled in this country.

The Massachusetts General Hospital has been enlarged by the addition of two spacious wings, which render it capable of containing more than double its former number of patients. And the increase of its permanent funds, from the numerous and large donations of the last few years, will enable the trustees to meet the expense attending their support.

The Lectures will begin at the new Medical College on the first Wednesday in November, and continue four months, as follows:

On Anatomy and Surgery,	by JOHN C. WARREN, M.D.
On Chemistry,	JOHN W. WEBSTER, M.D.
On Clinical Medicine and Materia Medica,	JACOB BIGELOW, M.D.
On Principles of Surgery and Clinical Surgery,	GEORGE HAYWARD, M.D.
On Obstetrics and Medical Jurisprudence,	WALTER CHANNING, M.D.
On Theory and Practice of Medicine,	JOHN WARE, M.D.

The students attend any or all the courses as they see fit. The collective fee for all the courses is $75. The fee for matriculation is $3, payable only by those who attend for the first time in this institution. The graduation fee is $20. The ticket for the dissecting room is $5. Admittance to the Hospital and the use of the Library are gratuitous.

Board is as low as in any of the Atlantic cities.

Practical anatomy is now amply provided for by law of this Commonwealth.

The vast increase which has lately taken place in the population of Boston, the numerous avenues and extensive commercial relations, by which it is now connected with all parts of the country, its extensive and unrivalled public charities, its Hospital, its Dispensary, its Eye and Ear Infirmary, its House of Industry, the Marine Hospital at Chelsea, the scientific collections of mineralogy and of pathological and comparative Anatomy, as well as the proximity of Harvard University, of which the Boston Medical School is a department—are circumstances which point to this city as a most convenient and profitable residence for the medical student, while the thorough and complete course of instruction given at the College and Hospital it is believed have distinguished the graduates of this University among those of the United States.

July 4.   July 15—t Nov 3   W. CHANNING, *Dean.*

CHARITABLE INFIRMARY.

Announcement of classes and faculty in the medical school (1834). Dr. Webster is listed as the professor of chemistry.
Boston Medical and Surgical Journal, 1834; 11: 20.

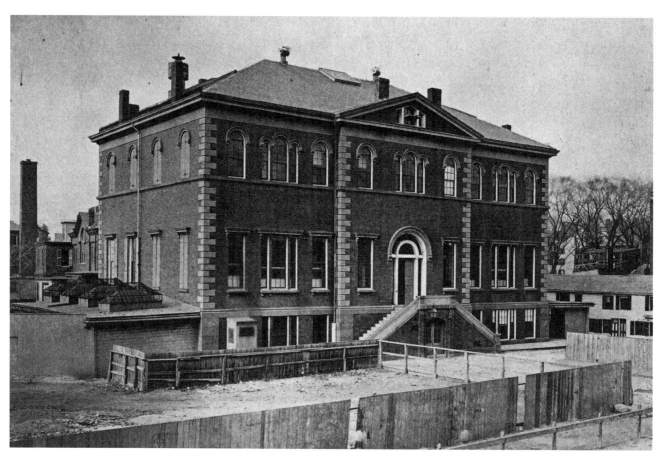

Exterior view of the Old Harvard Medical School, Boston, Mass, ca. 1880. Photograph by Baldwin Coolidge.
Courtesy of Historic New England.

33 years of marriage until Friday, November 23, 1849, which was just six days before Thanksgiving. "The Pedestrian" was last seen at about 1:00 p.m. that day walking up the steps to the Medical College on North Grove Street. He was never seen alive again.

DR. JOHN WHITE WEBSTER: THE CHEMIST

Like Parkman, John White Webster was an integral part of the Harvard Medical School community. He was born in Boston on May 20, 1793 (*Wikipedia*, n.d., under "John White Webster"). He was the only child of Redford and Hannah (White) Webster. His grandfather was a successful and wealthy merchant; his father made his fortune

as an apothecary. Webster's father was very involved in Boston's activities; he was a founding member of the Massachusetts Historical Society, the treasurer and trustee of the Boston Library Society, and a town official who represented Boston in the Massachusetts General Court. He was also elected a Fellow of the American Academy of Arts and Sciences. The family lived in the Clarke-Frankland Mansion in the fashionable North Square, which was close to where Paul Revere had lived. "Webster, indulged as a child and pampered in youth, had a petulant and fussy disposition but was known for his kindly nature" (*Wikipedia*, n.d., under "John White Webster"). The Websters were friends with the influential Prescotts, Shaws, and Parkmans. George Parkman's brother, Reverend Francis Parkman, was their Unitarian pastor.

John Webster was three years younger than George Parkman. Parkman graduated from Harvard College in 1809, Webster in 1811, and they were at Harvard two years together as undergraduates. "In 1814 he [Webster] was among the founders of the Linnaean Society of New England" (*Wikipedia*, n.d., under "John White Webster"), and in 1815 he graduated from the Massachusetts Medical College at Harvard University, which was located at 49 Marlborough Street. The Medical College didn't move to its new location on Mason Street until 1816. His thesis requirement for graduation was entitled, "On the Diagnosis Between Hydrocephalus, Worms, and Foulness of the Stomach and Bowels." After he received his medical degree, Dr. Webster spent approximately two years at Guy's Hospital in London in three training positions: "a surgeon's pupil, a physician's pupil and a surgeon's dresser. He then went to São

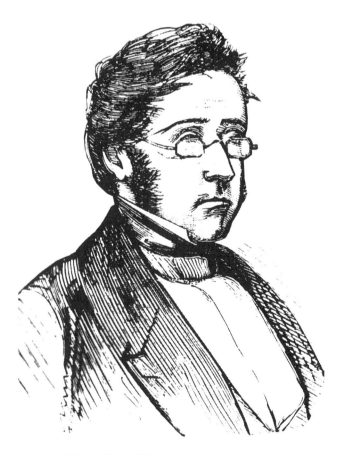

Drawing of John White Webster. U.S. National Library of Medicine.

Miguel Island in the Azores (1817–1818). There he practiced medicine, published his first book, and met the daughter of the American vice-consul on the island, Harriet Fredrica Hickling, whom he married on May 16, 1818; they had four daughters" (*Wikipedia*, n.d., under "John White Webster"). He demonstrated wide scholarly interests, including in geology, with the publication of his first book at age 28 in 1821, *A Description of the Island of St. Michael, Comprising an Account of Its Geological Structure with Remarks on the Other Azores or Western Islands*. In the preface he stated: "I have thought it would be useful to point out the rocks of some well known European locality, which many specimens from St. Michael resemble" (Webster 1821).

After returning to Boston, Webster started a private practice, but he was unsuccessful (*Wikipedia*, n.d., under "John White Webster"). With Parkman's assistance, he obtained a teaching position at the Medical College. In 1826, he was a resident lecturer on chemistry at the University in Cambridge; Dr. Gorham was still the lecturer on chemistry for the medical students. By 1830, Webster had replaced Gorham as the lecturer on chemistry, a position associated with Dr. John C. Warren (anatomy and surgery), Dr. Jacob Bigelow (*materia medica*), Dr. Walter Channing (midwifery and jurisprudence) and Dr. James Jackson (theory and practice of physic). Interestingly, along with Drs. Warren, Jackson and Ware, Dr. Webster charged $15 for his 13-week course of lectures; whereas the other professors charged $10. In 1826, Webster published his second book, *A Manual of Chemistry, on the Basis of Professor Brande's*. It was designed as a textbook for students attending his lectures, and it was arranged in the order of his lectures. He published several editions of his *Manual of Chemistry*. One reviewer wrote: "After a very careful perusal of the work, we strenuously recommend it, as containing the most complete and excellent instructions for conducting chemical experiments" (*Boston Medical and Surgical Journal* 1828).

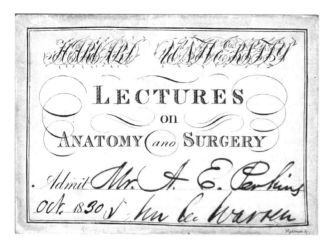

Ticket for Dr. Warren's lectures, October 1830.
University Archives and Records Center, University of Pennsylvania.

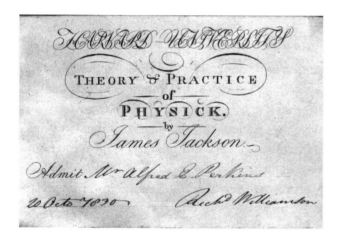

Ticket for Dr. Jackson's lectures, October 1830.
University Archives and Records Center, University of Pennsylvania.

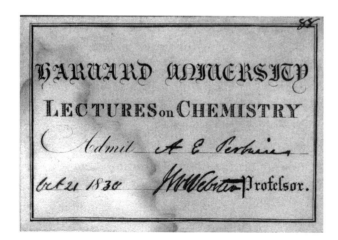

Ticket for Dr. Webster's lectures, October 1830.
University Archives and Records Center, University of Pennsylvania.

By 1828, Webster had been promoted to the Erving Professorship of Chemistry at Harvard University. He was a

popular lecturer at Harvard College…described by Oliver Wendell Holmes, Sr. as "pleasant in the lecture room, rather nervous and excitable." Many of Webster's class-room demonstrations involved some of the latest chemical discoveries…Michael Faraday's liquefaction of the common gasses…George F. Hoar mentioned that Webster's lectures were "tedious," at least for a non-chemistry major, but that: [Webster] was known to the students by the sobriquet of Sky-Rocket Jack, owing to his great interest in having some fireworks…when President Everett, his former classmate, was inaugurated…Many anecdotes suggest his classroom demonstrations were livened by polytechnic drama…reports written [later]…criticized his teaching ability: for instance, the *Boston Daily Bee* described him as "tolerated rather than respected, and has only retained his position on account of its comparative insignificance. As a lecturer he was dull and common-place and while students took tickets to his lectures, they did not generally attend them." (*Wikipedia*, n.d., under "John White Webster")

In 1830, a national committee was formed to revise and publish the new *Pharmacopoeia of the United States.* From Boston, both Jacob Bigelow and John Webster were appointed to the committee. Recognized as an expert, Webster was asked by the physician of the Massachusetts State Prison to examine remnants of food eaten the previous day by the inmates. On August 5, 1833, 196 prisoners had become very ill with abdominal pain, vomiting, and diarrhea. After a careful analysis of the articles of food remaining, Webster reported that he discovered nothing poisonous. Candidates for the examination before the Censors of the Massachusetts Medical Society were required to provide evidence that they had read and studied books on

A

MANUAL OF CHEMISTRY,

ON THE

BASIS OF PROFESSOR BRANDE'S ;

CONTAINING

THE PRINCIPAL FACTS OF THE SCIENCE, ARRANGED IN THE
ORDER IN WHICH THEY ARE DISCUSSED AND ILLUS-
TRATED IN THE LECTURES AT HARVARD
UNIVERSITY, N. E.

COMPILED FROM THE WORKS OF

BRANDE, HENRY, BERZELIUS, THOMSON AND OTHERS.

DESIGNED

AS A TEXT BOOK FOR THE USE OF STUDENTS, AND PERSONS
ATTENDING LECTURES ON CHEMISTRY.

BY
JOHN W. WEBSTER, M. D.
Lecturer on Chemistry in Harvard University.

BOSTON :
PUBLISHED BY RICHARDSON AND LORD.

J. H. A. Frost, Printer.
1826.

Title page of Dr. Webster's book, *Manual of Chemistry*, 1826.
New York Public Library.

a long list (33 books); included on that list was Webster's *Manual of Chemistry*. In 1842, Webster was asked to edit an American edition of Professor Liebig's book *Animal Chemistry*, which was translated by Professor Gregory in England. Another American version was published at the same time in New York. The *Boston Medical and Surgical Journal* published a review of both and recommended the Cambridge edition by Webster writing: "it was deemed advisable to introduce new matter… by withdrawing portions and substituting the new matter…both the portions…. were forwarded by the translator for the use in the present edition"

(*Boston Medical and Surgical Journal* 1842). Webster corrected "errors that had crept into the transatlantic publication. It is, therefore, clear that the Cambridge edition has manifest advantage over the New York one, and should have the preference…of medical purchasers. From Dr. Webster's acknowledged accuracy in the department of chemistry, being the University Professor, we cannot admit that his revisions of a book are inferior, or unworthy of entire confidence" (*Boston Medical and Surgical Journal* 1842). Professor Gregory, who held the chair of chemistry at the University of Edinburgh, rewrote his book *Chemistry for Students* which "is to appear in Boston, under the editorial supervision of Prof. Webster, well known for his labors in the chair of Chemistry at the University in Cambridge. Just such an assistant will find a market in the New England colleges" (*Boston Medical and Surgical Journal* 1846).

In a second legal case, a murder case, Professor Webster was called to testify as an expert witness in a trial of a man accused of murdering his wife 15 years ago (1834). In February 1848, the family of the deceased woman requested that her body be removed from her tomb and examined for the presence of arsenic because part of her body remained "in an unusual state of preservation" (Hitchcock 1849), specifically the abdomen and its contents. Arsenic had been commonly used as a preservative by taxidermists. It was also a common poison in the nineteenth century. Webster was asked to examine the abdomen, stomach, intestines, and all contents for the presence of arsenic. When stating his qualifications at trial, he noted "that in the course of the preceding three months no fewer than four cases were submitted to my examination in two of which arsenic was found" (Hitchcock 1849). He then described in great detail the various methods that he used to detect arsenic in the abdomen and its contents, especially recognizing the importance of his findings because he knew of no case where arsenic had been detected after such a long period of time. He concluded that arsenic was present. "A very large number of medical witnesses were called for the government, and also for the defense. No exceptions were taken to Dr. Webster's chemical evidence, and no attempt was made to discredit the results of his analysis. There was a concurrence of opinion with the physicians that the symptoms of which Mrs. Cook died were consistent with poisoning by arsenic...The Chief Justice charged the jury favorably for the prisoner. After deliberating 40 minutes, the jury returned a verdict of Not Guilty" (Hitchcock 1849). Chief Justice Lemuel Shaw was the presiding judge.

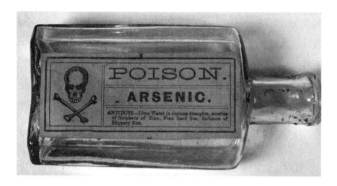

Arsenic bottle.
Massachusetts General Hospital, Archives and Special Collections.

In 1849, upon learning that George Hayward, the professor of surgery at Harvard (and MGH) was resigning, Webster, along with Walter Channing, Jacob Bigelow, John Ware, J. B. S. Jackson, and Oliver W. Holmes signed a letter to Dr. Hayward and published it in the *Boston Medical and Surgical Journal*. Recognizing his contributions, they stated that he was "a most acceptable and useful instructor... [and admired] your zeal for general interests, your efficient influence in the management of...affairs, and your liberality in contributing to...means of instruction...we remain, dear Sir, your friends" (*Boston Medical and Surgical Journal* 1849).

Webster appears to have habitually lived beyond what his means would permit. His annual income was between $1200 and $2000; in 2015, the approximate value would have been $38,000 to $63,000. He supplemented his professor's salary with fees from other lectures, chemistry books he edited or published, and as a frequent expert witness in trials. Although he had inherited some money from his father ($50,000) and his wife also had some inheritance, Webster squandered it all. He was personable and well-liked, but his penchant for the finer things in life did not pair well with his inability to manage household funds. He organized many musical events with his friend Henry Wadsworth Longfellow, his wife hosted fancy parties, and he purchased a home beyond his means. As a result, he eventually had to move, selling the property on Harvard Street and living in a leased home.

His leased home is now known as the Wyeth-Webster House, which is at 22 Garden Street, about three blocks north of Harvard Square. Webster and Parkman were friends; Parkman's brother had baptized the Webster children (four girls); and Mrs. Parkman and Mrs. Webster were close friends as well. However, as Webster incurred more and more debt, he teetered on the edge of bankruptcy. Eventually, after repeatedly borrowing from friends and family, his debt reached $4,500 or what would have been about $144,000 in 2015. Family often forgave his debts, but he owed more than half of this debt to Parkman ($2,432, which in 2015 would have been approximately $76,000) (Bahne 2012). Webster unscrupulously mortgaged the same asset, a mineralogical collection, to both

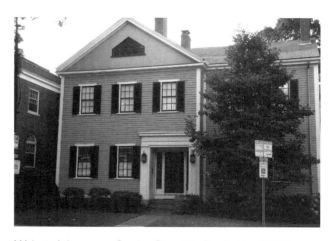

Webster's house on Garden Street in Cambridge (2018).
Photo by the author.

Parkman and Parkman's brother-in-law, Robert Gould Shaw. When Parkman learned of this second mortgage, "he declared at the time [April, 1848] that this was downright fraud and that Dr. Webster ought to be punished" (*Boston Medical and Surgical Journal* 1850a).

Webster knew that Parkman was becoming increasingly angry about his unpaid loan, which had been outstanding for a couple of years. He suggested a meeting to resolve things on Friday, November 23. That afternoon Webster was waiting for Parkman in his laboratory at the Medical School on North Grove Street.

EPHRAIM LITTLEFIELD: THE JANITOR

On Friday afternoon, November 23, 1849, Ephraim Littlefield was in his apartment at the medical school. He worked as the janitor at the Massachusetts

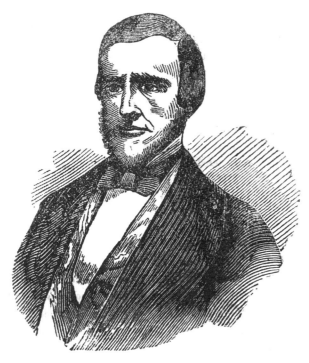

Portrait of Ephraim Littlefield. From *"Trial of Professor John W. Webster for the Murder of Dr. George Parkman."* Reported Exclusively for the N.Y. *Daily Globe*, 1850.
U.S. National Library of Medicine.

Medical College of Harvard University. He had worked for the medical school for eight years; six years while the school was located on Mason Street (1816–1847) and for the last two years in the new school on North Grove Street, which opened in 1847. He lived there in the basement with his family. In addition to cleaning the building, he started fires for the faculty and set up specimens for their lectures. "To supplement his income, he obtained cadavers for dissection…selling them to students and professors at a price of about twenty-five dollars [worth approximately $800 in 2015] a body" (*Wikipedia*, n.d., under "Parkman-Webster Murder Case"). Littlefield searched for and accepted cadavers using both above-board and unscrupulous means alike, obtaining them from both grave robbers and possible murderers.

THE MURDER CASE: TRIAL OF THE NINETEENTH CENTURY

Dr. Parkman was never again seen alive after entering the Medical School on North Grove Street. As a man of regular habits, his wife became concerned when he missed his first luncheon with her in their 33 years of marriage; she immediately suspected foul play. Obviously concerned, Mrs. Parkman spoke with her brother-in-law, Robert Gould Shaw, who posted flyers and published notices in the daily papers the next day on Saturday, November 24. They offered a substantial reward for tangible information supplied: $3,000 (a value approximately equal to $94,000 in 2015) (*Murder by Gaslight* 2010).

Meanwhile, Dr. Webster had eventually left his laboratory Friday evening. He attended a family party, and he discussed Parkman's missing person with others. The only variation in Webster's routine over the next few weeks was a discussion with Littlefield about Parkman's visit and a gift (a Thanksgiving turkey) that he gave to the janitor. Previously, he had talked with the janitor only

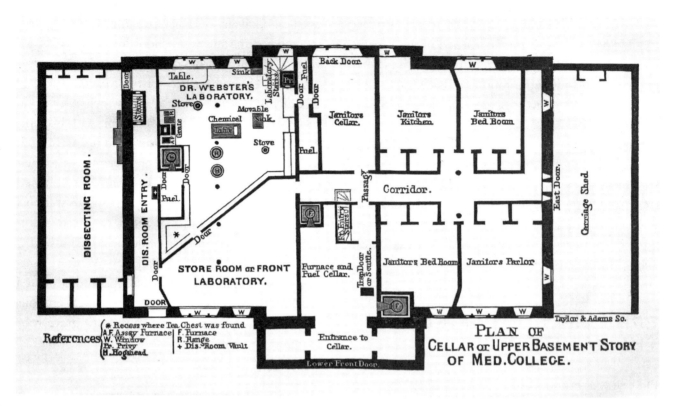

Floor plan of the medical school. Dr. Webster's lab is in the upper left. From *Report of the Case of John W. Webster Before the Supreme Judicial Court of Massachusetts* by George Bemis, Boston: Charles C. Little and James Brown, 1850.
U.S. National Library of Medicine.

in rare instances, and he had never before given him a gift.

The search for Parkman began without preamble with all hands-on deck, including all members of the police force in Boston led by Marshall Tukey. They searched all properties that Parkman had owned, distributed notices of his missing person both within and outside the city limits, and dredged the river. On Monday, November 26, the police searched Webster's laboratory and the other offices in the medical school. They found nothing. On Friday, November 30, Littlefield began his own search, including the crawl space below Webster's laboratory. Webster's privy emptied into this area and was contained within a brick wall which Littlefield broke through. He discovered human remains and immediately notified Marshall Tukey. After searching Webster's office and laboratory (also called his apartment), the police discovered both a human thorax in a tea chest and false teeth

in a stove. They also found other body parts in the privy vault and charred bones (including parts of a skull and jaw) in Webster's furnace. At Webster's trial, Tukey testified:

On the evening of Friday, 30th November, I…in company with Dr. Henry J. Bigelow…went to a trap-door in Littlefield's apartment near the lower laboratory, which allowed passage into the cellar below; in the brick wall at the corner of the cellar was found a hole 18 inches square, newly broken. I took a lamp and reaching into the hole, perceived what I thought to be pieces of flesh; the sea-water was flowing in and out, but nothing else could pass out. I directed Mr. Trenholm to take out the remains; they were three pieces, apparently a portion of a body, a part of a thigh and leg. Dr. Bigelow said they were human, but not a dissection subject.
(*Boston Medical and Surgical Journal* 1850a)

That Friday evening, the day after Thanksgiving, the police picked up Webster at his home under the pretense of conducting an additional search of his laboratory. Instead they stopped at the Leverett City Jail where they arrested him for the murder of Dr. Parkman. After entering his cell, Webster took a strychnine pill that he had made, but his suicide attempt failed. After a few days, a notice appeared in the *Boston Medical and Surgical Journal* (1849b):

> Never has this community had a severer shock than is now agitating it. Geo. Parkman, M.D., a very wealthy and well-known physician of this city, was unaccountably missing after Friday, November 23rd. To the astonishment of every one, on Friday evening last, November 30th, the remains of a human being, singularly mutilated, were found in and about the private apartments of Dr. John W. Webster, at the Medical College in Grove Street—some of the remains bearing evident marks of being partly burnt…He [Webster] is now in prison, and the public mind is in the highest state of excitement…circumstances have led to the horrible idea that the remains, found in the professor's room, were those of Dr. Parkman. It is singular, among other things, that Dr. Parkman generously gave the land, a few years since, on which the Medical College stands in which he is supposed to have been murdered. Dr. Parkman has long been in the habit of occasionally employing some of his few leisure moments in preparing brief articles for this Journal. These were mostly condensed statements of medical facts, divested of every extraneous word or sentence…He had given notice, a few days before his disappearance, that he should soon have a paper ready for the Journal, on the value of electricity in producing active ejection from the bowels. Prof. Webster has also, in former years, been a contributor to the Journal.

Circumstances had progressed from that of a missing person to a probable murder, prompting an immediate scandal with prolific and dramatic press coverage. The *Herald* produced the first drawing of Webster in their issue on December 4, 1849; the image differed sharply from Webster's usual amiable appearance and depicted him as

THE REMAINS FOUND IN THE MEDICAL COLLEGE.

No. 1.—Represents the vertebræ and thoracic cavity which is charred, and contains the lungs.
No. 2.—Represents the pelvic cavity, covered by flesh in its lower part.
No. 3.—The right thigh disarticulated from the pelvis.
No. 4.—The left thigh disarticulated from the pelvis.
No. 5.—The left leg disarticulated from the thigh and foot.

Drawing of the human remains found in the medical school. From "Trial of Professor W. Webster for the Murder of Doctor George Parkman." Reported exclusively for the N.Y. *Daily Globe.* New York: Stringer & Townsend, 1850. U.S. National Library of Medicine.

menacing—even demonic. Fanny, wife of the well-known American poet Henry Wadsworth Longfellow, wrote:

> Boston is at this moment in sad suspense about the fate of poor Dr. Parkman…You will see by the papers what dark horror overshadows us like an eclipse. Of course, we cannot believe Dr. Webster guilty, bad as the evidence looks… Many suspect the janitor, who is known to be a bad man and to have wished for the reward offered for Dr. Parkman's body. (Bilis 2015)

A coroner's jury was convened. Articles found in Webster's furnace were given by the jury to Drs. Charles T. Jackson, Jeffries Wyman, and Martin Gay. These three physicians assumed a role that we look back upon as that of early forensic science. They examined the remains to determine if they were human and, if they were, whether or not they were embalmed and may have been part of a cadaver from the lab. They also analyzed the remains for the presence of poison and proof of any attempts to destroy evidence. Jackson described this process and their findings when he wrote:

> Bones found in the cinders from the furnace [included]—right os calcis, right astragalus, tibia and fibula, phalanges, probably of the middle or ring finger. Coronoid process of lower jaw. Numerous fragments of a skull. A human tooth that had a hole in it as if once filled by dental operation. Three blocks of artificial mineral teeth were also found in the cinders, without the gold plate [and other]… various articles…such as needed chemical analysis were subsequently taken by Dr. Gay and myself [Jackson] and examined…I made some chemical examinations…on the chest and one thigh, and found that they had been imbued with a solution of potash…I observed that the hair on the left side of the thorax had been singed by fire…I dissected out portions of

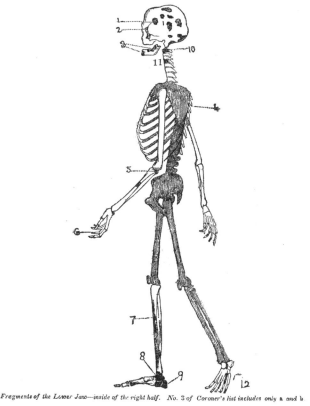

21

RESTORATION OF DR. PARKMAN'S SKELETON.
Designed by Rowse from a sketch by Dr. Jefferies Wyman, and engraved by Taylor & Adams

Fragments of the Lower Jaw—inside of the right half.   No. 3 of Coroner's list includes only a and b

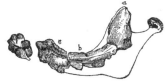

Drawing of the reconstructed skeleton of the remains by Dr. Jeffries Wyman. U.S. National Library of Medicine.

the femoral arteries and flesh of both thighs, and the artery and vein of the leg…to ascertain whether the body had been injected with the fluids used for preserving bodies in the dissecting room…[and] found no traces of zinc or arsenic substances used in the preservation of bodies…an attempt had been made to burn the thorax in the fire, but had not been preserved in. (Jackson 1850)

On December 13, 1849, the coroner's jury issued their final report, which stated:

1. The sparse human remains found in the medical school were the remains of Dr. Parkman.

2. George Parkman had come to his death by violence on the 23rd day of November 1849 at the Harvard Medical School.

3. The death of Parkman was caused "by blow or blows, wound or wounds" inflected upon him and said means were used by the hands of said John W. Webster by whom he was killed...

This startling and condemning report of the coroner's jury was published verbatim in the Boston and New York press. (R. Sullivan 1969)

Afterward, a grand jury of Suffolk County was convened and indicted Webster on January 26, 1850.

Webster's trial began on March 17, 1850, and lasted 12 days. The chief justice was Lemuel Shaw, before whom Dr. Webster had testified as an expert witness in previous murder trials. Attorney General John H. Clifford, who later became Governor of Massachusetts in 1853, turned over the major portion of the prosecution's case to George Bemis, a private attorney. Webster had asked Daniel Webster (no relation to him) and Rufus Choate, two prominent defense attorneys to represent him; both men refused. Phiny Merrick—who would be appointed to the Supreme Judicial Court in 1853—and his associate, Edward H. Sohier, agreed to represent Webster. They were both experienced civil case attorneys, but they had virtually no experience in criminal cases.

The trial took on circus-like attributes, with a crowd of approximately 300 buying tickets to the event. Once the trial began, crowds were managed in ten-minute shifts with about 60,000 Bostonians attempting to gain admittance. The second phase of press coverage included the trial itself, which reached beyond the local level to national and international news. The press

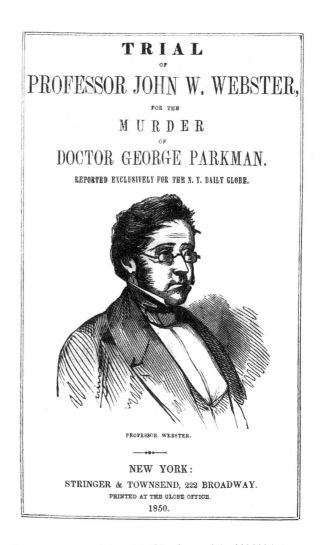

Announcement of the trial of Professor John W. Webster.
U.S. National Library of Medicine.

covered the case daily in every detail. They noted celebrities in attendance, including John C. Calhoun, a well-known southern statesman; Massachusetts Lieutenant Governor John Reed; speaker of the House, E. H. Kellogg; Harvard's librarian, John Sibley; the victim's brother, Reverend Francis Parkman; and many other respected clergy and public officials. Upon entering the courtroom each morning, Webster welcomed and embraced his friends in stark contrast to the serious setting.

After the Attorney General gave a three-hour opening address to the jury, George Bemis began calling witnesses for the prosecution. Much of the actual testimony was recorded phonographically by Dr. James Stone. The first witness was Robert Gould Shaw (Parkman's brother-in-law). He testified about Parkman's family, Parkman's invalid daughter, the anxiety of the Parkman family since the disappearance, his knowledge of Webster's sale of his mineral collection to another person, Parkman's generous contributions to Boston, and his own identification of the human body parts.

The next day, the jury toured the Medical School on North Grove Street. Afterward, they heard from the Medical Committee, which included three leaders of medicine in Boston: Drs. Winslow Lewis Jr., George H. Gay, and James W. Stone. All three knew Parkman, and they reported on the results of their examination of the body parts. Lewis, who chaired their committee, stated, "There was nothing in the appearance of the body that I should not have expected to have found in the body of Dr. Parkman; and I should think that the parts had been separated by some hand skilled in anatomy. It is my opinion that the five parts belonged to one and the same body" (*Boston Medical and Surgical Journal* 1850c). Their report was very detailed and described each anatomic part, stating that "Five portions of a human subject were examined; a thorax, a pelvis, two thighs, and a left leg...These portions appeared to belong to a person of between 50 and 60 years of age...total height, five feet ten and a half inches" (*Boston Medical and Surgical Journal* 1850a).

The most important witness was next, Dr. Nathan C. Keep—a surgeon and dentist who had made some false teeth for Dr. Parkman in 1846. He had kept a plaster cast that he made of Parkman's jaw and testified that the teeth, although damaged by the fire, were "the teeth I made for Dr. Parkman" (*Boston Medical and Surgical Journal* 1850e). Dr. James Wyman, a professor of anatomy who examined the bones and articles with questionable blood stains, testified that "on examining the thorax, I was struck with the fact that the sternum was removed in the manner usual in *post-mortem* examinations; as well as its

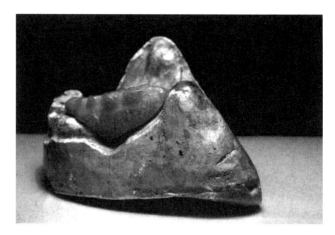

Dental casts of Dr. Parkman (1846).
Harvard Medical Library in the Francis A. Countway Library of Medicine.

separation from the collar-bone and the first rib. The route which the knife passes is such that a person unacquainted with the operation would have great difficulty. There is only one way" (*Boston Medical and Surgical Journal* 1850e). Dr. Wyman had also examined stains on some of Webster's clothing and the walls of his laboratory stairs. He concluded his testimony by stating:

> I examined certain spots on the sides of the stairway leading from the upper to the lower laboratory. Some...were tobacco spittle. But there were others higher up, of which I discovered nothing definite. On Sunday, these were moist...[and] to be nitrate of copper...[which can cause] the discs of blood...[to have] disappeared. There were brought to me a pair of slippers, and a pair of pantaloons...where I cut out certain spots...I have satisfied myself that these spots were blood...Dr. Webster's name is marked upon them...[On cross-examination he stated] I should think nitrate of copper effectual to remove blood...the spots it examined... can by the microscope distinguish human blood from that of some animals, but not many. (*Boston Medical and Surgical Journal* 1850b)

Dean Oliver W. Holmes, the Parkman Professor of Anatomy who followed Dr. Wyman on the stand, agreed that the body parts "had been dissected by a hand experienced in the field of anatomy…that having known Dr. Parkman…for many years, he saw nothing about the remains dissimilar from Dr. Parkman's person" (R. Sullivan 1969). Later, Dean Holmes testified for the defense as a character witness for Webster, one of Harvard Medical School's six professors. Interestingly, Holmes was giving a lecture in the room above Webster's lab at the same time Webster and Parkman met that fateful day. Holmes testified: "My lecture room is over Dr. Webster's, and I never was disturbed by a noise from the room below, chemical explosion or other. The rooms are very high. The seats of the students are raised above the main floor, but I stand upon it" (*Boston Medical and Surgical Journal* 1850b).

Ephraim Littlefield was in the witness box for the next two days. He gave a detailed description of his observations of Webster after Parkman's disappearance; his concern about the extreme heat he felt on the outside wall of Webster's laboratory (next to Webster's furnace); and the fact that he couldn't enter Webster's lab the Friday afternoon of Parkman's disappearance because the door was locked from the inside. Littlefield had the only key to the basement under the dissecting room where human parts were discarded, and he let the police in to search the area; no suspicious human remains were found. Littlefield described how—because he was suspicious—he broke through the brick wall of Webster's privy to discover human remains and then notified the police. Some, including Webster, had raised suspicion that Littlefield may have been involved; they argued he may have obtained Parkman's body from someone on the street who had killed him, and then upon learning it was Parkman's body, tried to dispose of it in the Medical College. In response, Littlefield claimed during his testimony that he "never told anybody I meant to get a reward and I defy anyone to prove it" (*Boston Medical and Surgical Journal* 1850b).

During the trial, Marshall Tukey received many letters and comments, but three letters were of particular concern. All were signed using the name *Civis*, meaning citizen. All were attempts to shift the suspicion away from Webster. In response, the prosecution called upon an expert to analyze the handwriting on these three letters; they selected Nathaniel D. Gould, an instructor of penmanship

guise blended in the " Civis" letter ; I cannot describe the whole of the points of resemblance observed by me in these letters and the writing known to be that of Professor Webster's without sitting down and looking at my notes.

The letters were then read by Mr. Bemis, junior counsel for the Government. We give them verbatim :

Directed to **Mr**. Tukey, City Marshal.

(VERBATIM COPY.)

BOSTON, Nov. 31st, 1849.

" **MR**. TUKEY—*Dear Sir :*—I have been considerably interested in the recent affair of Dr. Parkman, and I think I can recommend means, the adoption of which may result in bringing to light some of the mysteries connected with the disappearance of the fore-mentioned gentleman. In the first place, in regard to the searching houses—and I would recommend that particular attention be paid to the appearance of cellar-doors—do they present the appearance of having been freshly covered by the piling of wood? Have the houses and necessaries being carefully examined? Probably his body was cut up into small pieces and placed in a stout bag, and thrown into the river from Craigie's Bridge, and I would recommend the firing of cannon from some of these bridges, and various parts of the harbor and river, in order to cause the body to rise to the surface of the water. This, I think, would be the last resource, and it should be done effectually, and I recommend that the cellars of the houses in East Cambridge be examined.

Yours respectfully, CIVIS."

Copy of one of the letters written by "CIVIS" to Marshall Tukey. From "Trial of Professor W. Webster for the Murder of Doctor George Parkman." Reported exclusively for the N.Y. *Daily Globe*. New York: Stringer & Townsend, 1850. U.S. National Library of Medicine.

for over 50 years who was also familiar with the handwriting of all six professors at Harvard Medical School because each was required to sign diplomas of the graduates. "Gould opined that all the letters were written by Webster and the handwriting showed that Webster had attempted to disguise his own handwriting" (*Boston Medical and Surgical Journal* 1850b).

On March 27, 1850, the eighth day of the trial, the defense attorney, Edward D. Sohier made his opening statement. Sohier "began with a fiery plea to the jurors to put prejudice against the defendant from their minds…[then closed by conceding] 'that there would not be an acquittal and that he was arguing for the lesser of the two alternatives—guilty of manslaughter [and not murder]'" (*Boston Medical and Surgical Journal* 1850b). Nevertheless, Webster continued before and throughout the trial to proclaim his innocence. That same day the defense called 16 witnesses to testify, "All of whom swore that Webster had been known to them for many years and that his reputation in the community was that of a mild, placid, peaceable, quiet, and humane gentleman" (*Boston Medical and Surgical Journal* 1850b). The mayor of Cambridge and Jared Sparks, the president of Harvard College, were included in this group.

A total of 26 witnesses testified for the defense. Three of Webster's daughters testified, as well as a housekeeper for the Webster family. The most effective witness was Dr. William T. G. Morton, the dentist who three years before the trial had given ether anesthesia to a patient of Dr. John Collins Warren at the Massachusetts General Hospital. He was very well known in Boston. Dr. Morton testified that he

> was familiar with Dr. Keep's artistry in dentistry in the manufacture of artificial teeth…there were no marks about the teeth…identified by Keep as Dr. Parkman's by which it would be possible for Dr. Keep, or anyone else, to identify them…the teeth which Keep identified as

being those made by him for Parkman had been subjected to such ferocity of heat that they had been fused and…therefore, quite impossible to identify them. Next, taking the mold which Keep claimed he had used in the manufacture of Parkman's teeth in 1846…Dr. Morton proceeded to fit into this mold false teeth, which he had in his pocket, teeth entirely unrelated to the case…Morton said, "I could take this mold and find teeth which would better fit the mold then these [pointed to the teeth found in Webster's furnace]." (*Boston Medical and Surgical Journal* 1850b)

Following Morton's dramatic testimony, the defense called on six witnesses, all of whom knew Dr. Parkman and stated they had seen or passed by him (sometimes nodding) between 2:00 p.m. and 5:00 p.m. on Friday, November 23, 1849. The defense rested. "On March 30, after the defendant's closing remarks were concluded… the prosecution's closing remarks…[lasted] nearly five hours" (*Wikipedia*, n.d., under "Lemuel Shaw").

Before charging the jury, Chief Justice Shaw "informed Dr. Webster of his privilege of making any remarks" to the jury (*Boston Medical and Surgical Journal* 1850e). It was unusual for a defendant to speak during his own case, and defendants did not have a right to testify in their own defense until 16 years after the Webster case. However, precedent had emerged allowing a defendant to address the jury as long as the jury was instructed not to include it among evidence considered. Webster's lawyer advised against this action, but Webster nevertheless seized the opportunity to speak for about 15 minutes. He said:

> In nine cases out of ten, I could have given a satisfactory explanation of the circumstances which have been so unfortunately and completely distorted against me here…I was in the hands of counsel, who were highly recommended to me, and I deferred to their

superior judgment, and they did not think to act upon my suggestion. I have placed in their hands the testimony necessary to explain very many things which have pressed most against me, but they have judged proper, in some cases, to disregard my wishes and instructions. (*Boston Medical and Surgical Journal* 1850e)

Webster then proceeded to refute some of the allegations and evidence against him. He concluded with a comment about the three letters signed by Civis, asserting: "I declare I never wrote those letters" (***Boston Medical and Surgical Journal*** 1850e).

It was time for the jury to deliberate. In 1850 "the leading authorities upon the law of criminal evidence...made it quite clear that the fact of the *corpus delecti*, or the commission of a homicide, had to be proven to an absolute certainty or beyond the least doubt. After this... the burden of proof of the prosecution was to show that the defendant had committed the crime beyond a reasonable doubt" (R. Sullivan 1969). Shaw's charge to the jury, accepted today, was not agreed to by everyone in 1850. Many people then and even today challenge the judge's charges and therefore the verdict at the conclusion of the trial; "the learned judge says, 'for concealment implies guilt, a depraved heart, and presupposes malice'" (***Boston Medical and Surgical Journal*** 1850f). Regarding the testimony of the witnesses who claimed to have seen Dr. Parkman late afternoon the day of his disappearance, the judge stated:

Perhaps no man was better known in the city than the deceased. It is obvious that if Parkman was seen by the witnesses at the times and places stated by them...hundreds or perhaps thousands of persons would have seen him and would have come forward to declare it. The absence of such testimony is to be weighed and "considered." (R. Sullivan 1969)

At 8:00 p.m. on Saturday, March 30, 1850, Chief Justice Shaw completed his charge to the jury; he asked them to begin their deliberations immediately, and:

Less than three hours later, at 10:50 p.m. the jury returned to the Court with their decision..."Guilty"...Webster shut his eyes, his hands convulsively clutched the bar before him and he sank into his chair in tears. The terrible gloom which swept the courtroom and the galleries manifested the great sympathy felt, in Boston, for Webster...On the twelfth and last day of the trial [Monday, April 1]...Chief Justice Shaw...[read] these words: "and then be hanged by the neck until you are dead—And may God, in his Infinite Goodness, Have mercy on your Soul!" Webster leaned against the bar, placed his handkerchief to his face, and burst into tears. (R. Sullivan 1969)

By the conclusion of the trial, the entire city was in shock.

AFTERMATH

The number of people who had attended the trial equaled almost half the population of Boston (130,000); the crowds included international press from London, Paris, and Berlin. The entire city responded in shock because

a man who had been in the highest walks of society, esteemed one of the pillars of science, and a professor in Harvard University, the first and oldest institution of learning in America, must suffer death, for the horrible crime of murdering a fellow being—a member of the same profession with himself. The trial may be considered as one of the most important on record, and possesses a painful interest to the medical profession. (*Boston Medical and Surgical Journal* 1850c)

During the first week of April, the medical school opened for anyone to tour through the site of the murder in response to the tremendous curiosity of the public. Five thousand people visited Webster's laboratory and office on the second day of that week.

Entering its third phase, the press now focused on Webster's family. Newspapers such as *The New York Star* labeled Webster's wife and four daughters "the real suffers in this unhappy case" (quoted in Chaney 2004). Now lacking Webster's income and left with his debts, they had to take in sewing and perform other jobs. Many family and friends assisted them with both the financial and emotional fallout of the tragedy. One friend (Samuel Cunningham) supplied Mrs. Webster with a house located on Mt. Auburn and Ash streets, close to her previous home on Garden Street and near Harvard Square. In addition, Mrs. Parkman quite magnanimously became one of their greatest benefactors.

In the ensuing months, numerous petitions were "presented to the Executive [Governor Briggs] for the full pardon of said Webster, founded upon the belief and presumption that he never committed even a homicide" (*Boston Medical and Surgical Journal* 1850h). However, the Reverend George Putnam, a clergyman who had never met Webster before the trial, began to frequently visit him in jail in the hope of providing some comfort as Webster's spiritual advisor. In the course of these meetings, Webster confessed his crime to Reverend Putnam. Webster described the meeting with Dr. Parkman in his laboratory:

> He [Parkman] immediately addressed me with great energy; "Are you ready for me, Sir? Have you got the money?" I replied "No, Dr. Parkman" and was then beginning to…make my appeal to him. He would not listen to me… He called me "scoundrel" and "liar" and went on heaping upon me the most bitter taunts and opprobrious epithets…"I got you into your office and now I will get you out of it"…the torrents of threats and invectives continued…at

first I kept interposing, trying to pacify him…But I could not stop him, and soon my own temper was up. I forgot everything. I felt nothing but the sting of his words…and while he was speaking and gesticulating in the most violent and menacing manner…I seized what ever thing was handiest—it was a stick of wood—and dealt him an instantaneous blow, with all the force that passion could give it…on the side of his head… He fell instantly upon the pavement…He did not move…Blood flowed from his mouth…I got some ammonia and applied it to his nose, but without effect. Perhaps I spent ten minutes in attempts to resuscitate him; but I found that he was absolutely dead. In my horror and consternation, I ran instinctively to the doors and bolted them…I saw nothing but…the concealment of the body…[or total] destruction I took off the clothes, and began putting them into the fire…I [removed] the watch…and threw it…over the bridge as I went to Cambridge. My next move was to get the body to the sink…[where] it was entirely dismembered…The head and viscera were put into that [lower basement] furnace… Some of the extremities I believe were put in there…the pelvis and some of the limbs… were put under the lid of the lecture room table in…a deep sink…the thorax was put in a similar well in the lower laboratory, which I filled with water, and threw in a quantity of potash…I left the college to go home, as late as six o'clock… My single thought was concealment and safety…After the first visit of the officers, I took the pelvis and some of the upper limbs from the upper well and threw them into the vault under the privy. I took the thorax from the well below and packed in the tea-chest as found [with tan]. (Webster 1850)

With this confession and additional details, Reverend Putnam submitted a petition on Webster's behalf that the death sentence be commuted to life imprisonment, arguing that the murder was not premeditated but was instead a crime of

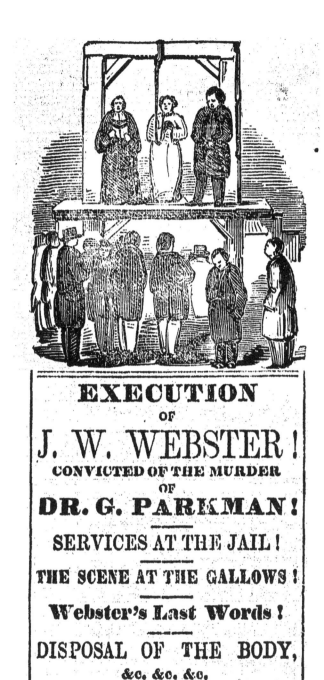

Announcement of the execution of John W. Webster.
Boston Herald, August 31, 1850.

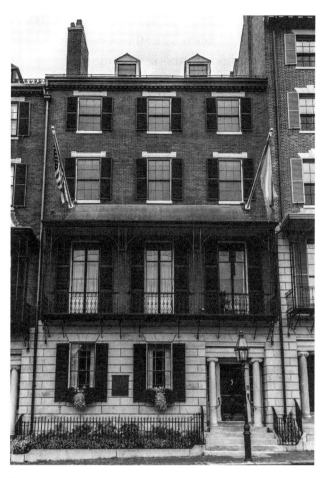

Parkman House at 33 Beacon Street.
Kael E. Randall/Kael Randall Images.

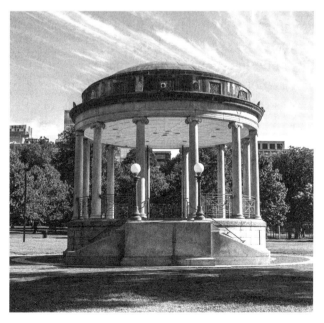

Parkman Bandstand. Built 1912. Named for George F. Parkman, who died in 1908. Kael E. Randall/Kael Randall Images.

passion. Reverend Putman appeared before the Committee on Pardons on July 2, 1850, and read Dr. Webster's confession. The committee decided: "that they cannot, consistently with what they conceive their duty, recommend a commination of the sentence…but to advise your Excellency to decide upon that day [August 30] as the time for the execution of John W. Webster" (*Boston Medical and Surgical Journal* 1850h). Governor Briggs found no reason to authorize a pardon.

On Friday, August 30, 1850, Dr. Webster was publicly hanged in the Leverett Street jail yard at 9:30 a.m. According to the *Boston Medical and Surgical Journal* (1850i):

> After being suspended half an hour, his body was lowered into the coffin beneath, which was immediately removed to [his] cell. There were some two hundred persons present...His remains were taken to the residence of his family in Cambridge on the same evening.

That same night, Webster's family and friends secretly buried him in Copps Hill Burying Ground in the North End. Webster had wanted to be buried in his family plot in Mt. Auburn Cemetery, but the cemetery refused.

Three years after her husband's death, Mrs. Parkman and her two children moved into a mansion on 33 Beacon Street overlooking the Common. After Mrs. Parkman's and her daughters' death, her son George F. Parkman lived alone in the mansion until his death in 1908. He was a lawyer and, as his father, a philanthropist and a member of the Somerset Club. He left his 9,000 square foot mansion—known as the Parkman House—to the City of Boston, along with a $5 million trust for the preservation and maintenance of the Common. On the eastern side of the Boston Common is a bandstand built after George's death and named for him (Parkman Bandstand) in recognition of his generous donation. The mansion has been used for city government functions and was the home of Mayor Menino in 2013 during his long convalescence.

LASTING SIGNIFICANCE

During and after Dr. Webster's trial, many were divided as to his guilt. This uncertainty provoked further scandal and intrigue, capturing the minds of all those who have attempted to tell the tale—so much so that even Charles Dickens asked to visit the site of the murder when he visited the United States. On April 10, 1850, only 11 days after the verdict, an article was published in the *Boston Medical and Surgical Journal* by Dr. A. C. Castle of New York, entitled, "Fallibilities of Scientific Evidence in Medical Jurisprudence." I was unable to discover any information about Dr. Castle, but in his article he wrote:

> The fallibilities of scientific evidence is a subject of highest importance...The trial of Webster offers the same ground for argument as its predecessors. We will commence with that essential piece of humbug and superlation, the proving of human blood in contra-distinction to the blood of animals...One witness in Webster's case states that the microscope is the best, the safest and the most certain method of detecting human blood...Now in the case of Webster, we have, in addition to...scientific tests, the all-faithful and never-to-be-mistaken microscope...Yet as we have the conviction of a man on trial for a capital offense resting upon the judgment—yes, we repeat, resting on the judgment of one man, and that judgment dependent perchance, upon an imperfect test...The prisoner has no chance in such cases, for whoever heard of a chemist discovering any other poison than that poison which he was directed to search for?...We have a witness that the skull of Parkman was fractured before death. He states that such fractures cannot take place after the bone has been burned...It is all insufficient, and it only requires an eminent name to establish a theory for a fact, and to impress the assumption of a truth. The next scientific evidence is that of Dr. Keep. This gentleman stands high as a mechanical dentist; but is he an anatomical, medical and surgical dentist as well?...To upset this evidence, one dentist, only, is brought forward to prove the contrary...Dr. Morton's evidence

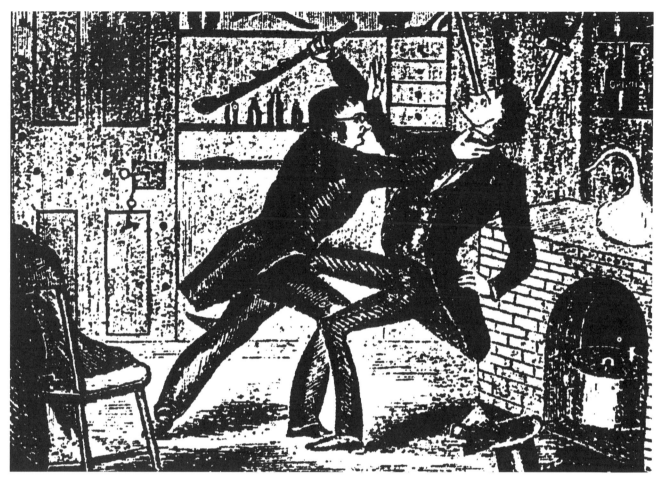

Drawing of Webster and Parkman fighting in Webster's lab. Widener Library/Associated Press.

was professionally correct, with proper incontrovertible truths capable of practical proofs. Yet four or five dentists were thought necessary to rebut Dr. Morton's testimony. Were these gentlemen anatomical surgical dentists…By a most singular omission…wherein science could have been triumphantly made use of…to bear with singular fatality upon Mr. Littlefield's evidence with regard to the sink was altogether omitted or lost sight of…but the really available portion of science fails, or is lost sight of, or when brought into requisition in nine cases out of ten has proved but a doubtful corroborative at best. (Castle 1850a)

The following week (18 days after the verdict) a second article appeared in the *Boston Medical and Surgical Journal* by "A Medical Witness"

(anonymous) entitled, "Accuracy of the Scientific Evidence in the Trial of Professor Webster" (*Boston Medical and Surgical Journal* 1850d). The medical witness stated:

"Sir.—The flippant and careless manner in which remarks have been made in some of the newspapers of other States, concerning the evidence in the Webster trial, has excited some surprise and regret in this city, and the errors into which some of the writers in question have been led have been charitably referred to their want of adequate knowledge on the subject upon which they have written. It is highly probable that a hasty reading of partial or incorrect reports, imperfectly transcribed into the newspapers of other States, may have caused some persons to fall into error; but it would have been wiser, we deem, for such persons to have examined authentic documents before venturing to question the decision of our highest judicial tribunal…Attempts have been made in other States to show that Prof. Webster was sacrificed to mere local prejudice existing against him in Boston. This seems wholly unjustifiable; for if there was any bias in public sentiment here, it was in his favor…I would now call your attention to some very erroneous and as I think unjustifiable strictures published in the last number of the Medical and Surgical Journal by A.C. Castle, M.D. of New York…I was surprised, Mr. Editor, that you admitted such an article…when you had already, in the heading…shown that the writer knew little concerning the persons whose evidence he presumed to criticize, and did not know enough of the localities to distinguish between a locked-up dissecting room vault, a 'sink,' and Dr. Webster's privy; and was not aware that Drs. Wyman, Keep, Harwood, Tucker and Codman, are all well-educated medical gentlemen, familiar with human anatomy, and that 'Dr. Morton' is not universally regarded 'as a well-educated medical man' or a 'talented dentist'…My object at present is to show Dr. Castle that he is in error concerning the testimony of that distinguished anatomist, Dr. Jeffries Wyman, and that of the corroborating witnesses whose opinions coincided with his in relation to the method of detecting the presence of blood. If Dr. Castle is…a well-educated medical man, he must have learned,…that blood is…as readily detected by…the microscope…and that the size of the blood globules or discs varies with the species of the animal from which the blood is taken… Dr. W. [Wyman] did examine all the spots in question, and…discriminated at once between tobacco spittle and blood, pointing out with faithful accuracy which spots were blood and which tobacco spittle, and showing…

that the spots on Dr. Webster's pantaloons and slippers were really well-characterized blood, having its perfect organic structure. He proved beyond question that the microscope did afford the most conclusive evidence with regard to the presence of blood…But really, Mr. Editor, I cannot divine what Dr. C. is driving at in all this parade of chemical learning. What has it to do with the trial of Dr. Webster? I do not find any such count in the indictment…in nine out of ten cases, when the chemist searches for poisons in suspected poisoning, he reports that no poison is discovered…I would next invite your attention to the misrepresentation which has been made concerning Dr. Wyman's testimony respecting the fractured skull bones found in Dr. Webster's furnace. Dr. Wyman never testified that the skull had been broken during life, but that the skull appeared to have been broken before it was calcined…As to the recognition of the artificial teeth of Dr. Parkman by Dr. N.C. Keep, I would remark that it is believed no possible mistake could have taken place… The teeth were in blocks of peculiar form, and exactly fitted the mould on which they were originally prepared…everyone in the courtroom…was perfectly convinced that Dr. Keep could not be mistaken in the fact that those were the teeth he made for Dr. Parkman… In conclusion, Mr. Editor, let me advise those who live at a distance from the scene of this dreadful murder, not to meddle with the facts that they have but a very imperfect knowledge of. They do not help Dr. Webster's case by their lucubrations, but only make it worse. Dr. W. [Webster] has friends here, who will do all for him that is in their power to do, and every one would be delighted to learn any fact that would tend to mitigate the crime of which he is convicted…the general wish of all the medical witnesses…that evidence should be discovered which would exculpate him from the dreadful charge made against him."

Dr. Castle replied to the medical witness's article with a second publication, "The Fallibilities of Scientific Evidence in Medical Jurisprudence— No. II" (Castle 1850b). After a long historical essay on medical science, he voiced his disagreements with the medical witness's arguments:

I do not agree with "A Medical Witness"...I do without hesitation deny the powers of the microscope to distinguish one blood from another...So much, I repeat, for the humbug and superlation of testing human blood...I claim it as a right...to express my opinions, and to expose those things which, in my mind, may be based on errors, prejudices or scientific theories; and, where a fellow-being's life is jeopardized, common humanity, if not the higher feeling, duty, demands it...I do not deem that medical and chemical science has yet arrived at the point of absolute perfection...I am at a loss to account for "A Medical Witness's" irritability, in the matter of Dr. Morton's evidence...what does he [A Medical Witness] mean by "They...do not help Dr. Webster's case by their lucubrations, but only make it worse?" If this sentence...[does] not excite surprise, it is because the records of Massachusetts show that not more than eight or ten capital punishments have taken place during the last twenty-five years; otherwise, the above sentence would lead the distant reader to suppose that prejudice, not justice; vindictiveness, not mercy; were the characteristics of the State, which only required opposition or contradiction to give them still greater tenacity...the character of the American people... [is that] their instinctive aspirations soar too high in the cause of truth, justice and liberty, to permit them to stoop and pour out "lucubrations"...their motto is..."God and my right"...They were not born, much less educated, to bow to a powdered wig...God grant that such lucubrations ever will characterize the American people.

There were no further editorial comments from the "Medical Witness" or Dr. Castle in the *Boston Medical and Surgical Journal*.

However, over the more than 150 years since the trial, many articles, books, and even plays have been written or performed about this infamous case. Such writers have come down on both sides: Dr. Webster was the murderer or Dr. Webster was convicted on circumstantial evidence and may not have been the killer despite his later confession. Two diametrically opposite but intriguing books were published in 1971; one by Helen Thomson, a historian, and the other by Robert Sullivan, a Massachusetts superior court judge. In his review of these two books, Robert Ireland, a historian at the University of Kentucky, wrote that Thomson, in accepting the truth of prosecutor George Bemis' official report, assumed that Webster was guilty. However, Sullivan argued that Webster was victim to political and monetary ambitions of those involved and the incompetence of his own counsel. Sullivan even expresses his concern that George Putnam, Webster's spiritual advisor, produced a fake confession and was in league with the attorney general. However, despite the faults of the trial itself, evidence continues to point toward Webster's guilt. His unusual behavior after the murder, including his premediated suicide attempt all point toward an accurate verdict. Richard B. Morris (1952) agreed that although the trial was unfair and faulty, the verdict was still sound. The *Boston Medical and Surgical Journal* wrote a defense of the medical profession:

The intelligent portion of the community know full well the importance of the study of anatomy, and that for any other purpose than the benefit of science dissections of dead bodies would ever be made...that the statements alluded to [Dr. Putman's explanation that medical men have little feeling in dissecting human bodies] misrepresent the character and feelings of the profession entirely. The whole fault in this melancholy case lies at the door of the one who now confesses that he perpetrated the tragedy. If this same confession [Webster presented three months after his conviction] had been immediately after the homicide, no one can for a moment doubt that the result would have been entirely different from what it now is. (*Boston Medical and Surgical Journal* 1850g)

Today, readers and writers alike continue to be intrigued by a case fraught with scandal—one filled with the horrors of dismemberment and the inclusion of upstanding and well-known members of the community as both suspect and victim. It was a case that highlighted the divisive role of testimony, one in which the accused was not permitted to testify on his own behalf, and in which the same witness (Holmes) could be called upon by both the defense and the prosecution. The case provides insight into the role of early forensic science, underscoring the complex process of determining guilt without the assistance of modern sophisticated medical tests.

Index

West Roxbury Veterans Admin-
istration Hospital and,
4: 378–379
Orthopaedics Today, 2: 281
Orthopedic Nursing (Funsten and
Calderwood), 3: 303
Orthopedic Surgery (Bradford and
Lovett), 4: 318
Orthopedic Surgery (Jones and
Lovett), 2: 69, *69*, 166
*Orthopedic Treatment of Gunshot
Injuries, The* (Mayer), 3: 156*b*
L'Orthopédie (Andry), 3: 90
orthoroentgenograms, 2: 171
os calcis fractures, 4: 313, 314*b*,
335–336
Osgood, John Christopher, 2: 113
Osgood, Margaret Louisa, 2: 138
Osgood, Martha E. Whipple, 2: 113
Osgood, Robert B. (1873–1956),
1: *193, 194*; 2: 113, 118, 125, 140,
222, 255; 4: *404, 417*
adult orthopaedics and, 2: 157
on AEF medical care organization, 4: 417
AEF splint board, 4: 416
American Ambulance Hospital
and, 2: 117–123; 4: 386,
389*b*, *390*, 392–393
on Andry's *Orthopaedia*, 1: xxii
AOA preparedness committee,
4: 394
on arthritis and rheumatic disease, 4: 58
back pain research and, 3: 203
Base Hospital No. 5 and, 4: 420,
421*b*, 422, 422*b*, *422*
Beth Israel Hospital and,
4: 208*b*, 247
Boston Children's Hospital and,
1: 192; 2: 16, 40–41, 114,
132–133, 140, 247, 274, 282;
3: 99
Brigham and Women's Hospital
and, 4: 195*b*
British Expeditionary Forces and,
4: 420
Burrage Hospital and, 4: 226
Carney Hospital and, 2: 116
as chief at MGH, 1: 151, 192
chronic disease treatment and,
4: 52
as clinical professor, 1: 158
curative workshops and,
4: 403–404
death of, 2: 140
Department for Military Orthopedics and, 4: 405
Diseases of the Bones and Joints,
2: 117; 3: 81–82

education and training,
2: 113–114
on Edward H. Bradford, 2: 44
elegance and, 2: 138–140
end-results clinics and, 1: 194
European medical studies, 2: 116
faculty salary, 1: 177, 179
on FitzSimmons, 2: 258–259
on foot problems, 2: 56,
123–124
foot strength apparatus and,
2: 101–102
*Fundamentals of Orthopaedic Sur-
gery in General Medicine and
Surgery*, 2: 135–136
George W. Gay Lecture, 4: 324
Georgia Warm Springs Foundation and, 2: 78
hand-washing policy, 1: 193
Harvard Unit and, 2: 119–121,
123–124; 3: *180, 369, 370*;
4: 386–387, 421*b*
HCORP and, 1: 192–195
as head of HMS orthopaedic surgery department, 1: 174–175,
177, 192
HMS appointment, 2: 116,
133–135
honorary degrees, 2: 137
House of the Good Samaritan
and, 2: 113–114
identification of Osgood-Schlatter
disease, 2: 115, *116*, 117
John Ball and Buckminster
Brown Professorship, 2: 133;
4: 195*b*
Journal of Bone and Joint Surgery
editor, 2: 130
Katzeff and, 2: 275
King Manuel II and, 4: 401
on Legg-Calve-Perthes disease,
2: 105
Lovett Fund and, 2: 82
marriage and family, 2: 138
MGH and, 2: 116–117, 129–
134; 3: 67
MGH crystal laboratory, 2: 322
MGH Fracture Clinic and,
3: 313; 4: 464
as MGH orthopaedics chief,
3: 11*b*, 227, 266, 268; 4: 472*b*
MGH surgical intern, 1: 189
military orthopaedics and,
2: 124–128; 4: 403, 406–407,
412, 417–419, 423*b*, 453
on mobilization of stiffened
joints, 4: 27*b*
"Nation and the Hospital, The,"
2: 137–138, 138*b*–139*b*

New England Surgical Society
president, 2: 136
Ober on, 2: 148
as orthopaedic chair, 2: 15*b*
orthopaedic research support,
1: 193, 195
orthopaedic surgery and, 1: xxiii;
2: 79, 106, 116–117, 132, 140
"Orthopaedic Work in a War
Hospital," 2: 120
orthopaedics education and,
1: 152; 2: 133–136
Orthopedics and Body Mechanics
Committee, 4: 235
poetry of, 2: 128–129, 129*b*,
140
poliomyelitis treatment, 2: 77,
264
on preventative measures,
2: 122–123
private medical practice and,
1: 176; 3: 338
professional memberships,
2: 136–137
as professor of orthopaedic surgery, 1: 172
"Progress in Orthopaedic Surgery" series, 2: 43, 297
publications and research,
2: 135–137; 4: 32, 65, 421*b*
as radiologist, 2: 114–115
RBBH and, 4: 25–26, 28, 31, 56
on rehabilitation of wounded
soldiers, 4: 451
roentgenograms and, 2: 54, 116
on sacroiliac joint fusion,
3: 184–185
scoliosis treatment, 2: 87
on synovial fluid diagnosis,
3: 175
on transformation of orthopaedic
surgeons, 2: 130*b*–131*b*, *132*
treatment of fractures, 3: 61
US Army Medical Corps and,
3: 61
on visceroptosis, 3: 87–88
war injury studies and,
2: 128–129
World War I and, 2: 65, 117–
128; 3: 157, 166; 4: 403,
406–407, 412, 417, 421*b*
World War II volunteers and,
4: 363
Osgood Visiting Professors, 2: 141*b*
Osgood-Schlatter disease, 2: 89,
115, *116*, 117
Osler, Sir William, 1: 1, 185, 275;
3: 2; 4: vii, *6*
osteoarthritis

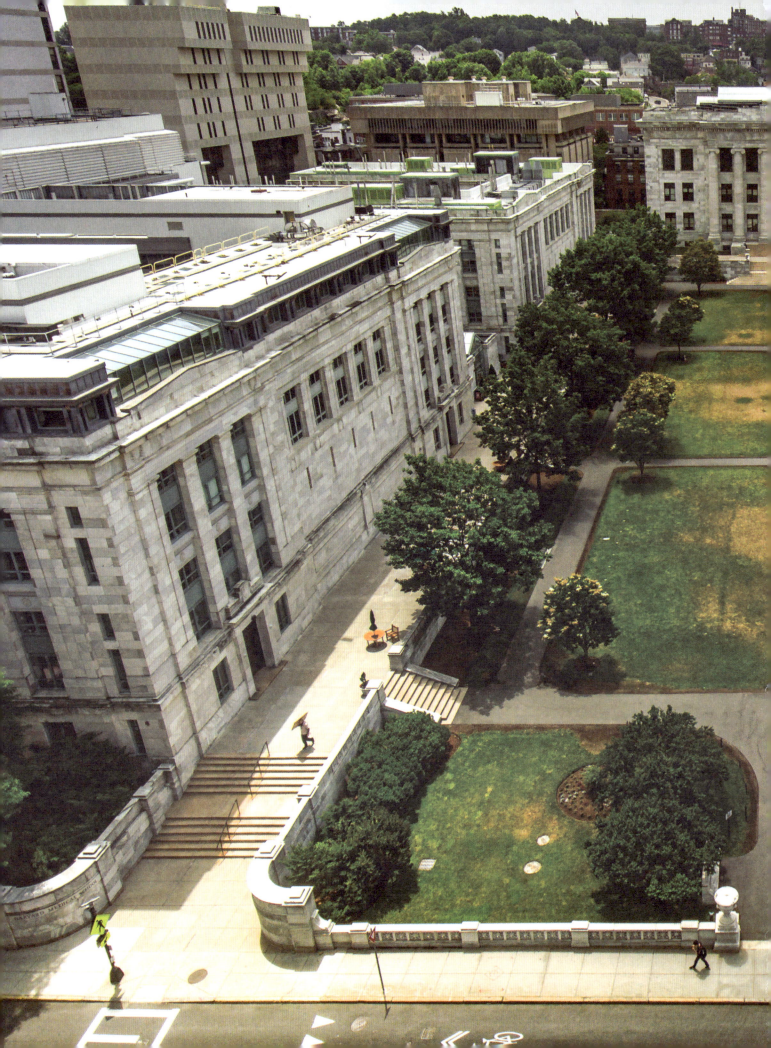